SAVING LIVES, BUYING TIME

Economics of Malaria Drugs in an Age of Resistance

Committee on the Economics of Antimalarial Drugs
Board on Global Health

Kenneth J. Arrow, Claire B. Panosian, and Hellen Gelband, *Editors*

INSTITUTE OF MEDICINE
OF THE NATIONAL ACADEMIES

THE NATIONAL ACADEMIES PRESS
Washington, D.C.
www.nap.edu

THE NATIONAL ACADEMIES PRESS   500 Fifth Street, N.W.   Washington, DC 20001

NOTICE: The project that is the subject of this report was approved by the Governing Board of the National Research Council, whose members are drawn from the councils of the National Academy of Sciences, the National Academy of Engineering, and the Institute of Medicine. The members of the committee responsible for the report were chosen for their special competences and with regard for appropriate balance.

This study was supported by Contract No. HRN-A-00-00-00012-00 between the National Academy of Sciences and the U.S. Agency for International Development (USAID) and the Bill and Melinda Gates Foundation. Any opinions, findings, conclusions, or recommendations expressed in this publication are those of the authors and do not necessarily reflect the views of the organizations or agencies that provided support for this project.

Library of Congress Cataloging-in-Publication Data

Saving lives, buying time : economics of malaria drugs in an age of resistance / Committee on the Economics of Antimalarial Drugs, Board on Global Health ; Kenneth J. Arrow, Claire Panosian, and Hellen Gelband, editors.
    p. ; cm.
  Includes bibliographical references and index.
  ISBN 0-309-09213-2 (hardcover)
  1. Antimalarials—Economic aspects. 2. Pharmaceutical policy. 3. Drug resistance in microorganisms.
  [DNLM: 1. Malaria—drug therapy. 2. Antimalarials—economics. 3. Antimalarials—therapeutic use. 4. Drug Costs. 5. Drug Resistance. WC 770 S267 2004] I. Arrow, Kenneth Joseph, 1921- II. Panosian, Claire. III. Gelband, Hellen. IV. Institute of Medicine (U.S.) Committee on the Economics of Antimalarial Drugs.
  RC159.A5S28 2004
  616.9'362061—dc22

                           2004017959

Additional copies of this report are available from the National Academies Press, 500 Fifth Street, N.W., Lockbox 285, Washington, DC 20055; (800) 624-6242 or (202) 334-3313 (in the Washington metropolitan area); Internet, http://www.nap.edu.

For more information about the Institute of Medicine, visit the IOM home page at: **www.iom.edu.**

The serpent has been a symbol of long life, healing, and knowledge among almost all cultures and religions since the beginning of recorded history. The serpent adopted as a logotype by the Institute of Medicine is a relief carving from ancient Greece, now held by the Staatliche Museen in Berlin.

Cover photograph by Claire B. Panosian. Mkuranga, Tanzania, November 2002. Family and neighbors of Amina Selemani, including her daughter and newborn grandchild. Another grandchild, Zulfa Mshamu (not shown) received ACT treatment for malaria through a clinical research trial co-sponsored by the Ifakara Health Research and Development Centre and the U.S. Centers for Disease Control and Prevention.

"Knowing is not enough; we must apply.
Willing is not enough; we must do."
—Goethe

INSTITUTE OF MEDICINE
OF THE NATIONAL ACADEMIES

Adviser to the Nation to Improve Health

THE NATIONAL ACADEMIES
Advisers to the Nation on Science, Engineering, and Medicine

The **National Academy of Sciences** is a private, nonprofit, self-perpetuating society of distinguished scholars engaged in scientific and engineering research, dedicated to the furtherance of science and technology and to their use for the general welfare. Upon the authority of the charter granted to it by the Congress in 1863, the Academy has a mandate that requires it to advise the federal government on scientific and technical matters. Dr. Bruce M. Alberts is president of the National Academy of Sciences.

The **National Academy of Engineering** was established in 1964, under the charter of the National Academy of Sciences, as a parallel organization of outstanding engineers. It is autonomous in its administration and in the selection of its members, sharing with the National Academy of Sciences the responsibility for advising the federal government. The National Academy of Engineering also sponsors engineering programs aimed at meeting national needs, encourages education and research, and recognizes the superior achievements of engineers. Dr. Wm. A. Wulf is president of the National Academy of Engineering.

The **Institute of Medicine** was established in 1970 by the National Academy of Sciences to secure the services of eminent members of appropriate professions in the examination of policy matters pertaining to the health of the public. The Institute acts under the responsibility given to the National Academy of Sciences by its congressional charter to be an adviser to the federal government and, upon its own initiative, to identify issues of medical care, research, and education. Dr. Harvey V. Fineberg is president of the Institute of Medicine.

The **National Research Council** was organized by the National Academy of Sciences in 1916 to associate the broad community of science and technology with the Academy's purposes of furthering knowledge and advising the federal government. Functioning in accordance with general policies determined by the Academy, the Council has become the principal operating agency of both the National Academy of Sciences and the National Academy of Engineering in providing services to the government, the public, and the scientific and engineering communities. The Council is administered jointly by both Academies and the Institute of Medicine. Dr. Bruce M. Alberts and Dr. Wm. A. Wulf are chair and vice chair, respectively, of the National Research Council.

www.national-academies.org

Reviewers

This report has been reviewed in draft form by individuals chosen for their diverse perspectives and technical expertise, in accordance with procedures approved by the NRC's Report Review Committee. The purpose of this independent review is to provide candid and critical comments that will assist the institution in making its published report as sound as possible and to ensure that the report meets institutional standards for objectivity, evidence, and responsiveness to the study charge. The review comments and draft manuscript remain confidential to protect the integrity of the deliberative process. We wish to thank the following individuals for their review of this report:

Umberto d'Alessandro, Prince Leopold Institute of Tropical Medicine, Belgium
Scott Barrett, The Johns Hopkins University
Mohamud Daya, Oregon Health and Science University
Peter Heller, International Monetary Fund
Tran Tinh Hien, Hospital for Tropical Diseases, Ho Chi Minh City, Vietnam
Alison Keith, Consultant, Health Economist, Springdale, UT
T.K. Mutabingwa, Gates Malaria Partnership & National Institute for Medical Research, Muheza, Tanzania
François Nosten, Shoklo Malaria Research Unit Hospital for Tropical Diseases, Bangkok, Thailand

Jeffrey D. Sachs, Columbia University
Terrie E. Taylor, Michigan State University

Although the reviewers listed above have provided many constructive comments and suggestions, they were not asked to endorse the conclusions or recommendations, nor did they see the final version of the report before its release. The review of this report was overseen by **Robert E. Black,** The Johns Hopkins University and **Charles Phelps,** University of Rochester. Appointed by the National Research Council and Institute of Medicine, they were responsible for making certain that an independent examination of this report was carried out in accordance with institutional procedures, and that all review comments were carefully considered. Responsibility for the final content of this report rests entirely with the authoring committee and the institution.

Preface

Let me use this preface to share some of my own learning experience over the course of this study. At first blush, recommending appropriate therapy for malaria, as for other diseases, might seem a matter for medicine, pharmacology, and other branches of biology. Indeed, as this report will show, while biological and pharmacological details are of utmost importance, malaria policy also requires the best economic understanding we can muster. Anyone conscientiously engaged in practical policy making is painfully aware of the limitations of our understanding of the economic system. In the course of developing this report, I also became increasingly aware of our limited understanding of natural systems, a fact of life that my biological and medical colleagues on our committee candidly acknowledged.

Economics is the study of the allocation of scarce resources among competing ends. It is not surprising, therefore, that economic considerations should loom large in health policy, including the provision of effective pharmaceuticals. Today, the richer countries of the world are devoting an ever-growing proportion of resources to health care. In the United States, how to finance therapeutic drugs for the elderly is an ongoing political debate. If countries in which scarcity is least felt must still devote major attention to medical economics, how much more is this likely to be true of those countries, especially in Africa, where per capita incomes are 5 percent or less of the U.S. level?

It was clear before this IOM Committee met that the existing antimalarial drug supply was starting to fail. For more than 40 years, the system had been largely based on a single agent—chloroquine—which was at one time very effective and remarkably cheap. Even in the poorest countries, at 10 cents per retail course, most people can still afford it. Moreover, the drug is familiar to the populace, and has been used—both within and outside of organized health care systems—well enough to prevent many malaria deaths and suppress (if not completely cure) acute attacks of the disease. For lack of an affordable alternative, chloroquine remains the most frequently used antimalarial in Africa. Chloroquine is distributed mainly through private economic channels, eventually reaching consumers via the local stores and drug sellers that are ubiquitous in poor countries. The private sector has, in this case, filled a niche left open by public and private health care systems that are neither sufficiently accessible nor affordable to serve much of the population—particularly, the rural poor.

Over time, however, resistance to chloroquine emerged worldwide, first leading to treatment failures in Southeast Asia, then to treatment failures in large parts of east Africa. It is now believed that chloroquine will be useless against most life-threatening falciparum malaria infections in fairly short order. In the meantime, replacement drugs have been introduced, but they too have quickly lost ground. The main exception is a family of antimalarials derived from sweet wormwood (*Artemisia annua)*. Over the last 25 years, artemisinin derivatives have proved highly effective in Thailand, Vietnam, and other Asian countries while no artemisinin resistance has surfaced. Partnering artemisinins with a second drug confers even greater protection against the development of drug-resistant mutants. Two- or three-drug treatments—now commonly called artemisinin combination therapy, or ACT—also offer therapeutic advantages over single antimalarial drugs.

In short, the occurrence of a medical difficulty is offset by an opportunity. An economist does not expect a free lunch, as the cliché goes, and this lunch is not free. In fact, it is relatively, though not absolutely, expensive. At present, ACTs cost about US$2 a treatment, roughly twenty times the price of chloroquine. By any reasonable standards, their cost per individual course is not large and will decline even further with competition and economies of scale. As best we can estimate, the total drug cost of ACTs for worldwide treatment of falciparum malaria is likely to be about $500 million a year—barely noticeable on the scale of the budget of any major developed country. Nevertheless, this is an unmanageable cost for countries with per capita incomes of $2,000 a year or less. Subsidies are needed.

Having said this, multiple economic issues arise. What is the justification for subsidies targeted to specific kinds of expenditures? Why is there not a whole series of new antimalarial drugs coming on line (as there is, for example, for HIV/AIDS or depression)? How do we measure the benefits of curing a case of malaria against the increased costs of treatment? If we agree on the necessity of subsidies, how can we maintain an efficient system of distribution?

We discuss all of these issues in one way or another in the report, but I will make a few brief comments here. ACTs (compared with monotherapies) serve to avoid the emergence of resistance worldwide. This equals, in economists' jargon, the avoidance of negative externalities, or the creation of global and intertemporal public goods. Preventing or delaying the emergence of resistance will save lives in future generations. Even if artemisinin resistance eventually emerges, slowing down its appearance increases the chance that high-risk individuals will have access to new and improved drugs when that time arrives.

The historical slowness in producing new antimalarials reflects the way in which new drugs are developed in a market system. Research, development, and testing of drugs engender a large upfront cost. In a private enterprise system, the incentive to make this expenditure is the monopoly mark-up over the relatively low manufacturing costs, a monopoly conferred by intellectual property rights. This incentive, however, depends on the economic strength of the market. When a large market exists in rich countries, drugs are developed. When the market mainly consists of poor people, however, the incentive is weak and drug development usually founders.

In fact, the original development of artemisinins did exemplify an alternative path to pharmaceutical innovation. The first artemisinins were developed by Chinese medical researchers who claimed no intellectual property rights. Not even fame, the scientist's alternative motivation to money, was involved; the original paper was published under the name of a collective. However, today, if artemisinin production is to expand and ACTs are to become the global norm, the international community must take the initiative and fuel a series of actions to ensure this outcome.

Economic evaluation of a new antimalarial treatment requires an analysis of its respective costs and benefits, or at least a comparison of its reduction of malaria morbidity and mortality vis-à-vis other therapies. In the case of ACTs, the costs were so low and the relative efficacy so high that inquiring into the benefits in greater detail was hardly worthwhile.

Perhaps the knottiest issue we faced was how an ACT subsidy might be administered. It was hard to conceive that subsidizing ACTs at a local level, say through vouchers, would be compatible with a market-driven distribution system. Although public health systems have succeeded in distributing antimalarials in Thailand and Vietnam, the consensus of our experts was that such systems would not work equally well in Africa. We want to disturb the existing market system as little as possible. Therefore, we urge that the subsidies enter at a high international level.

Another lesson of medical economics is the importance of recognizing the specific character of the disease under consideration. The policy challenges that arise in treating malaria are simply very different from those attached to other major infectious scourges. For example, speed of treatment is much more important in malaria than in TB or HIV/AIDS, and reliance on sophisticated diagnosis necessarily reduced. Malaria's distinctive mode of transmission (via mosquitoes) suggests additional environmental control measures. High mosquito breeding rates and the special "homophilia" of the major vector species in Africa also carry important policy implications.

In the course of the study, I learned that the challenge of controlling malaria involves far more than identifying and treating individual victims one at a time. Malaria exists as an entire ecology for which real control requires a complement of measures, chief among them, effective antimalarial drugs. Our charge was the study of the economics of drugs; we could not have done justice to other antimalarial measures. But I came away with the clear understanding that interventions such as insecticide-treated bednets and other, broad environmental strategies offer great potential for synergy when effective drug therapies are available.

Finally, this report consciously refrains from the frequent recommendation by committees such as ours for more research. Nonetheless, it must be said that resources devoted to gathering malaria data are grossly inadequate. For one thing, we were not able to determine clearly the number of malaria deaths worldwide, where the error may be 25 percent either way. Such an elementary fact as the current number of treatments taken per year (a very important figure when estimating the cost of changing the drug of choice) seems not to be known within a factor of three. One could go on, but these examples are illustrative. The information gaps and vast uncertainties made this committee's task more difficult, but not impossible. The scientists, physicians, and economists who compose the committee are unanimous about the correctness of the solutions proposed in our recommendations. We need not—and cannot—wait for better information to meet the current crisis.

Kenneth J. Arrow, Ph.D., Chairman
Professor Emeritus, Department of Economics, Stanford University

Acknowledgments

The committee gratefully acknowledges the contributions of many individuals who provided information and insights for the study. Those listed below assisted in particular ways—participating in workshops, helping to arrange field visits, providing unpublished materials or data, or simply being available for consultations on salient topics.

Salim Abdulla, Ifakara Health Research and Development Centre
Irene Agyepong, Ghana Health Service
David Alnwick, Roll Back Malaria, WHO
Lawrence Barat, The World Bank
Joel Breman, U.S. National Institutes of Health
Denis Broun, Management Sciences for Health
Dennis Carroll, USAID
Yann Derriennic, Abt Associates
Mary Ettling, USAID
David Evans, WHO
Catherine Goodman, London School of Hygiene and Tropical Medicine
William Haddad, Biogenerics, Inc.
Ian Hastings, Liverpool School of Tropical Medicine and Hygiene
Carolyn Hicks, University of Oxford
Gerald Keusch, Boston University School of Public Health
Rashid Khatib, Ifakara Health Research and Development Centre

Patience Kuruneri, Roll Back Malaria Partnership
Jo Lines, London School of Hygiene and Tropical Medicine
Francesca Little, University of Capetown
Ellis McKenzie, U.S. National Institutes of Health
Kamini Mendis, Roll Back Malaria, WHO
Wilbur K. Milhous, WRAIR
Dr. Abdulnoor Mulokozi, Ifakara Health Research and Development
  Centre
Vinand Nantulya, The Global Fund to Fight AIDS, Tuberculosis and
  Malaria
Ok Pannenborg, The World Bank
Christopher Plowe, University of Maryland School of Medicine
Wirichada Pongtavornpinyo, Mahidol University
Magda Robalo, WHO-AFRO
A. Ebrahim Samba, WHO-Afro
Allan Saul, U.S. National Institutes of Health
Thomas E. Wellems, U.S. National Institutes of Health
Shunmay Yeung, Mahidol University

PROJECT CONSULTANTS AND COMMISSIONED AUTHORS

Karen Barnes, Division of Pharmacology, University of Cape Town, South Africa

Paul Coleman, London School of Hygiene and Tropical Medicine, London, England

Don De Savigny, Swiss Tropical Institute, Basel, Switzerland; Tanzania Essential Health Interventions Project (TEHIP), and International Development Research Centre (IDRC), Canada

David Durrheim, James Cook University, Australia

Edward Elmendorf, The World Bank, Washington, DC

Catherine Goodman, London School of Hygiene and Tropical Medicine, London, England

Patricia Graves, Independent Consultant in International Health, Fort Collins, Colorado

Jean-Marc Guimier, Management Sciences for Health, Arlington, Virginia

Steven Hoffman, Sanaria, Gaithersburg, Maryland

John Horton, Department of Pharmacology and Therapeutics, Liverpool University, England, and WHO/TDR, Geneva, Switzerland

Barbara Jemelkova, Resources for the Future, Inc., Washington, DC

Harun Kasale, International Development Research Centre (IDRC), Canada, and Ministry of Health, Tanzania

Ramadhan Madabida, Tanzania Pharmaceuticals Industries Limited

Honrati Masanja, International Development Research Centre (IDRC), Canada, and Ifakara Health Research and Development Centre, Tanzania

Charles Mayombana, Ifakara Health Research and Development Centre, Tanzania

Conrad Mbuya, International Development Research Centre (IDRC), Canada, and Ministry of Health, Tanzania

Di McIntyre, Health Economics Unit, University of Cape Town, Cape Town, South Africa

Abdulatif Minhaj, Rufiji Demographic Surveillance System, Tanzania

Yahya Mkilindi, Rufiji Demographic Surveillance System, Tanzania

Devota Momburi, Rufiji Demographic Surveillance System, Tanzania

Chantal Morel, London School of Hygiene and Tropical Medicine, England

Charlotte Muheki, Health Economics Unit, University of Cape Town, Cape Town, South Africa

Eleuther Mwangeni, Rufiji Demographic Surveillance System, Tanzania

Clive Ondari, World Health Organization, Geneva, Switzerland

Graham Reid, Tanzania Essential Health Interventions Project (TEHIP), and International Development Research Centre (IDRC), Canada

Sam Shillcutt, Health Economics Research Centre, University of Oxford, Oxford, England

Rima Shretta, Management Sciences for Health, Arlington, Virginia

Robert Snow, The Wellcome Trust / KEMRI Collaborative Programme, Nairobi, Kenya, and Centre for Tropical Medicine, University of Oxford, John Radcliffe Hospital, Oxford, England

Alan Tait, Consultant, Sandwich, Kent, England

Jean-Francois Trape, IRD, Dakar, Senegal

David Ubben, Medicines for Malaria Venture, Geneva, Switzerland

Holly Anne Williams, Malaria Epidemiology Branch, Centers for Disease Control and Prevention, Atlanta, Georgia

Virginia Wiseman, London School of Hygiene and Tropical Medicine, London, England

Contents

PART 3
ADVANCING TOWARD BETTER MALARIA CONTROL

SAVING LIVES, BUYING TIME

Economics of Malaria Drugs
in an Age of Resistance

Executive Summary

INTRODUCTION

For more than 50 years, chloroquine silently saved millions of lives and cured billions of debilitating episodes of malaria. Falciparum malaria has always been a major cause of death and disability—particularly in Africa—but chloroquine offered a measure of control even in the worst-affected regions. At roughly 10 cents a course and readily available from drug peddlers, shops, and clinics, it reached even those who had little contact with formal health care.

Now chloroquine is increasingly impotent against falciparum malaria, and malaria's death toll is rising. Yet desperate patients still turn to chloroquine and other failing, low-cost malaria medicines because they lack the few dollars needed to buy new, potentially life-saving treatments. Chief among these new treatments are the "artemisinins," paradoxically both an ancient and a modern class of drug that can still cure any form of human malaria. If falciparum malaria sufferers had the same broad access to artemisinins that currently exists for chloroquine, the rising burden of malaria in the world today would halt or reverse.

The crisis is both economic and biomedical. On the economic side, to state the obvious, the era of cheap and effective antimalarial treatment may have ended, but poverty in sub-Saharan Africa and malarious countries elsewhere, has not. Thus, although artemisinins at a dollar or two per course are both inexpensive by U.S. or European standards and highly cost-effective by any norm, neither national governments nor consumers in most

1

malaria-endemic countries can afford them in quantities that remotely approach the world's current consumption of chloroquine—roughly 300-500 million courses of treatment per year.[1]

Biomedically, today's malaria situation also is precarious. The artemisinins are the *only* first-line antimalarial drugs appropriate for widespread use that still work against all chloroquine-resistant malaria parasites. If resistance to artemisinins is allowed to develop and spread before replacement drugs are at hand, malaria's toll could rise even higher.

The challenge, therefore, is twofold: to facilitate widespread use of artemisinins while, at the same time, to preserve their effectiveness for as long as possible. The central recommendation of this report—*a sustained global subsidy of artemisinins coformulated with other antimalarial drugs*—is the most economically and biomedically sound means to meet this challenge.

Two caveats must accompany this report and its recommendations. Even in the best of times when chloroquine was still effective, it did not reach everyone. As a result, at least one million people died each year from malaria, most of whom could have been saved by adequate treatment. Merely substituting artemisinin combination therapies (ACTs) for chloroquine is not the whole answer. *Expanded access* to effective treatment will also be needed if we are to gain ground against malaria.

Second, malaria control requires a suite of interventions to *prevent* disease: insecticide-treated bednets, environmental measures to limit mosquito breeding, and intermittent preventive treatment of high-risk asymptomatic individuals (eventually, malaria vaccines will join the armamentarium). If proven preventive interventions are combined with ACTs, we can expect even greater progress generally, while, in some areas, good drugs plus good control can actually reduce malaria transmission to near zero. Commitments of international funding substantially greater than the sums needed for an antimalarial drug subsidy but still modest in terms of their return on investment are therefore needed to advance malaria control overall.

However, this report does not address malaria control comprehensively; that is a task for others. This committee was asked to recommend economic mechanisms to make effective antimalarial drugs widely accessible in order to stem the deaths from drug-resistant malaria that now occur day in, day out. When it comes to saving lives, effective drugs will always be a mainstay while malaria continues to threaten humankind.

---

[1]It should be noted that the price of artemisinins is based on the costs of production and not added premiums to recoup research and development costs, which were borne largely by the public sector.

THE CURRENT MALARIA SITUATION

Although malaria was once a global scourge, by the mid-20th century it was eliminated as a major health problem in much of the world. The hard core remained, however, and in many parts of sub-Saharan Africa, malaria still is the largest contributor to the burden of disease and premature death. To a lesser degree, malaria also remains an important health problem in parts of south Asia, South America and other tropical regions of the world.

Chloroquine began losing its effectiveness against falciparum malaria in Asia during the 1960s and 1970s. Looking back, we know that mutant parasite strains with genetically-mediated chloroquine resistance initially arose in areas of low malaria transmission (Asia and South America) and reached east Africa by the 1980s. Over the next 2 decades, sub-Saharan Africa—where real malaria control had never been achieved, yet chloroquine was effectively treating illness and preventing deaths, especially among children—was hard hit. After declining from post–World War II through the mid-1990s, death rates from malaria are now increasing in Africa. The failure of chloroquine, followed by the waning efficacy of other low-cost drugs such as sulfadoxine-pyrimethamine (SP), appears to be the main cause.

It was the original emergence of drug resistance in Asia that inspired development of the artemisinins, an extraordinarily effective family of antimalarials derived from a traditional Chinese medicinal herb. Although they are nonproprietary, artemisinin compounds still cost more to produce than chloroquine because plants must first be cultivated and harvested and the drugs then extracted and processed rather than simply synthesized from inexpensive chemicals.

Over the past 2 decades, the use of artemisinins in Asia has grown continuously, but demand in Africa has remained negligible. At first the reason was that chloroquine and SP were still effective in Africa, but now the reason is strictly economic: artemisinins cost about 20 times more than chloroquine, and African countries and their citizens cannot afford their higher price tag. The lack of global demand for artemisinins has, in turn, led to a desultory pace of production and impeded the economies of scale and improved production methods that would substantially reduce prices, were larger markets and competition in place.

This is the crux of the current crisis: African countries are increasingly adopting artemisinin combination therapies (ACTs) for first-line treatment of uncomplicated malaria; however, without external funding neither governments nor consumers—who bear most of the cost—can afford them.

The IOM committee took these realities into account in devising a concrete plan for reversing the trend of increased malaria morbidity and mortality while preserving effective drugs for the future. To understand the reasoning behind the recommendations of the committee, it is important to appreciate certain biological aspects of malaria, particularly as they relate to the development and spread of drug resistance.

DRUG RESISTANCE AND THE NEED FOR COMBINATION THERAPY FOR MALARIA

The evolution of drug resistance is an inevitable consequence of genetics and natural selection when drugs are used against microbial pathogens, including the protozoan parasites that cause malaria. As effective and robust as the artemisinin drugs are today, it is only a matter of time before genetically resistant strains emerge and spread. However, practical steps can be taken to push that day further into the future. The logic is as follows.

In the case of any antimalarial drug, the new development of drug resistance is a rare event: a chance genetic change in a single parasite in a single patient.[2] But once that single malaria parasite generates multiple descendants, the math changes. Now, mosquitoes can acquire resistant parasites from a single individual and transmit them to other people. The subsequent spread of a *robust, resistant clone* would be similar to the spread of any malaria strain.

The way around this dismal scenario derives from the fact that a nascent resistant parasite will *not* survive and proliferate in an infected person's bloodstream if a *second* effective antimalarial drug *with a different mechanism of action* is simultaneously present. The key, therefore, to preserving the artemisinins is to eliminate their routine use as "monotherapies," and to treat patients with uncomplicated malaria (the vast majority of cases) with "artemisinin-based combination therapies" (ACTs) instead. ACTs equal an artemisinin derivative plus *another unrelated* antimalarial drug, ideally coformulated in a single pill so that individual drugs cannot be knowingly or inadvertently used as monotherapies. Combining drugs in this way—already an accepted practice in the treatment of tuberculosis and HIV/AIDS infection—minimizes the likelihood that a single parasite with drug resistance will propagate and spread. Since all drug-resistant microbes are capable of crossing national borders, delaying the development of resistance through this strategy creates a benefit, otherwise

---

[2]This discussion is simplified to basic concepts. In fact, the rate at which resistant parasites emerge varies tremendously by drug, which explains why chloroquine remained effective for decades (the known instances of new chloroquine-resistant strains developing are fewer than 10), whereas resistance to SP arises much more quickly (SP-resistant strains have developed de novo dozens or hundreds of times).

known as a "global public good," for people living both within and beyond malaria-endemic areas.

Although still relatively new to malaria, combination therapy is no longer controversial: within just the past few years, it has been endorsed by the World Health Organization, the Global Fund to Fight AIDS, Tuberculosis and Malaria, and by malaria experts worldwide. In addition, combinations are not only good for preventing resistance, they also confer advantages to patients. In the case of the artemisinins, the treatment regimen is shortened from 7 days using monotherapy to 3 days using a combination.

In order for antimalarial combination treatment to keep drug resistance at bay over the long term, however, it must be used as first-line treatment for uncomplicated falciparum malaria as widely as possible. Should monotherapies persist in some locales and drug resistance result, there would be no way to contain the resistant parasites to one country or continent. Artemisinin monotherapy is, in fact, widely used in Asia today in the same areas where resistance to chloroquine and SP originally surfaced not that long ago. There is an urgent need for Asian-based production of artemisinin monotherapy to convert to ACT production, aided by a global subsidy. The window of opportunity to create a global public good—years of extended effective antimalarial drug life—is open now, but it may not remain open very long.

The equal urgency for change in Asia and Africa may seem counterintuitive but antimalarial drug resistance historically has emerged in areas of low transmission—mainly Southeast Asia and South America—and then spread to high-transmission areas, mainly Africa. This pattern fits with current understanding of the biology of drug resistance in low- and high-transmission areas. As a practical matter, it is therefore essential that ACTs quickly dominate the market in low-transmission areas in Asia and Africa, as well as penetrate Africa's most endemic locales.

"Market penetration" will occur in a meaningful way only if the brunt of the increased cost of the drug is not borne by consumers—many of whom earn less than $1 per day. As the most practicable way to achieve this end, this report recommends a large subsidy near the top of the distribution chain, which will lower the price to consumers at all points of sale.

THE ECONOMICS OF ARTEMISININS AND ACTs

By Western standards, artemisinin derivatives are already inexpensive. They also are well within the bounds of what is internationally acknowledged as cost effective for health care interventions in low-income countries. With the incentive of a secure and large market, producers already are promising that wholesale prices for a course of ACTs will fall to US$ .50-1.00 (or possibly lower) within 2 years. However, that projected price is still 5 to 10 times higher than the price of chloroquine or SP in Africa, making artemisinins essentially unaffordable for most sub-Saharan governments and individuals, especially the poor, rural families whose children are most likely to die from malaria.

Without substantial and sustained subsidies, in some countries well over half of all malaria patients needing treatment—including most who currently are able to acquire chloroquine and SP—will not have access to artemisinin-based drugs. Children will die and many more will suffer.

Priming the Market for ACTs

Once scaled up, the additional cost of ACTs versus currently failing drugs for the world is expected be US$ 300-500 million per year (a closer approximation is difficult because estimates of malaria cases—or fevers assumed to be malaria—are imprecise). This cost estimate assumes that ACTs will be used to treat up to half a billion episodes per year, which roughly equals the number currently treated by chloroquine or SP. The estimate also assumes a competitive market in which ACT prices fall over time.

In the meantime, there is a chicken-and-egg dilemma surrounding ACT supply and demand. Without an assured market, potential manufacturers will not commit to adequate ACT production, nor will farmers expand the cultivation of *Artemisia annua*, the source plant.[3] There is a critical need to jump-start ACT production. To do this, the global community must provide sufficient funds to encourage investments by manufacturers, guarantee purchases of ACTs and generally stimulate a robust world market. This must be done through a visible, centralized mechanism, ideally using existing national and international organizations (e.g., UNICEF, WHO), which can quickly take on the task.

THE CASE FOR A GLOBAL SUBSIDY FOR ANTIMALARIAL DRUGS: THE CORE RECOMMENDATION OF THIS REPORT

The global community can take definitive action by subsidizing the difference in cost between inexpensive but ineffective antimalarials, and effective ACTs. For ACTs to reach most consumers, the subsidy must first bring the price of ACTs down to about the price of chloroquine (even at those prices, the poorest in society will need assistance to make them af-

---

[3]On average, one hectare of *A. annua* produces enough raw material for about 25,000 adult courses of an ACT. This equates to 20,000 hectares (200 km^2) for 500 million courses (Personal communication, J.M. Kindermans, Médecins Sans Frontières, June 8, 2004).

fordable). Then the subsidy must be sustained, at least over the medium term, until either economic conditions improve in the endemic countries, or the price of effective antimalarials comes down significantly. Furthermore, for consumers to *preferentially* choose ACTs over monotherapies, they must cost no more than the least expensive monotherapy available (whether an artemisinin or another drug). Otherwise, simple economics will dictate that a vulnerable monotherapy will be chosen over an ACT, and the global benefits of combination treatment in countering the emergence of resistance will not be achieved. (This report recommends specific measures to keep unneeded monotherapies off the market, as well.)

The subsidy must be applied in a way that does not diminish access to antimalarials. The routes through which people obtain antimalarials vary from place to place, but overall in Africa, upwards of 70 percent of these drugs reach consumers through the private sector, particularly small pharmacies, street side drug peddlers, and general store kiosks.

The importance of drug availability "close to home" cannot be overemphasized: if not treated, malaria can kill a small child within 24 hours of the onset of fever. Delayed consultations and referrals and correspondingly slow access to treatment can work for chronic infectious diseases such as tuberculosis, but not for malaria. Of course, public sector and nongovernmental organizations are important sources of health care, especially where they do reach populations as the village level, but frequently they are restricted to towns and cities.

Recognizing the many pathways by which antimalarials flow to consumers leads inevitably to the conclusion that external financing should be injected at a point very high in the purchasing chain—above the level of individual countries. It is widely recognized—including by this committee—that existing drug distribution is not optimal. As a result, overtreatment, undertreatment and other poor prescribing practices are rife, drugs (mainly chloroquine) have been wasted, malaria episodes left uncured, and other health conditions untreated. Clearly, public sector systems and regulatory oversight must be improved and sustained. *However, it is equally clear that private sector distribution systems reach millions of people with no other practical alternative.* Efforts to improve drug delivery—utilizing better information, technology (e.g., rapid diagnostic tests tailored to sub-Saharan Africa), and support for health systems generally—must continue. Such changes will realistically evolve over a longer time frame, however, than is currently available for the switch to ACTs, which is urgent.

A global subsidy near the top of the distribution chain will stabilize demand and create incentives for ACT production, resulting in lower prices. A global antimalarial subsidy also will accomplish the following for the global community:

- with the assent of individual countries, it will allow ACTs to flow through existing public- and private-sector channels even in remote places, without disrupting existing market structures;
- it will allow all countries to adopt the most appropriate malaria treatment policies, including ACTs as first-line treatment, without concern over the sustainability of external funding for their purchase and without forcing countries to choose between effective antimalarials and other malaria control measures;
- it will provide equity of access to inhabitants of all endemic countries, including those countries that, for whatever reason, may not receive sufficient external funds to purchase ACTs at market prices;
- it will give the global community leverage to dissuade artemisinin manufacturers who wish to sell through the subsidized system from producing artemisinin monotherapy;
- it will minimize administrative costs of applying the subsidy;
- it will minimize the incentives for counterfeit ACT production;
- it will minimize incentives for diversion and smuggling of ACTs, which would exist with differential subsidies and pricing; and
- as new drugs with appropriate characteristics to save lives and counter resistance are developed, it will provide a mechanism of integrating them into an existing distribution system.

Funding a Global Antimalarial Subsidy

Countries with the greatest malaria burdens are least able to cover the added cost of ACTs, either through public or private sector budgets. Governments and citizens of endemic countries will contribute something, but most of the shortfall must come from external sources. This does not mean altogether *new* funding, however. Substantial amounts of committed but unspent monies—especially from the World Bank's International Development Association—could be tapped to support ACT purchases. Other likely sources are bilateral aid programs from the United States and other countries. The Global Fund to Fight AIDS, Tuberculosis and Malaria is in a good position to solicit contributions from around the world and earmark substantial amounts for this purpose.

One issue to be raised up front is historical precedent: in the past, major development institutions and aid agencies have allocated funding almost exclusively at the country level. Although this approach is appropriate for the majority of projects, it is not ideal for programs involving global public goods. Putting together a global subsidy for ACTs will require creativity and flexibility from these funders, but it is possible. Structuring an antimalarial subsidy supranationally is also consistent with recent efforts to increase global funding for the major diseases of poor countries.

Some may argue that a subsidy for ACTs can stop the current backslide, but it will do nothing to solve the many other problems that allow malaria to thrive. However, the availability of very effective drugs is likely to inspire increased country- and local-level malaria control efforts that previously may have seemed futile when programs were saddled with ineffective drugs. It is vitally important that funding for ACTs not be diverted from other malaria control measures.

How Much Money Is Needed?

If 300-500 million episodes are treated annually worldwide, and US$1 is the incremental cost per ACT course, an adequate ACT global subsidy would be US$300-500 million. This would constitute drug costs for the entire world. Although the sum is substantial, it is less than will be spent every year on antiretroviral drugs to treat a fraction of the people in Africa infected with HIV. And rather than continuing to increase each year, the demand for antimalarials should, in the worst case scenario, stay roughly stable. In the best case, demand will decline as better treatment and other control measures take effect.

The Need for a Centralized Procurement System

A mechanism for centralized procurement of antimalarial drugs (analogous to the process by which many nations now obtain subsidized tuberculosis drugs and childhood vaccines) should be established. This responsibility could reside with an existing organization or with a new one (for example, a program currently being explored by WHO, similar to the recently-established "Global Drug Facility" for tuberculosis). The functions of a centralized procurement agency would be: 1) to help keep prices low and production high through multiple producers; 2) to monitor quality control; and 3) to structure incentives to assure that individual countries follow the most prudent malaria treatment policies. The procurement agency must be empowered to make multiyear commitments toward the purchase of ACTs. The agency also could provide technical assistance to countries on internal regulatory matters, and surveillance and monitoring activities.

The Specifics of Procurement Nationally and Internationally

In effect, the procurement agency would buy ACTs directly from manufacturers at competitive prices, then resell them to countries at a lower, subsidized price (this process would ideally occur through a "virtual" rather than a physical warehousing system). Although decisions regarding the allocation of ACTs within countries would remain under the control of national governments, ACTs must flow into both the public and private sectors in every country for the subsidy to achieve its goal. In addition, governments will need to oversee price controls in the private sector in order to assure that the subsidy truly reaches consumers and that profit margins are not excessive. Pricing rules do exist in most countries, but they can be difficult to enforce. Improved packaging and labeling (which could include a printed price), and consumer education will facilitate both price controls and the rational use of antimalarial drugs, and should be supported internationally and nationally.

The need for action is urgent, but optimal levels of financing and procurement will likely take 2 to 5 years to ramp up. During this "phasing-in" period imposed by limited financing or drug supply, priorities should reflect global humanitarian need. Currently, East and Southern Africa and parts of Southeast Asia are the regions with the highest burden of chloroquine-resistant malaria coupled with the least access to ACTs.

THE NEED TO MAINTAIN RESEARCH AND DEVELOPMENT FOR NEW ANTIMALARIAL DRUGS

Managed well, artemisinins could remain the first-line antimalarial for many decades. Resistance has not yet developed in Asia, even following extensive monotherapy use. Eventually, however, the artemisinins will begin to lose effectiveness and new drugs will be needed. Even before that happens, drugs that can be manufactured more cheaply, or are superior to artemisinins (e.g., effective in a single dose) could supplant or join artemisinins on the front line.

For the first time in decades, the R&D pipeline for antimalarials has been invigorated through the Medicines for Malaria Venture (MMV), a public-private partnership begun in 1998. MMV, the WHO Special Programme on Research and Training in Tropical Diseases (TDR) and the Walter Reed Army Institute of Research (WRAIR) are the main innovators in antimalarials. Current annual funding needs for these organizations total an estimated US$60 million dollars, rising another US$20 million per year as more drugs reach the stage of clinical and field trials. These projected investments represent only a small addition to the cost of supplying artemisinins globally, but are several times the current collective budgets. Agencies supporting malaria control should allocate sufficient funds to these organizations to meet the MMV goal of one new antimalarial drug every 5 years, and WRAIR's similar target.

IMPROVING ACCESS AND THE PROMISE OF
INTEGRATED MALARIA CONTROL

Additional themes that run through this report are *access* and *integrated malaria control*. Even during the decades when chloroquine was effective, about one million Africans—mainly children—died of malaria every year. Lack of access to health care and inadequate preventive measures in Sub-Saharan Africa remain ongoing challenges. With comparably priced *effective* antimalarials, the access problem will not worsen, but neither will the full benefits of effective combination treatments be realized. This will require strengthened health care systems, better patient education regarding combination antimalarial treatment, and further innovations in antimalarial tools and access to them.

On the positive side, there is every reason to believe that effective drugs combined with other control measures in well-designed, locally appropriate programs can lower the malaria burden close to zero in some places. Insecticide-treated bednets can reduce child mortality substantially, given sufficient coverage of households. Environmental measures—spraying interior walls and rafters with insecticide, reducing mosquito breeding sites near houses—also work. These measures alone are worthwhile, but partnered with effective treatment, they are synergistic, especially in areas of relatively low malaria transmission. Witness the transformation recently brought about in KwaZulu Natal province, South Africa. This program combined the first internationally available ACT (artemether-lumefantrine or Coartem™, prescribed after a positive rapid diagnostic test), indoor house spraying and insecticide-treated bed nets. The result was dramatically reduced malaria transmission within the space of 2 years. Despite the program's relatively high initial costs, South Africa is now reaping real cost *savings* that will continue to accrue indefinitely. Similar programs utilizing multiple tools are not immediately feasible in all locales, but by targeting areas where transmission has already decreased somewhat, packaged interventions can achieve additional progress and valuable lessons applicable to high-transmission areas in the future.

In summary, over time, malaria can be contained through strategic deployment of ACTs and other control measures, which should lead to improved economic opportunities for people held back by the disease for generations. Effective malaria control also frees up national health care to tackle other pressing problems, and global resources to counter the disease in yet more places. The prospect of new tools such as a malaria vaccine for endemic areas—although very unlikely within 10 years—is another reason for long-term optimism.

THE CURRENT CHOICE

What is the current choice? In the view of the IOM Committee, it is unacceptable that cheap, effective drugs with a single medical purpose are currently unavailable to people whose lives would be saved by them. Failure to prevent the premature loss of our relatively few effective drugs through the simple expedient of coformulated drugs (currently, ACTs) also is unacceptable. The strategy offered in this report is a way to preserve the effectiveness of antimalarials for all global citizens—a true global public good. With coordinated policies, funding, and implementation, progress can be made. Without rapid adoption of ACTs, we will only continue to lose lives and lose ground.

RECOMMENDATIONS

At the Global Level

1. Within 5 years, governments and international finance institutions should commit new funds of US $300-$500 million per year to subsidize coformulated ACTs for the entire global market to achieve end-user prices in the range of US$0.10-.20, the current cost of chloroquine.

The subsidy must be applied high up in the ACT supply chain, above the level of individual countries. To assure the greatest international access, the public and private sectors of all endemic countries should be eligible to purchase ACTs at low, subsidized prices. In the future, subsidies could apply to other new combination antimalarials that meet technical criteria and are considered equivalent in their therapeutic promise to ACTs.

2. Artemisinin production should be stimulated in the short term by assuring and stabilizing demand through funding of at least $10-30 million per year from governments and international finance institutions.

Funds must be committed toward the global purchase of artemisinins in the 2- to 5-year time frame to encourage new companies to begin and producing companies to ramp up production. Once funds are committed and the conditions of purchase developed, potential producer companies should be actively solicited and provided with information and, if needed, technical assistance. If upgraded production facilities are needed, the International Finance Corporation (a sister institution of the World Bank) could provide needed funds. WHO should be prepared to assist companies in making their products "pre-qualified" and eligible for purchase through an international procurement process.

3. A centralized process for organizing ACT procurement should be established.

In the short term, procurement should take place within an existing organization with the capacity to manage the task. This organization must have the authority to make multiyear commitments to purchase ACTs from manufacturers. In the medium term, procurement could remain with the original organization or it could move. The aim is to maintain a healthy, competitive market with adequate production capacity and low prices. The organization also could monitor quality control of ACT manufacture and provide technical assistance on regulatory matters. Access to the procurement organization should be available to all countries, subject to conditions related to rational drug use. Conditions of participation for both countries and manufacturers would be aimed at assuring access to high-quality ACTs and minimizing the availability of unnecessary monotherapies.

4. Monotherapies for routine first-line treatment of falciparum malaria should be discouraged through a range of actions by the centralized procurement organization and governments of malaria-endemic countries, assisted by Roll Back Malaria and other global partners.

Monotherapy with oral drugs as first-line treatment will be discouraged by the availability of lower-priced ACTs, but this should be reinforced by other disincentives. Countries that obtain subsidized ACTs through the centralized procurement organization should neither register nor allow domestic production of artemisinin monotherapies or other drugs that are or would be effective partners to artemisinins. Companies selling through the subsidized system could be required to forgo producing these same monotherapies. Exceptions may be necessary, e.g., if particular monotherapies are needed to treat or prevent malaria in pregnant women. Artemisinins are not recommended during the first trimester of pregnancy, but are under evaluation. The current standard for preventive therapy during pregnancy is SP, which will not be used as a partner drug in an ACT. There is also a case for producing and distributing artesunate suppositories as an emergency stopgap treatment for children with severe malaria who cannot take oral drugs.

At the Country Level

5. All countries receiving subsidized ACTs should facilitate access to the drugs, especially among the poorest segments of society, and improve their effective use. Countries and funding organizations should support research toward these ends.

Countries should build on the malaria control impetus that widespread access to ACTs will create by:

• expanding access to ACTs (including treatment in or near the home) by decreasing geographic and financial barriers to drugs; and

• improving adherence to treatment schedules through public education, provider training, labeling, packaging, and dispensing.

6. Countries should be encouraged to carry out intensive integrated control programs in low-transmission areas where transmission may be dramatically reduced or eliminated within a few years.

Successful programs integrating household spraying with insecticides or insecticide-treated bednets, environmental management, and treatment with effective drugs, such as in KwaZulu Natal and Vietnam, should be encouraged in other low-transmission areas.

Monitoring, Evaluation, and Research

7. All countries should be encouraged to monitor public and private drug distribution systems to assure that subsidized antimalarials reach their intended targets at least as well as chloroquine has. Technical and financial assistance should be made available to carry out these tasks.

The procurement organization (in consultation with national and international bodies) should specify the monitoring information to be collected and help to ensure the availability of funds and technical assistance to accomplish this activity. Information should be collected, e.g., on the state of antimalarial packaging when drugs reach end users (whether the drugs are in their original packaging or have been repackaged in single doses, for example) and end-user prices. The availability of monotherapies also should be tracked.

8. Two different types of monitoring and surveillance should be made a routine part of every national malaria control plan: 1) monitoring the effectiveness of drug regimens, treatment failures and the emergence of resistant strains; and 2) surveillance for adverse antimalarial drug effects. Both should be required as a condition of access to subsidized antimalarials.

The best antimalarials for a country or region—in particular, partner drugs for artemisinins—must be selected based on accurate surveillance of individual drug efficacy, as close as possible to real time. Early warning systems that identify drug resistance, if acted upon in a timely way, could lead to the replacement of a failing ACT partner drug. This action, in turn, could protect the artemisinin component of a given ACT *and* save lives. Models for resistance monitoring exist in the multicountry networks already operating in various parts of Africa. Regarding safety, no major problems associated with ACT use have yet appeared, but widespread use in Africa is still pending. Surveillance, particularly in the early years, will be needed to quickly identify potential problems. The requirement for monitoring and surveillance cannot be absolute, however, in cases where it would impede access to effective, combination antimalarials. Countries in or just emerging from conflicts, or those dealing with natural or manmade disasters, for example, may not have the administrative capacity to monitor drug resistance. The enforcement of this recommendation will necessarily lie in the hands of the international organization in charge of procurement.

9. The global R&D investment should quickly rise to $60-80 million per year to guarantee the ongoing development of new antimalarials. Half of this amount should go to MMV from its regular funders, and half should be provided by the U.S. government to WRAIR and its public sector research partners.

Governments and other organizations that support malaria control activities should assure sufficient levels of funding to the major organizations behind antimalarial R&D, namely, MMV and WRAIR, to achieve the MMV target of one new antimalarial every 5 years, with similar progress expected from WRAIR.

PART 1

A Response to the Current Crisis

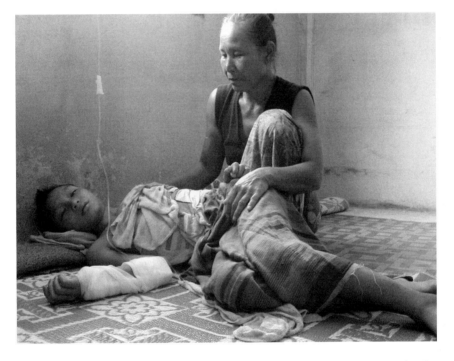

Treatment of multi-drug resistant falciparum malaria on the North-Western border of Thailand. Photo credit: Dr. Francois Nosten.

1

Malaria Today

INTRODUCTION TO THE STUDY

Chloroquine, after decades of use as the first-line drug for uncomplicated falciparum malaria, is failing. But it is still the most widely used antimalarial because a newer safe and effective alternative—artemisinin combination therapy (ACT) at a few dollars per course—has been considered unaffordable by national governments. As a result, illness and deaths from malaria are on the rise. Most fatalities occur among children in Africa, but failing drugs also account for a vast and largely unrecorded morbidity in people of other ages and demographics, not only in Africa, but in Asia and to some extent, everywhere that falciparum malaria (the most severe form) occurs. There also is evidence that drug resistance is leading to epidemics in fringe areas where malaria was previously well controlled when chloroquine was effective.

The IOM Committee on the Economics of Antimalarial Drugs was constituted to study the economics of making effective antimalarials accessible to those who could benefit from them. The Committee had two main tasks: 1) to recommend global actions to ensure the broadest possible access to effective antimalarial drugs, thus halting the accelerating loss of life (and malaria's attendant health and economic burdens) as quickly as possible; and 2) to consider some economic aspects of longer-term global malaria drug policy.

Genesis of the Project

The U.S. Agency for International Development (USAID) has a strong history and current portfolio in bilateral and multilateral assistance projects in malaria. USAID represents the United States in the "Roll Back Malaria" (RBM) partnership, centered in the World Health Organization (WHO), and including malaria-endemic countries, their bilateral and multilateral development partners, the private sector, nongovernmental and community-based organizations, foundations, and research and academic institutions. It was largely in connection with its leadership role in RBM that USAID approached the Institute of Medicine for independent advice and economic recommendations to counter the current global crisis in antimalarial drug resistance. The Bill and Melinda Gates Foundation later joined as a study cosponsor.

Charge to the Committee

The charge to the committee from USAID was the following:

> The committee will recommend steps that could be taken to maximize the influence of both new and established antimalarial drugs while postponing the development of drug resistance. The immediate focus will be on the class of artemisinin derivatives and other drugs with which they are (or could be) coformulated or paired, but the methodology developed should be generally applicable to new agents still in the pipeline.

The statement of task emphasized the fact that that influence would be maximized to the extent that: 1) new and established antimalarial drugs were affordable to the people who needed them; and 2) the antimalarial drugs were engineered and packaged, and delivered in ways that encouraged adherence to prescribed regimens. The Committee applied its energy mainly to the first point, while reviewing relevant information and making some recommendations on the second.

About This Report

The crisis of spreading resistance to antimalarial drugs has biomedical origins, but the inability of affected countries to respond by changing national treatment policies and making effective artemisinin-based drugs widely available is rooted in economics. The recommendations in this report were developed in light of the biomedical, social and cultural, and economic realities that define the burden of malaria and how it is addressed

---

BOX 1-1
Structure of This Report

Part 1: A Response to the Current Crisis

Chapter 1.	Malaria Today
Chapter 2.	The Cost and Cost-Effectiveness of Antimalarial Drugs
Chapter 3.	The Case for a Global Subsidy of Antimalarial Drugs
Chapter 4.	An International System for Procuring Antimalarial Drugs

Part 2: Malaria Basics

Chapter 5.	A Brief History of Malaria
Chapter 6.	The Parasite, the Mosquito, and the Disease
Chapter 7.	The Human and Economic Burden of Malaria
Chapter 8.	Malaria Control
Chapter 9.	Antimalarial Drugs and Drug Resistance

Part 3: Advancing Toward Better Malaria Control

Chapter 10.	Research and Development for New Antimalarial Drugs
Chapter 11.	Maximizing the Effective Use of Antimalarial Drugs

---

in endemic countries today. We attempt to draw together all these threads to present the reader with a complete and coherent set of facts from which to draw conclusions.

The report is in three parts (Box 1-1). Part 1 focuses on the immediate financing problem and proposes a global solution. Part 2 gives a foundation for understanding malaria as a disease, the tools we have to control it, and the burden it imposes on affected populations. The chapters that make up Part 2 are intended as both background for the nonspecialist and updates for those with a basic knowledge of malaria. They lay groundwork for the policy discussions and recommendations, but the reader may choose to pass by some of this material. Part 3 stresses the need to make further inroads against malaria by investing in the development of better antimalarial drugs and finding ways to better use new and existing tools.

The remainder of this chapter describes the extent of malaria in the world (with the greatest focus on Africa), how people deal with the disease on an individual level, how nations deal with it as a public health problem, and major global initiatives dealing with malaria control. It begins with a discussion of why this report focuses on artemisinin derivatives and artemisinin combination therapies (ACTs), and the roles of other antimalarial drugs.

THE ROLE OF THE ARTEMISININS IN MALARIA CONTROL

Artemisinins are the focus of international attention, and the center-piece of the recommendations in this report. Their full story—from discovery onward—is recounted in Chapter 9, as are the properties, advantages, and disadvantages of other currently effective antimalarials, and those of historic importance. Because the artemisinins figure so prominently, a few lines of explanation are in order to justify the primacy given to this family of compounds in the current circumstances.

It already has been said that chloroquine—after a remarkable period of effectiveness—no longer works against falciparum malaria in much of the world. The only other drug that has had relatively widespread use in Africa—sulfadoxine-pyrimethamine (SP)—worked as first-line therapy for a much shorter period than chloroquine before being evaded by resistant malaria organisms in many places. Continued use of SP would foster additional resistant strains and the drug would become largely ineffective, probably within several years. This should not be allowed to happen because SP has a very specific and important role, at least for the time being. It is the agent of choice for intermittent preventive therapy (IPT) for pregnant women. Next to children, they are the individuals most vulnerable to malaria, particularly in Africa.

One further idea must be introduced, and this is the global shift in strategy toward simultaneous treatment with two different antimalarials, adopted as a means to delay the development and spread of drug-resistant malaria. Combination treatment is not specific to artemisnin combinations but will become the standard henceforth, involving other drugs in the future.

The question remains as to why artemisinins are considered essential components of combinations, over the other currently effective antimalarials with which they would be paired: amodiaquine, mefloquine, and the most recent addition, Lapdap.[1] In fact, other combinations of drugs from different classes could be developed, but they are unlikely to be better than ACTs and would lack some of the benefits of a combination with an artemisinin. The main reasons for endorsing artemisinin-containing combinations are:

- the artemisinins represent a new family of compounds, with a novel mode of action, and faster antimalarial activity than any of the other drugs;
- they have proven themselves robust over at least a decade of consistent use in Asia, both in terms of effectiveness and safety and in the lack of any documented drug resistance (at least in part because they have a re-

---

[1]SP and Lapdap both are made up of two drugs but are not considered combinations in the sense of ACTs because the mechanisms of action of the two drugs are linked, and the individual drugs are not fully effective antimalarials.

markably short half-life, so subtherapeutic levels in the body, which promote resistance, are fleeting);

- in places where the level of transmission is low, they may play a role in reducing transmission because they act against the gametocyte (sexual) stage of the malaria parasite, as well as the asexual forms responsible for malaria symptoms; and finally,
- they have proven effective at the individual level in every transmission zone in Africa and elsewhere.

In contrast, the "companion" drugs are all related to earlier drugs, and there is either already documented resistance to them in some places, or the presumption that cross-resistance to the related drugs could compromise them. (The choice of which companion drug should be used in a given area will depend largely on the existing or potential resistance to each one.) In addition, any cautions applied to ACTs because of the lack of widespread use in Africa apply equally to these drugs, since none of them has been used extensively in high-transmission settings.

Can we be absolutely sure that widespread use of ACTs will halt the rising malaria mortality in Africa now resulting from the use of ineffective drugs? Not by direct evidence, although current evidence points in that direction. The truth is that they have not been deployed on a large scale in the highly endemic parts of Africa. Determining their overall impact will require years of surveillance, which should be carried out as conscientiously as possible. But there is no rationale for delaying actions to move ACTs into the hands of the greatest number of consumers, as quickly as possible, to replace the failing drugs now being used.

MALARIA TODAY

The Extent and Effects of Malaria

There is no time in memory when malaria was not a global health problem. It was common in many parts of the world until well into the 20th century. It was eliminated in Europe, North America, and parts of other continents through deliberate programs of mosquito control and clinical treatment, as well as through generally improved social and living conditions. The muscle behind eradication efforts elsewhere was never applied in Africa's highly endemic areas, however (Breman, et al., 2001). Today, sub-Saharan Africa remains the area of greatest malaria concentration, but significant problems exist in Asia, in Latin America, and focally in other areas. At least 85 percent of deaths from malaria occur in Africa, 8 percent in Southeast Asia, 5 percent in the Eastern Mediterranean region, 1 percent in the Western Pacific, and 0.1 percent in the Americas.

Now, at the beginning of the 21st century, there is good reason to believe that inroads against malaria can be made in Africa and elsewhere, using the control measures described in this report, if effective combination antimalarials are made widely available.

Malaria in Africa

The extent of the challenge is illustrated by the map of Africa (Figure 1-1), showing a vast swath between the northern coastal countries and the most southerly ones (excluding most of the horn of Africa) where malaria transmission is intense and malaria is ever-present. This area is ringed by a region prone to seasonal malaria transmission or periodic epidemics—with often devastatingly high mortality rates. More than half a billion people—more than two-thirds of the African population—live with malaria year in, year out, most of them where transmission is intense. The vast majority of the million or so deaths from malaria occur in Africa, mostly among children who have yet to acquire sufficient immunity to protect them from heavy malaria infections. The prevalence of malaria varies with levels of endemicity, but it averages to at least one acute clinical episode per year for which some treatment is sought, or on the order of half a billion treated episodes.

It is worth remembering that the malaria map would have looked very different half a century ago, and that control measures are largely responsible for shrinking the highly-endemic zone. The low- and no-transmission areas of southern Africa (including Namibia, Swaziland, South Africa, Botswana, and Zimbabwe) were previously highly endemic—and could become so again, if control measures fail.

The map lays out the boundaries of a very large problem, but does not tell the whole story. Who becomes sick and who dies is what is important. Once the discussion moves beyond acknowledging that malaria is a "big" problem, however, estimates of the relevant numbers—malaria cases, deaths from malaria—and the distribution among the population, geographically and by age, vary so widely that they can appear unusable for policy and planning. This lack of specificity is at least part of what makes tackling the problem so unsettling.

Malaria in Asia

There are about 27 million cases and 30,000 deaths from falciparum malaria in Southeast Asia each year, with no perceptible decline over the last decade (WHO Regional Office for South-East Asia,). Unlike Africa, where acquired semi-immunity protects most adults from severe clinical disease and death, intermittent infections in Asian endemic areas are usu-

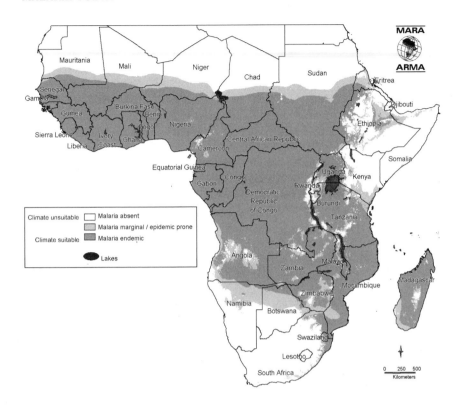

FIGURE 1-1 Distribution of Endemic Malaria in Africa.
SOURCE: Reprinted with permission from MARA/ARMA, Copyright 2001. Taken from Craig, MH, Snow RW, le Sueur D. 1999. A Climate-Based Distribution Model of Malaria Transmission in Sub-Saharan Africa. *Parasitology Today* 15(3):105-111.

ally symptomatic, not uncommonly with very high parasitemias (parasite numbers in the blood) and a risk of death. Apart from the sheer numbers— not approaching African levels, but substantial—Southeast Asia has been the epicenter of drug-resistant malaria precisely because of this pattern of infection and treatment of nonimmune individuals with heavy parasite loads. Some of the most difficult problems arise in border areas, where refugees have gathered after political conflicts. Isolated tribal groups in various countries, with little or no access to health care, also suffer disproportionately from malaria.

Malaria in the New World

North America and most of the Caribbean are free from malaria transmission, a result of eradication efforts that began in earnest in the 1950s. But 200 million people live where there is still some risk of transmission, in 21 countries of Central and South America, and the Caribbean, about 20 percent of them in areas considered "high risk" for the region. About one million cases and 200 deaths were recorded in 2001. Drug resistance is becoming widespread, and changes in drug policy have already been made in some places. And the same factors that can disrupt control in Africa and Asia—migration, civil unrest, poor economic conditions—occur in the Americas.

The Varied and Far-Reaching Effects of Malaria[2]

Malaria is not simply a matter of episodes of illness and deaths, as enormous as those burdens are. Effects vary from place to place, but nearly all people living in endemic areas will at some stage in their lives become infected with malaria through the bite of a mosquito, and after the parasite has multiplied in numbers, they will suffer an attack of fever and other symptoms when large numbers of parasites are released into the bloodstream. Untreated, these episodes may progress in severity and naturally resolve, or the person may become overwhelmed and die. Or antimalarial drugs may be used to quell the infection. Functional immunity develops in those who survive the early episodes, if they are continually exposed to malaria from birth, preventing most symptomatic recurrences at older ages.

But that is not the whole story. There are less obvious, but equally serious, consequences of the chronic infections and repeated reinfections that characterize life in high-transmission areas, including most of sub-Saharan Africa. Chronic, subclinical infections can cause anemia and predispose to undernutrition. These processes may further increase the chances of severe malaria developing with a subsequent infection, and possibly of more severe outcomes of infections with other pathogens. Unlike other adults in endemic areas, pregnant women are themselves more susceptible to malaria's most severe effects—including death—and asymptomatic infection of the placenta significantly reduces the weights of their newborn children, reducing their chances of surviving infancy.

Some proportion of those who survive severe malaria—with or without effective treatment—are left with permanent, serious effects, including epi-

---

[2]Chapter 6 gives a detailed account of the disease and its effects, which are summarized briefly here.

lepsy and spasticity. More subtle consequences have also been described and include behavioral disturbances and cognitive impairment. Currently, it is not possible to do much more than mention this spectrum of effects. They cannot yet be quantified, which is not surprising when even the most concrete of end points—the number of deaths from malaria—is only roughly estimated (see Chapter 7).

What People Do When They Suspect Malaria

Where malaria is common, a child may have four or five bouts of fever, and an adult one or two each year, all presumed to be malaria. People live with malaria in their midst in a variety of ways, but not infrequently with a compromised quality of life. Families do make efforts and spend precious resources to prevent malaria (in part, by eliminating nuisance insects), but most of the readily accessible methods, such as burning mosquito coils or leaves, are only partially effective. Insecticide-treated bednets—the most effective single preventive intervention—are still relatively rare, though coverage is increasing (see Chapter 8). In the absence of effective prevention, treatment of symptomatic cases is the most common form of malaria control.

Decisions about whether and what kind of treatment to seek depend, first, on whether the patient or caregiver thinks that malaria is the cause of the illness. A host of considerations—specific symptoms, personal and family history, season of the year—factor into this judgment. Unfortunately, the symptoms of severe malaria—convulsions, loss of consciousness—often are ascribed to other causes, so malaria treatment is not sought, at least initially. When a decision is made to seek treatment for what is presumed to be malaria, what actually happens reflects both the demand side—what people want—and the supply side—what is available to them. It is, in many ways, more complex than a parallel decision to seek treatment for a febrile illness in the United States or Europe, where there would be no need to worry, for instance, about whether a clinic or hospital actually has the drug needed to treat the disease. The costs of treatment in money, time, travel, and otherwise, in general, are more onerous for a poor rural African, Asian, or South American family than for their poor counterparts in richer countries. Decisions may be delayed while options are weighed, funds gathered, and arrangements made. People know that children die of malaria, but they also know from experience that most episodes resolve uneventfully. An unfortunate reality is that in the cases when children do die from malaria, it can happen very quickly, especially for the very young: one day the child has a mild fever and then one of a number of serious symptoms appear, and the child is dead. In those cases, the consequences of waiting are severe and irreversible.

The topic of this report demands some understanding of where patients go for malaria treatment (if they go), and in the case of drug treatment, the path drugs follow to get to the varied outlets in the public and private sectors. As is the case for a number of the key issues (e.g., the quantitative burden of malaria), there are many generalizations but frustratingly little solid information. What we really need to know is how to intervene to reduce the morbidity, shrink the overall malaria burden, and prevent the deaths. A starting point is knowing what people do when they or their children have malaria, whether they think it is malaria or something else. When this has been studied it has been almost exclusively among the survivors. Certain patterns emerge, as reviewed later in this chapter. The question that remains almost entirely untouched is what chain of treatment-seeking events took place for those who eventually died from malaria. A preliminary analysis of the most extensive such study undertaken has been completed recently by the Tanzania Essential Health Interventions Project (TEHIP) (de Savigny et al., 2003). (Appendix 1A is a detailed account of the study and its results to date.)

The TEHIP Study: Preliminary Findings

Study Description

TEHIP studied the circumstances leading to deaths from malaria in the stable perennial malaria transmission belt that runs along the coast of Tanzania and up the Rufiji and Kilombero River basins, from January 1999 through the end of 2001. The Rufiji Demographic Surveillance Site (DSS) covers 85,000 people in 17,000 households in 31 villages, registering all births, deaths, in-migrations, out-migrations, pregnancies and other vital events. A "verbal autopsy" is conducted for each person who dies in the population. Following routine DSS procedures for verbal autopsy,[3] a trained health officer interviews the next of kin (or other close "informant") about the person who died and the events leading to the death. Questions are asked about the use of health facilities during the fatal illness, reasons for using or not using a particular health facility, and confirmatory evidence of cause of death, if available. The interviewer assesses the information and assigns a tentative cause of death. A physician reviews the entire record and assigns the final cause.

From the full details of each case, treatment can be divided broadly into "modern care"—which includes biomedical, Western, pharmaceutical, pro-

---

[3]Not all verbal autopsies use the exact method described here. Procedures for gathering information and for assigning the recorded cause of death may differ.

fessional, official or formal health care—and "traditional care"—which includes traditional medicine, traditional healers, traditional providers, lay providers, traditional practices, or folk care. (Use of "modern care" does not necessarily mean that the care was appropriate, or used correctly.)

Results

Over the 3-year period, 3,023 people died and 2,953 (97.7 percent) verbal autopsies were conducted. Out of these, 722 were suspected to be directly or indirectly due to malaria. Just under half (46 percent) of the 722 who died were male, 44 percent were under 5 years of age, and 39 (5 percent) had had convulsions indicating possible cerebral malaria. Findings of particular interest include:

- Treatment most often started at home using antipyretics and antimalarials from local shops or left over from previous episodes.
- 626 (87 percent) sought care at least once before death, while 96 (13 percent) did not, or could not, seek care. These figures were similar for those under and over age 5.
- Of the group that did *not* have convulsions, 91 percent used modern care first, and by the second treatment, more than 99 percent had used modern care. Hence, traditional care delayed modern care for 9 percent of cases.
- Of those who did have convulsions, a similar proportion (90 percent) used modern care first, but only 63 percent continued with modern care for a second treatment when the first had failed.

This pattern is considerably better than was seen in the mid-1980s in Bagamoyo, when 55 percent of children who died had not utilized any modern care (Mtango et al., 1992).

TEHIP is continuing to refine the information from this study and will be analyzing the narrative portion of the verbal autopsy questionnaires to look at some specific aspects of the health care received, including:

- reasons for delay in *seeking* modern care (e.g., tried to treat at home without antimalarials, no transport, poor recognition of severity, lack of confidence in modern care, no power to decide, insufficient finances);
- reasons for delay in *receiving* modern care (e.g., arrived after working hours or on the weekend, long queues); and
- reasons modern care was ineffective (e.g., poor communication, no referral, drugs not available, abusive health worker, noncompliant providers, poor adherence of patients).

Decisions to Seek Malaria Treatment and Beliefs about the Disease: The Knowledge Base[4]

Adults sense when they have a fever, and mothers know when their children are sick. Where malaria is common, people generally associate it with febrile illness, but this varies from place to place depending on cultural practices and beliefs, education and experience, and individual characteristics.

When malaria is suspected, people may go to one of a wide range of places (although in a given place, the choices may be few), including modern health providers in public clinics or health centers of various sizes in private facilities run by religious groups or other nongovernmental organizations; or the commercial private sector, which includes traditional healers, pharmacies, shops, markets, and drug peddlers. It is these latter outlets—mainly shops and drug peddlers, often referred to as the "informal private sector"—that provide antimalarial drugs for more than half of all treated episodes in sub-Saharan Africa (Mwabu, 1986; Deming et al., 1989; Ejezie et al., 1990; Snow et al., 1992; Mnyika et al., 1995). It also is common for people to get drugs from more than one source: people often begin with self-treatment using drugs from the informal sector, and then seek care from formal providers (McCombie, 1996).

But people have varied beliefs about the causes of disease and what treatments are appropriate. In the few places where it has been studied both in Africa and Asia, mild and severe malaria often are considered distinct diseases, with different words to describe them and different beliefs about how to treat them. Severe malaria with convulsions may be perceived as involving supernatural intervention, such as spirit possession or magic spells (Mwenesi et al., 1995; Winch et al., 1996; Ahorlu et al., 1997; Muela and Ribera, 2000), and as a consequence, people may be more likely to go to a traditional healer for treatment, such that the most dangerous cases are least likely to get effective antimalarial drugs. It is not uncommon in Africa for mothers to believe that "modern" treatment, injections in particular, are dangerous for children with convulsions (Mwenesi et al., 1995; Makemba et al., 1996; Ahorlu et al., 1997) even though injections often are preferred over tablets for other conditions. Alternatively, both traditional and Western medical providers may be consulted in turn.

Treatment through the Formal Sector

Most malaria treatment takes place at home with drugs from the informal sector, but formal facilities bear a substantial burden. In sub-Saharan

---

[4]This section is drawn largely from an in-depth review by Hanson et al. (2004).

Africa and rural Asia, fever is the reason for 20 to 40 percent of all clinic and dispensary visits. These outpatient facilities generally do not offer the life-saving emergency treatments required when severe malaria develops, however. Only hospitals or health centers with inpatient facilities—where malaria's share of admissions ranges between 0.5 and 50 percent (Chima et al., 2003)—are able to provide this care.

The pattern of treatment-seeking and treatment itself is different in countries outside of Africa—mainly Asia and the Latin America/Caribbean region. Malaria is a significant problem in a number of countries, but it is generally more localized to specific areas, and everywhere is much less common than in Africa. Therefore, the burden on individuals as well as the health care system is much less. In Asia and Latin America, people with malaria are treated in general medical facilities, or in special malaria clinics. Laboratory diagnosis is much more widely used, and where these facilities are not available on-site, patients with suspected malaria often are treated presumptively for the immediate symptoms, and given further treatment if their malaria is confirmed.

Treatment through the Informal Sector

Use of the informal sector for malaria treatment is very common throughout the world, even where malaria is less common. Most of this involves the purchase of antimalarials from shops, where people may ask for a "product" by name, rather than a "service" including diagnosis and advice. In Thailand, for example, "ya chud"—a packet with a mixture of medicines including antimalarial drugs sold in private outlets—is used frequently (one study found that around 90 percent of respondents had used ya chud at least once in their lifetime) (McCombie, 1996).

The role of traditional healers and the use of traditional medicines for uncomplicated malaria varies, but generally is considered to be of less importance than other sources of care (McCombie, 1996), though people may underreport use of these services because of perceived disapproval. However, in various parts of Africa, traditional healers often may be consulted for severe malaria. In one site in rural Tanzania in the early 1990s, 90 percent of the children under 5 who died from acute febrile illness with seizures, died at home. Most (85 percent) had been seen by some kind of traditional healer, and only about half had been to a formal health facility before they died (de Savigny et al., 1999).

Weaknesses of Malaria Treatment

People seeking treatment for malaria through any of the channels described here often are frustrated by their experiences. In both the public and private sectors, patients may be faced with low quality of care, lack of drugs or poor quality drugs, and unpredictable costs, to name just a few of the problems. All of these problems affect patients, but they also are concerns for health care systems. Some of the key problems are enumerated below.

Issues in Diagnosis

- Where diagnosis is based on symptoms alone, overdiagnosis, with resultant overuse of antimalarial drugs and real causes of illness possibly left untreated (Stein and Gelfand, 1985; Olivar et al., 1991; Guiguemde et al., 1997).
- Where parasitologic diagnosis is attempted, poor equipment, lack of supplies, limited training and supervision of laboratory staff, and inapropriate use of diagnostic results in treatment choices (Palmer et al., 1999; Barat et al., 1999).
- Lack of accurate microscopy, and for rapid diagnostic tests, the difficulty of determining whether a parasitic infection that is detected is the cause of the current illness. Especially in highly endemic areas, diagnosis based on symptoms may be equally valid.

Lack of Effective Drugs and Inappropriate Use of Drugs

- Chloroquine remains the first-line drug, and sometimes the only antimalarial stocked in health centers and hospitals, even in some countries with very high rates of chloroquine resistance.
- Health facilities frequently are out of stock of essential drugs including antimalarials, and the malaria peak in some countries coincides with the end of the financial year, exacerbating the problem at a key time.
- Second- and third-line drugs may not be made available to lower level health facilities, despite the high frequency of treatment failure with the first-line remedy.
- "Polypharmacy"—prescribing of multiple, unnecessary drugs in addition to the antimalarial is common. As well as being wasteful, it may increase the risk of side effects.
- Where patients have to pay for drugs, they may buy only some of the products prescribed, or incomplete doses, including the antimalarial itself. They may buy a complete course, but take only the first part (particularly if they feel better), storing the remainder for a subsequent episode, leading to systematic underdosing and encouraging the emergence of resistance.
- Expensive (and possibly more dangerous) formulations may be used in place of cheaper ones: in a study in Ghana, 42 percent of chloro-

quine prescribed to outpatients was administered by injection rather than orally (Ofori-Adjei and Arhinful, 1996).

- Poor quality drugs are common in retail pharmacies in Africa and Asia, due both to lack of quality control in manufacture and to degradation during storage (Shakoor et al., 1997; Maponga and Ondari, 2003).
- Counterfeit drugs are an enormous problem in tropical countries. Fake antimalarials have been a particular problem recently in Southeast Asia. For example, until a recent publicity campaign, more than half of the antimalarial drugs available in the private sector in Cambodia were fake. Widespread counterfeiting of artesunate has led to erroneous reports of resistance (Newton et al., 2001).

When patients buy their own drugs through shops or drug sellers, they may use their own judgment about how much to take (or how much they can afford to buy), and they also may get information from the sellers which may or may not be accurate. As an example of what takes place:

- In a survey in Kenya, only 4 percent of children given store-bought chloroquine got an adequate dose, and only half of those children received this dose over the recommended 3-day period (Marsh et al., 1999).
- In the same survey, aspirin was widely used and 22 percent of children received potentially toxic doses (Marsh et al., 1999).

How Quality Issues Affect Patients

Patients factor in what they know from past experience and general community knowledge when they decide on malaria treatment. In one rural area in Tanzania, the most common reason people gave for not using government services was the poor drug supply. At the same time, people report that public clinic staff are often rude and insensitive, and there are long waiting times to be seen. The facilities themselves often are in poor condition, discouraging people from coming (Gilson et al., 1994).

Costs are sometimes unpredictable in public facilities. Providers may add on charges for drugs that ought to be covered by the consultation fee. If there are no drugs in the clinic, the patient may have to pay for the consultation, and then be told to purchase the drugs privately.

Private clinics and other outlets have their problems too. While staff attitudes may be better and waiting times shorter, private facilities may not have as wide a range of equipment or trained staff as in the public sector (Silva et al., 1997; Mutizwa-Mangiza, 1997). And patients are aware they are paying higher prices for private services, which may make them skeptical about the motivations of private providers, balancing the welfare of patients against their own profits (Silva et al., 1997; Smithson et al., 1997).

DRUG FLOWS AND PRICING OF ANTIMALARIALS

Examples from Senegal, Zambia, and Cambodia

It is easy to find out that the prices people pay for drugs in many countries vary tremendously, but not so easy to know the pathways that drugs travel and the costs incurred along the way. Descriptions of the flow of drugs from manufacturer to consumer, and the price mark-ups that accompany each transaction, are scarce or nonexistent for Africa and Asia. The IOM Committee asked Management Sciences for Health (MSH) to document the flow and prices of antimalarial drugs in a sample of countries. The information summarized here is taken from their report (Shretta and Guimier, 2003).

MSH gathered information directly for this report in Senegal, Zambia, and Cambodia, all poor countries where malaria is a major health problem (see Table 1-1 for basic economic and health indicators for the three countries).

Malaria in Senegal, Zambia, and Cambodia

The entire population in Senegal is considered to be at risk of malaria; the disease is mesoendemic in some areas to hyperendemic in others. Malaria is the leading cause of morbidity, in 1996, the reason for 32 percent of outpatient consultations (27 percent for those under 5 years age, 39 percent for those over 5 years).

Malaria is endemic throughout Zambia and continues to be the leading cause of morbidity and mortality, especially among pregnant women and children under age 5. Malaria accounts for 36.7 percent of all outpatient attendance, 62.1 percent of inpatient admissions, and 10.3 percent of pregnant women seen at health facilities.

About two million of Cambodia's 12 million population are at risk of malaria. The worst affected are ethnic minorities, temporary migrants, settlers in forested areas, plantation workers and others who live in the country's hilly forested environments and forest fringes. In 1995, malaria and fever accounted for a quarter of outpatient attendances (42 percent in highly malarious areas), 6 percent of hospital admission (over 30 percent in malarious areas), and 15 percent of reported deaths (over 50 percent in endemic areas).

Drug Flows

In all three countries—and typical of most other malaria-endemic countries in Africa and Asia—drugs flow into the country and to consumers

TABLE 1-1 Economic and Health Indicators in Senegal, Zambia, and Cambodia

	Senegal	Zambia	Cambodia
Economic Indicators			
Gross National Income (GNI) per capita, 2001, US$	490	320	270
% population below US$1 per day	26 (1995)	64 (1998)	not available
% population below national poverty line	33 (1992)	73 (1998)	36 (1997)
Total health expenditures as % GDP (1997-2000)[a]	4.6	5.6	8.1
Public health expenditures as % of total (1997-2000)[a]	56.6	62.1	24.5
Private health expenditures as % of total (1997-2000)[a]	43.4	37.9	75.5
Health expenditure per capita, US$ (1997-2000)[a]	22	18	19
Health and Population Indicators (2001)			
Total population, millions	9.8	10.3	12.3
Under 5 mortality rate (per 1,000)	138	202	138
Infant mortality rate (per 1,000 live births)	79	112	97
Life expectancy at birth (years)	52	37	54
Pharmaceutical Market (2001)			
Total value of pharmaceutical sales (US$ millions)	$50	$20	$50

[a]For most recent year available.
SOURCE: World Bank, 2003; Shretta and Guimier, 2003.

through the usual public and private sectors, and also through various illegal channels. In each sector, drugs flow into the system from large importers and some local manufacturers, who supply outlets lower down in the chains. Drug flows in each country are depicted schematically in Figures 1-2, 1-3, and 1-4.

Public Sector Drug Flows

Senegal

The Senegalese Pharmacie Nationale d'Approvisionnement (PNA), a state-owned enterprise, is responsible for importing, storing, and distributing the drugs on the national essential drug list. The drugs flow from the PNA downward through several levels of the public sector and are accessible to consumers in a variety of places, but always involve interactions with health care providers (physicians, midwives, nurses, or health workers.

The PNA supplies five regional stores (Pharmacie Regionale d'Approvisionnement [PRA]), which in turn supply the district depots, which then provide drugs to the health facilities. Similarly, health centers and health posts are supplied by the district depot. Health huts obtain their supplies from the posts. Overall, the public sector accounts for about 35 percent of the sales value of antimalarials.

Zambia

Most pharmaceuticals are imported from India (some also come from Zimbabwe, Tanzania, Kenya, and South Africa) and most come in as finished products, which are exempt from import duties and taxes. Six local companies manufacture generic essential drugs in Zambia (one meets international Good Manufacturing Practice standards). No multinational pharmaceutical companies produce drugs in Zambia.

All drugs on the national essential drug list, including antimalarials, are procured by the Central Board of Health, either by international competitive bidding or by selective tender. Preference (including a 15 percent price advantage) is given to locally manufactured or procured drugs. Local companies are rarely awarded large tenders, however, because they cannot meet some of the conditions.

All drugs procured by, or on behalf of, the government are delivered to Medical Stores Ltd. (the country's Central Medical Stores). Public sector drugs and medical supplies are delivered to all districts, nine general hospitals, and four specialized hospitals. When Medical Stores Ltd. cannot supply all the needs of districts, they purchase their own drugs to fill gaps.

The public sector is more important in Zambia than in many other countries. Up to 70 percent of people seeking treatment for malaria go first to the public sector. However, private sector use is increasing and use of public health facilities is decreasing, in part due to only partially effective exemption mechanisms for the poor and frequent drug shortages in the public sector.

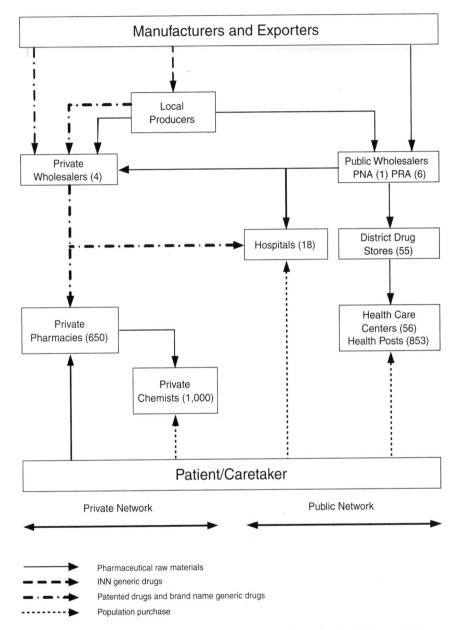

FIGURE 1-2 Organization of distribution networks for antimalarial drugs in Senegal, excluding the parallel market.

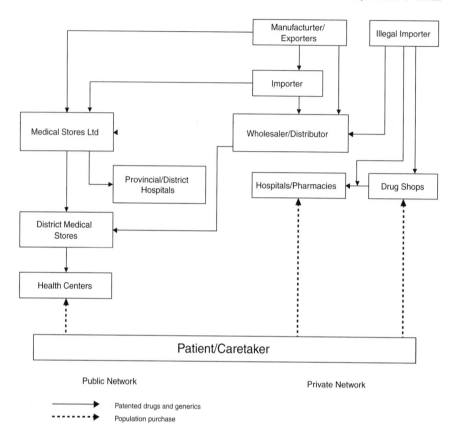

FIGURE 1-3 The distribution of pharmaceuticals in Zambia.

Cambodia

Most pharmaceuticals (public and private sector) are imported, with some manufactured locally. About 25 percent of all legal pharmaceuticals imports come in through the public sector (through 14 companies in 2001) (SEAM, 2001). Six local manufacturers produce more than 26 essential drugs, including chloroquine. Blister packaging of A+M tablets and Malarine (a coformulation of the same two drugs, artesunate and mefloquine) is carried out by Cambodian Pharmaceutical Enterprise with support from WHO.

Public sector drug procurement and distribution are centralized and, since 2002, procurement has been through an open tender system. Drug needs for malaria are determined by the National Malaria Center (CNM),

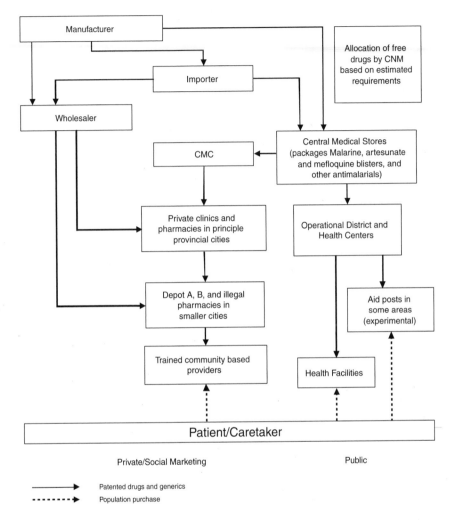

FIGURE 1-4 Flow of drugs in Cambodia, including public and private sectors.

which informs the Central Medical Stores how much of each drug to send to each province. Drugs are supplied quarterly to all 73 referral hospitals and more than 700 health centers across the country. They are distributed by motor vehicles and in areas isolated during seasonal flooding, by boat. Road conditions generally are poor, which impedes distribution.

Private Sector Drug Flows

Senegal

Four private wholesalers feed into 650 pharmacies that sell drugs to consumers and also, in rural areas, to private chemists who sell, officially, a limited line of medications to consumers (however, much more variety is usually available). These networks represent nearly 65 percent of the total sales value of antimalarials in the country (excluding the illegal market). The private market is efficient at maintaining stocks, especially for urban pharmacies, which may be supplied daily.

Most of the products in the private sector come from France and are marketed under brand names, but essential generic medications—mostly locally produced—are sold under standard International Nonproprietary Names (INNs). Since June 2003, private networks also have distributed generic medications under INNs that they purchase at the PNA, which appear on the limited list of thirty medications, including three antimalarials (chloroquine tablets and two dosages of injectable quinine).

Zambia

About 50 registered pharmaceutical wholesalers and distributors import drugs into Zambia to supply the private market, which consists of private clinics, hospitals, and retail pharmacies. Unlike the situation in Senegal, the private sector cannot purchase drugs from the public sector to sell in private outlets.

Private distributors deliver drugs only within Lusaka, the capital, and to towns on the railway line to the Copper Belt and the Southern province. Depending on the location of the provider, a drug may go through two or three wholesalers before it arrives at its final place of sale.

Drug Flow through the Churches Health Association of Zambia

The Churches Health Association of Zambia (CHAZ)—the largest private not-for-profit organization in Zambia—includes more than 100 church-administered hospitals, health centers, and community programs, which operate as part of the public health system. Mission hospitals serve as district hospitals where there is no Ministry of Health hospital, mostly in poor rural areas.

CHAZ procures drugs quarterly, using a restricted tender system from suppliers pre-qualified by WHO. CHAZ is exempt from registration fees and various duties on imported drugs and medical equipment. The main suppliers are the International Dispensary Association in the Netherlands and Mission Pharma, in Denmark. CHAZ handles about 90 products, all of them on the Zambian National Formulary. About 55 of the 100 mission hospitals and health centers in Zambia regularly procure drugs from CHAZ, which they purchase directly from the warehouse in Lusaka.

Cambodia

The private sector—particularly drug sellers—are the first point of contact for more than 70 percent of the population when they are ill (Ministry of Health of Kingdom of Cambodia, 1998), and 75 percent of legal antimalarials are sold through the private sector. Self-treatment is common among the poor, and for many people indigenous or traditional healers remain the first point of contact. The private sector is largely unregulated for price and quality, and there are no accurate records of volumes of antimalarials (or other drugs) sold.

Social Marketing

A social marketing program for blister-packed mefloquine plus artesunate, branded as "Malarine," and a "dipstick" diagnostic test for *P. falciparum*, has been scaled up across the country (in all but two provinces), following a European Union pilot program in selected areas. Vendors who have signed a franchise agreement are provided with promotional posters, package dispensers, and a start-up supply of free packages and tests. A suggested retail price of R7,900 (price printed on the package) includes a profit of R1,000 for the franchiser. In practice, higher prices are charged. The blister-packed drugs are sold on the basis of a positive dipstick test available for US$0.55. The dipstick price was designed to be included in the price for Malarine, but it is sold separately by retail outlets.

Drug Flows through the Illegal Sector

Senegal

Parallel to the public and private legal networks is a large, thriving illegal market, believed to account for millions of dollars worth of drugs. The components of the illegal market are the traditional market ("sidewalk medication") found in cities in the interior and the Touba market, a highly organized illegal market providing pharmaceuticals at a wholesale and retail level. The illegal market is allegedly supplied from many sources, including organized smuggling networks, the private sector, leakage from the public sector, occasional diversions from the Dakar port or airport, illegal or declared imports of donations collected in France and in other countries in Europe by nongovernmental organizations (NGOs), and resale of prescribed medications not taken by patients (full or partial doses). Prices in the illegal market can be 30 percent lower than in the private sector, which makes them attractive to middle class as well as poorer customers, with or without a prescription.

Zambia

Apart from the registered suppliers, drugs are also supplied by some "cross border" traders (usually illegally) within the Common Market for Eastern and Southern Africa (COMESA) and the Southern African Development Cooperation Conference (SADCC) region.

Cambodia

The illegal market is supplied largely by pharmaceuticals smuggled across the border from neighboring countries, sold by an estimated 2,800 illegal drug sellers nationwide (Ministry of Health of Kingdom of Cambodia, 2001b). In Phnom Penh, there are an estimated 495 illegal drug sellers, compared with 298 registered pharmacies and drug sellers.

Availability of Antimalarials

Senegal

The public network provides four antimalarial drugs (amodiaquine, chloroquine, quinine, and SP), which come in nine different presentations, forms, and dosages. In the private sector, there are 13 compounds sold in 89 presentations, forms, and dosages.

Zambia

In the face of widespread chloroquine resistance, in 2003, Coartem was named as the official first-line drug. Coartem has been introduced into pilot districts, but because of cost, SP (which is cheaper), is available in most other places. Although no longer provided through the public sector, there are still considerable sales of chloroquine in the private sector. In addition, more than a hundred different brands, presentations, and forms of antimalarials are available in the private market as branded products, generics, and branded generics, representing about 14 different compounds. Artemisinin products are freely available without prescription in this sector, as monotherapies and combinations.

Cambodia

More than 100 brands and forms of antimalarials are found in Cambodia's private sector outlets, where patients receive treatment based on their ability to pay. The public sector distributes mainly generic products, about 8 antimalarials in various forms and strengths. In total, 30 antimalarials are officially registered.

A combination of artesunate and mefloquine (A+M) was introduced as the first-line drug in 1999, with a recommendation that all first-line drugs be based on a diagnosis by either microscopy or a rapid dipstick test. The combination is available as "A+M" in the public sector and is socially marketed in the private sector as "Malarine." Dipsticks also are socially marketed in the private sector.

Drug Pricing

In all three countries, in addition to transport, clearing charges and any taxes that may be added to manufacturing prices (in Senegal this is 10 percent and 1.5 percent), drug importers add a margin, which includes distribution costs. In Senegal, the markup by the public wholesaler was 13 percent, and by the private wholesaler, 9.9-24.6 percent, depending on the type of medication. District store markup in the public sector was typically 15 percent. In Zambia, wholesalers usually added a markup of 20-30 percent, and in Cambodia, this ranged from 1.82-49.57 percent. In Senegal, the Bamako pharmacies add margins of 30.5 percent in the public sector, while pharmacies and retailers in the private sector add margins of 9.9-56.2 percent. In Zambia, private pharmacies and retailers generally add a margin of 30-40 percent; in Cambodia these ranged from 1.85-2300 percent. These mechanisms, based on cumulative margins, lead to an almost doubling of the cost of entry prices (Table 1-2 lists consumer prices for selected antimalarials in the three countries, in some public and private sector outlets.)

Drug Financing

Senegal

More than 90 percent of drug costs are paid by consumers, either directly, in the private pharmacies or in public health facilities through the cost recovery system, or indirectly, through mandatory or voluntary contribution systems.

TABLE 1-2 Consumer prices of selected antimalarials in three countries for a typical adult course of treatment (in US$)

	Senegal		Zambia		Cambodia	
	Public	Private Range (median)	Public	Private (median)	Public	Private
Chloroquine tablets (150 mg in Senegal, 250 mg in Zambia and Cambodia)	.16			.16		.10-30
SP tablets (500 mg + 25 mg)	.32			.32		
Amodiaquine (200 mg)	.39	.56		.33		
Mefloquine (250 mg)				8.32		1.25-3.45
Artesunate tablets (50 mg)		3.98		6.44 (CHAZ: 3.12)		1.00-3.00
Coartem (artemether + lumefantrine) (8 tabs) [16 = 9.29]		5.64		22.50		
Artesunate + mefloquine (blister)					.50-1.63	1.75-2.13

SOURCE: Shretta and Guimier, 2003.

Zambia

Drugs in the public sector are financed by a combination of government funds and user fees. The fees vary according to the type of facility, the area of the country, and the patient. The poor and certain population groups (children under 5, people over 65), as well as certain services (e.g., antenatal care, tuberculosis treatment, childhood vaccination) are officially exempt from fees in all health facilities, but the system is not implemented well. Where fees are paid, the usual markup on drugs is about 30 percent, similar to the private sector.

In public hospitals, consultation fees vary from free to ZK5,000 (about US$1). In Lusaka and other urban areas, health centers charge membership (averaging ZK5,000 in Lusaka and ZK1500 in Kafue), which entitles the payer to treatment without further charges. Health centers elsewhere usually provide consultation services and drugs free of charge.

During 2000/1 CHAZ procured drugs, medical supplies, and vaccines valued at ZK379 million (US$95,000) with its own funds, and received donations valued at ZK9.55 billion (US$2.5 million). User fees, similar to those charged at public facilities, are charged at various mission hospitals.

Cambodia

More than 80 percent of health care is paid for directly by households and about 45 percent of households borrow money to pay medical bills. Formal user fees have been in place since 1997, with a required exemption for the poor. Since user fees were introduced, the quality of the service has improved, and use by the poor has increased. The exemptions function relatively well at the health center level, but not at referral hospitals, where staff discourage their use (Wilkinson et al., 2000).

The government accounts for less than 5 percent of health sector financing (Ministry of Health of Kingdom of Cambodia, 2002a,b). Pharmaceutical expenditures by the Ministry of Health Procurement Unit for the public sector in 2000 was approximately US$14.2 million (SEAM, 2001).

Donor funding, from governments and NGOs, amounts to 15 percent of total health financing (Ministry of Health of Kingdom of Cambodia, 2001b), and 25 percent of pharmaceuticals (SEAM, 2001). Donor resources (as are other public-sector resources) are allocated disproportionately to the capital area, where relatively few of the poor live (World Bank, 1999).

Common Themes and Contrasts

A wide variety of antimalarial drugs—more than those officially registered—can be bought for a wide variety of prices in these countries. One way or another (whether through a consultation fee or direct purchase), consumers pay a large proportion of the cost of antimalarial drugs. The private market prices are invariably higher than those in the public sector. Prices in the illegal sector may be among the lowest. A factor not mentioned earlier is that counterfeit drugs of all types are also common, and they are found not only in the private and illegal sectors, but in public sector facilities.

In Senegal and Cambodia, the private sector dominates the provision of antimalarial drugs, but in Zambia, the public sector is the main source of care for malaria, including provision of drugs. International donors, church-based clinics and hospitals, and other not-for-profit organizations all are established and play varying roles in the health care systems of these countries, making the flow of drugs even more fragmented and complex.

The extent of the illegal sector, the presence of many unregistered products even in the legal private sector, and the widespread problem of counterfeit drugs gives some sense of the difficulty of regulating drugs in these countries and their neighbors in Africa and Asia. While governments work toward greater control—with the aim of more rational drug use by their citizens—the current mix of distribution systems will not be changed quickly.

INTERNATIONAL ORGANIZATIONS AND MAJOR INITIATIVES IN MALARIA CONTROL

Global health programs have recognized malaria as a priority for decades. The most visible efforts have come through national malaria control programs with international support centered around the World Health Organization and its regional offices, but with considerable bilateral assistance from a number of countries. Particular lines of research have been driven consistently by funding from a select group of national science agencies including those in the United States, United Kingdom, France, and China; and from foundations, in particular, the Wellcome Trust and the Rockefeller Foundation. With sponsorship from several U.N. agencies, the WHO-housed Special Programme for Research and Training in Tropical Diseases (WHO/TDR) has worked for the past 28 years to develop and promote the best use of pharmaceuticals and other malaria control measures. In the last 10 years or so, the number of organizations and collaborations devoted to malaria has grown impressively (Table 1-3). The boost in funding from the Bill & Melinda Gates Foundation has had a major impact on existing initiatives, in taking new directions in malaria research and control, and in raising the public profile of malaria. The Global Fund to Fight AIDS, Tuberculosis and Malaria has also provided a central focus for international funding.

The programs and initiatives most directly relevant to this study—related to the development and deployment of effective antimalarial drugs—are described briefly below.

TDR:
The Special Programme on Research and Training in Tropical Diseases

Since it was started in 1975, the Special Programme on Research and Training in Tropical Diseases (TDR; a joint program of UNICEF, the World Bank, the U.N. Development Program and WHO, and housed at WHO) has organized research and development for new antimalarials, as well as supported research on the best ways to encourage the use of effective interventions of all types. TDR has leveraged its own modest budget by recruit-

TABLE 1-3 Selected Organizations and Initiatives for Malaria Research and Control of Recent Origin

EMVI—European Malaria Vaccine Initiative	EMVI was established in 1998 by the European Commission and interested European Union Member States to address structural deficiencies in publicly funded malaria vaccine development. EMVI's aim is to provide a mechanism to accelerate the development of malaria vaccines in Europe and in endemic countries.
MVI—Malaria Vaccine Initiative	MVI was created in 1999 with a grant from the Bill & Melinda Gates Foundation to PATH (Program for Appropriate Technology in Health). MVI's mission is to accelerate the development of promising malaria vaccines, and to ensure their availability and accessibility in the developing world. MVI works with other vaccine programs, vaccine development partners, and the Global Alliance for Vaccines and Immunization (GAVI) to explore commercialization, procurement, and delivery strategies that will maximize public health sector availability in the countries most affected by malaria.
MARA—Mapping Malaria Risk in Africa	MARA is a pan-African collaborative network, initiated in 1997, to collect, collate, validate, and manage all available malaria data from Africa, and to map the distribution, intensity, and seasonality of malaria on the continent. Its primary objective is to support African control initiatives.
MMV—Medicines for Malaria Venture	MMV is a not-for-profit public-private partnership, launched in 1999. Its goal is to develop and manage a portfolio of malaria drug discovery and development projects that will yield one new product every five years appropriate for (and affordable to) malaria-endemic countries. The initiative arose from discussions between WHO and the International Federation of Pharmaceutical Manufacturers Associations (IFPMA). Early partners were the Rockefeller Foundation, the World Bank, the Swiss Agency for Development and

continued

TABLE 1-3 Continued

	Cooperation, the Association of the British Pharmaceutical Industry, and the Wellcome Trust (see chapter 10 for a detailed description of MMV).
MIM—The Multilateral Initiative on Malaria	"MIM is an alliance of organizations and individuals concerned with malaria. It aims to maximize the impact of scientific research against malaria in Africa, through promoting capacity building and facilitating global collaboration and coordination." http://www.mim.su.se/english/about/index.html
	MIM was launched in 1997 following the first Pan-African Malaria Conference (Dakar, Senegal), where researchers from all over the world identified important research priorities for future malaria research. A multilateral funding mechanism was set up at TDR where MIM partners could directly contribute money for Research Capability Strengthening in Africa in the form of peer-reviewed grants. MIM now includes representatives of industry and development agencies. http://www.mim.su.se/english/about/mim_folder_12p_eng.pdf

ing collaborators and orchestrating larger projects. Among their accomplishments related to malaria are:

- several antimalarials brought through the R&D process, including key work on artemisinins and ACTs. TDR brought partners together, funded preclinical work, and orchestrated clinical trials;
- pivotal field trials for insecticide-treated bed nets, supporting research on better methods for treating nets, and encouraging industry to develop longer-lasting treated nets; and
- research on treatment-seeking and demonstrating the value of home treatment.

TDR remains active in malaria research (one of 10 diseases in its portfolio) and is a partner in many of the newer initiatives, including the Medicines for Malaria Venture (MMV), which has now taken the lead in R&D for new antimalarials (discussed in detail in chapter 10).

Roll Back Malaria (RBM)

Malaria was a top priority of Dr. Gro Harlem Brundtland when she assumed the leadership of WHO in 1998, convinced by African leaders that malaria was a heavy burden on the health and economies of many countries. The Global RBM Partnership was created to "reduce the burden of malaria throughout the world." It was developed not as a WHO program, but as a loose confederation of endemic country governments, other UN organizations, bilateral aid donors, foundations, NGOs, community groups, research and teaching institutions, and others—all the relevant parties in malaria control. A small Secretariat within WHO was to serve the needs of RBM, with leadership drawn from the external partners. Although not without problems, RBM is the most significant development in consolidating worldwide efforts to control malaria since the end of the era of malaria "eradication" in the 1960s (which largely bypassed Africa).

The African summit on Roll Back Malaria, held in Abuja, Nigeria in April 2000 is an RBM milestone. The summit was attended by delegates from 44 of the 50 malaria endemic countries in Africa, including 19 heads of state and many other high-level officials of member countries. Top-level representation from WHO, the World Bank, the African Development Bank, and several other major donors helped to further raise the profile of the meeting and underscore the importance of tackling the malaria problem. Hundreds of millions of dollars in assistance were pledged (although most did not materialize). Ambitious, but potentially achievable targets for the year 2005 were adopted by the summit participants (Table 1-4).

The RBM External Evaluation

In early 2002, several of the "core" RBM partners commissioned an evaluation of the organization and its progress by a seven-member team of experts, led by Richard Feachem (who shortly thereafter was named head of the Global Fund for AIDS, TB and Malaria). The evaluation, published in August 2002 (Feachem, 2002), documented both achievements and "serious constraints" that threaten progress in phase 2, defined as mid-2002 to 2007.

The accomplishments include raising the profile of malaria and increasing global funding—funding for malaria control doubled in RBM's first 3 years. The constraints centered on a lack of progress in getting activities under way quickly at the country level. RBM may not be able to achieve a "significant reduction in the global burden of malaria by 2007" given the pace of progress, which could undermine the partnership if not rectified.

Three major reforms and two tactical changes were recommended:

TABLE 1-4 The Abuja Summit Targets, April 2002

RBM strategy	Abuja target (by 2005)
Prompt access to effective treatment	• 60% of those suffering with malaria should have access to and be able to use correct, affordable, and appropriate treatment within 24 hours of the onset of symptoms
Insecticide-treated nets (ITNs)	• 60% of those at risk for malaria, particularly children under 5 years of age and pregnant women, will benefit from a suitable combination of personal and community protective measures, such as ITNs
Prevention and control of malaria in pregnant women	• 60% of pregnant women at risk of malaria will be covered with suitable combinations of personal and community protective measures, such as ITNs • 60% of pregnant women at risk of malaria will have access to intermittent preventive treatment
Malaria epidemic and emergency response	• 60% of epidemics are detected within 2 weeks of onset • 60% of epidemics are responded to within 2 weeks of detection

Note: The original Abuja declaration included the recommendation for chemoprophylaxis as well, but current WHO and RBM policy strongly recommends IPT—and not chemoprophylaxis—for prevention of malaria during pregnancy.
SOURCE: WHO/UNICEF (2003)

Major Reforms

- Reorganization of the RBM Secretariat
- Creation of an independent governance board
- Reconstitution of the Technical Support Network

Tactical Changes

- Selection of 8 to 12 focus countries that show a high degree of commitment and can make rapid progress in the next 3 years
- Appointment of Country Champions to provide dynamic leadership in these focus countries

Even before the final report was issued in August 2002, RBM was reorganized along the lines recommended. It is too soon to know whether these changes will lead to the success envisioned by the evaluation team, but major efforts are being made toward that end. If the recommendations in this report are implemented, RBM's ability to make rapid progress will get a large boost, particularly in increasing access to effective drugs.

The United Nations Millennium Development Goals

At the United Nations Millennium Summit in September 2000, world leaders agreed to a set of goals and targets to combat the world's ills: poverty, hunger, disease, illiteracy, environmental degradation, and discrimination against women. All 189 Member States of the United Nations adopted the eight broad "Millennium Development Goals" (MDGs), with timetables for achieving them by 2015. One of the goals names malaria specifically, and two others are directly relevant. These MDGs are:

- Reverse the spread of diseases, especially HIV/AIDS and malaria.
- Reduce under-5 mortality by two-thirds.
- Reduce maternal mortality by three-quarters.

The UN secretary general and the administrator of the UN Development Programme created the Millennium Project to recommend the best strategies for achieving the MDGs. Ten task forces of global experts were established to identify operational priorities, organizational means of implementation, and financing structures necessary to achieve the MDGs. Task Force 5 is focused on HIV/AIDS, malaria, TB, other major diseases and access to essential medicines, and a subgroup focused specifically on malaria. Each task force is to complete its report by the end of 2004, and a final synthesis of recommendations will be presented to the UN secretary general and the chair of the UN Development Group by June 30, 2005.

The issues addressed by the IOM Committee on the Economics of Antimalarial Drugs are directly relevant to the MDGs, and should complement the work of the malaria subgroup of Task Force 5.

The Global Fund

The Global Fund to Fight AIDS, Tuberculosis and Malaria (the "Global Fund") began operation just 2 years ago, in 2002. The idea of a centralized fund to help combat the three most devastating infectious diseases in countries without the resources to do so was first raised at a meeting in July 2000 of the Group of Eight (G8) leading industrialized countries. It gained currency through further discussions and meetings, and was solidified by

United Nations Secretary-General Kofi Annan at the African Summit on HIV/AIDS in Abuja, Nigeria, in April 2001, who called for the creation of a global trust fund for the three diseases.

As of July 2003, total pledges by donors to the Fund amounted to US$4.7 billion. Forty governments have pledged 98 percent of the funds, and 2 percent come from the private sector. By February 2004, a total of US$245 million in Global Fund resources had been disbursed to about 120 countries. In the first two rounds of grants, 21 percent went for malaria programs (59 percent for HIV/AIDS, 19 percent for tuberculosis). Over the first three rounds, a minority of funding was destined for purchase of ACTs—less than US$20 million, and less than the amount allocated for purchases of chloroquine and SP (Attaran et al., 2004). This reflects the requests of countries to the Global Fund, which does not dictate how countries should approach malaria control. However, the international health financing community—of which the Global Fund is a major part—has significant influence on what countries plan by way of disease control and what they ask for. Given the level of funding of the Global Fund itself, countries have made realistic requests, which may not include large quantitites of ACTs, because the price would make such requests nonviable. Countries also are concerned about how sustainable a system built on ACTs would be after Global Fund grants run out (if not renewed).

A principle by which the Global Fund operates is that their grants are not fungible: they must *augment* existing funding for the three diseases and not *supplant* them. Evidence that allocations for malaria from other sources are being reduced is grounds for the Global Fund to terminate a malaria grant. This principle acknowledges the historic underinvestment in malaria and the other diseases. Strictly speaking, it also can be seen as limiting the endemic countries' ability to freely allocate resources according to their own priorities, while signalling the global acceptance—of both donor and recipient countries—that only with greater resources is there hope of making progress against these diseases. With continued and increasing donor contributions, the Global Fund has the potential to be a major positive force for malaria control.

REFERENCES

Ahorlu CK, Dunyo SK, Afari EA, Koram KA, Nkrumah FK. 1997. Malaria-related beliefs and behaviour in Southern Ghana: Implications for treatment, prevention and control. *Tropical Medicine and International Health* 2(5):488-499.

Attaran A, Barnes KI, Curtis C, d'Alessandro U, Fanello CI, Galinski MR, Kokwaro G, Looareesuwan S, Makanga M, Mutabingwa TK, Talisuna A, Trape JF, Watkins WM. 2004. WHO, the Global Fund, and medical malpractice in malaria treatment. *Lancet* 363(9404):237-240.

Barat L, Chipipa J, Kolczak M, Sukwa T. 1999. Does the availability of blood slide microscopy for malaria at health centers improve the management of persons with fever in Zambia? *American Journal of Tropical Medicine and Hygiene* 60(6):1024-1030.

Berman P, Nwuke K, Rannan-Eliya R, Mwanza A. 1995. *Zambia: Non-Governmental Health Care Provision.* Boston: Harvard University International Health Systems Program.

Breman JG, Egan A, Keusch GT. 2001. Introduction and summary: The intolerable burden of malaria: A new look at the numbers. *American Journal of Tropical Medicine and Hygiene* 64(1-2 Suppl):iv-vii.

Brugha R, Chandramohan D, Zwi A. 1999. Viewpoint: Management of malaria—working with the private sector. *Tropical Medicine and International Health* 4(5):402-406.

Chima RI, Goodman CA, Mills A. 2003. The economic impact of malaria in Africa: A critical review of the evidence. *Health Policy* 63(1):17-36.

De Savigny D, Setel P, Kasale H, Whiting D, Reid G, Kitange H, Mbuya C, Mgalula L, Machibya H, Kilima P. 1999. *Linking demographic surveillance and health service needs: The AMMP/TEHIP experience in Morogoro, Tanzania.* Presentation at MIM African Malaria Conference, Durban, South Africa.

De Savigny D, Mwageni E, Mayombana C, Masanja H, Minhaj A, Momburi D, Mkilindi Y, Mbuya C, Kasale H, and Reid G. 2003. Care seeking patterns in fatal malaria: Evidence from Tanzania. Paper commissioned by the Institute of Medicine, Washington DC.

Deming MS, Gayibor A, Murphy K, Jones TS, Karsa T. 1989. Home treatment of febrile children with antimalarial drugs in Togo. *Bulletin of the World Health Organization* 67(6):695-700.

Ejezie GC, Ezedinachi ENU, Usanga EA, Gemade EII, Ikpatt NW, Alaribe AAA. 1990. Malaria and its treatment in rural villages of Aboh Mbaise, Imo State, Nigeria. *Acta Tropica* 48(1):17-24.

Feachem R. 2002. *Final Report of the External Evaluation of Roll Back Malaria.* Liverpool: Malaria Consortium.

Gilson L, Alilio M, Heggenhougen K. 1994. Community satisfaction with primary health care services: An evaluation undertaken in the Morogoro region of Tanzania. *Social Science and Medicine* 39(6):767-780.

Guiguemde TR, Ouedraogo I, Ouedraogo JB, Coulibaly SO, Gbary AR. 1997. [Malaria morbidity in adults living in urban Burkina Faso]. [French]. *Medecine Tropicale* 57(2):165-168.

Guimier JM, Candau D, Garenne M. 2001. *Etude Sur L'Accessibilité Aux Médicaments Au Sénégal—LEEM (France)-Ministere De La Santé Du Sénégal.* Dakar: Ministry of Health.

Hanson K, Goodman C, Lines J, Meeks S, Bradley D, Mills A. 2004. *The Economics of Malaria Control Interventions.* Geneva: Global Forum for Health Research, World Health Organization

Makemba AM, Winch PJ, Makame VM, Mehl GL, Premji Z, Minjas JN, Shiff CJ. 1996. Treatment practices for degedege, a locally recognized febrile illness, and implications for strategies to decrease mortality from severe malaria in Bagamoyo district, Tanzania. *Tropical Medicine and International Health* 1(3):305-313.

Maponga C, Ondari, C. 2003. *The Quality of Antimalarials: A Study in Selected African Countries WHO/EDM/PAR/2003.4.* Geneva: World Health Organization.

Marsh VM, Mutemi WM, Muturi J, Haaland A, Watkins WM, Otieno G, Marsh K. 1999. Changing home treatment of childhood fevers by training shop keepers in rural Kenya. *Tropical Medicine and International Health* 4(5):383-389.

McCombie SC. 1996. Treatment seeking for malaria: A review of recent research. *Social Science and Medicine* 43(6):933-945.

Ministry of Health of Kingdom of Cambodia. 1996. *Health Policy and Strategies 1996–2000*. Presentation at the meeting of the Meeting on Malaria Programme. Brussels: Ministry of Health, Kingdom of Cambodia.

Ministry of Health of Kingdom of Cambodia. 1998. *National Health Statistics 1998*. Phnom Penh: Ministry of Health, Kingdom of Cambodia.

Ministry of Health of Kingdom of Cambodia. 2000. *Cambodia's Health Sector Performance Report 2000*. Phnom Penh: Ministry of Health, Kingdom of Cambodia.

Ministry of Health of Kingdom of Cambodia. 2001a. *Country Update on Malaria Control, Kingdom of Cambodia*. Presentation at the meeting of the 4th Global Partners Meeting, Washington, DC, April 18-19, 2001. Prepared by the National Malaria Control Programme, Ministry of Health, Kingdom of Cambodia.

Ministry of Health of Kingdom of Cambodia. 2001b. *Joint Health Sector Review Report*. Phnom Penh: Ministry of Health, Kingdom of Cambodia.

Ministry of Health of Kingdom of Cambodia. 2002a. *Health Sector Strategic Plan 2003-7*. Phnom Penh: Ministry of Health, Kingdom of Cambodia.

Ministry of Health of Kingdom of Cambodia. 2002b. *Ministry of Health Expenditure Report 2000*. Ministry of Economy and Finance statement to fiscal working group by Minister of Health, April 23, 2002; Cambodia Development Council (CDC) estimates of external aid, April 2002. Phnom Penh: Ministry of Health, Kingdom of Cambodia.

Ministry of Health of Senegal. 2000. *Senegalese Survey of Health Indicators*. Dakar: Senegal Ministry of Health.

Ministry of Health of Zambia. 2003. *Request for Proposals for the Management of MSL. TB/SP/029/03*. Lusaka: Zambia Ministry of Health.

Mnyika KS, Killewo JZJ, Kabalimu TK. 1995. Self-medication with antimalarial drugs in Dar es Salaam, Tanzania. *Tropical and Geographical Medicine* 47(1):32-34.

Mtango FDE, Neuvians D, Broome CV, Hightower AW, Pio A. 1992. Risk factors for deaths in children under 5 years old in Bagamoyo District, Tanzania. *Tropical Medicine and Parasitology* 43(4):229-233.

Muela SH, Ribera MJ. 2000. Illness naming and home treatment practices for malaria—an example from Tanzania. Paper presented at workshop on People and Medicine in East Africa. Basel, Switzerland: Swiss Tropical Institute.

Mutizwa-Mangiza D. 1997. The opinions of health and water service users in Zimbabwe. Working paper. International Development Department, University of Birmingham, Birmingham, UK. [Online]. Available: http://www.idd.bham.ac.uk/research/Projects/Role_of_gov/workingpapers/paper24.htm.

Mwabu GM. 1986. Health care decisions at the household level: Results of a rural health survey in Kenya. *Social Science and Medicine* 22(3):315-319.

Mwenesi H, Harpham T, Snow RW. 1995. Child malaria treatment practices among mothers in Kenya. *Social Science and Medicine* 40(9):1271-1277.

Newton P, Proux S, Green M, Smithuis F, Rozendaal J, Prakongpan S, Chotivanich K, Mayxay M, Looareesuwan S, Farrar J, Nosten F, White NJ. 2001. Fake artesunate in Southeast Asia. *Lancet* 357(9272):1948-1950.

Ofori-Adjei D, Arhinful DK. 1996. Effect of training on the clinical management of malaria by medical assistants in Ghana. *Social Science and Medicine* 42(8):1169-1176.

Olivar M, Develoux M, Chegou Abari A, Loutan L. 1991. Presumptive diagnosis of malaria results in a significant risk of mistreatment of children in Urban Sahel. *Transactions of the Royal Society of Tropical Medicine and Hygiene* 85(6):729-730.

Palmer K, Schapira A, Barat L. 1999. Draft position paper prepared for informal consultation on "Malaria diagnostics at the turn of the century." Presentation at the meeting of the role of light microscopy and dipsticks in malaria diagnosis and treatment. A joint meeting of TDR, Roll Back Malaria and USAID. Geneva, Switzerland.

SEAM. 2001. *Strategies for Enhancing Access to Medicines. Country Assessment: Cambodia.* Arlington, VA: Management Sciences for Health.

Shakoor O, Taylor RB, Behrens RH. 1997. Assessment of the incidence of substandard drugs in developing countries. *Tropical Medicine and International Health* 2(9):839-845.

Shretta R, Guimier J-M. 2003. Flow of antimalarial drugs in the public and private sector, affordability and discussions of potential strategies to improve financial access. Paper commissioned by the Institute of Medicine.

Silva T, Russell S, Rakodi C. 1997. The opinions of health and water service users in Sri Lanka. Working paper. International Development Department, University of Birmingham, Birmingham, UK. [Online]. Available: http://www.idd.bham.ac.uk/research/Projects/Role_of_gov/workingpapers/paper25.htm.

Smithson P, Asamoa-Baah A, Mills A. 1997. The case of the health sector in Ghana. Working paper. International Development Department, University of Birmingham, Birmingham, UK. [Online]. Available: http://www.idd.bham.ac.uk/research/Projects/Role_of_gov/workingpapers/paper26.htm.

Snow RW, Peshu N, Forster D, Mwenesi H, Marsh K. 1992. The role of shops in the treatment and prevention of childhood malaria on the coast of Kenya. *Transactions of the Royal Society of Tropical Medicine and Hygiene* 86(3):237-239.

Stein CM, Gelfand M. 1985. The clinical features and laboratory findings in acute *Plasmodium falciparum* malaria in Harare, Zimbabwe. *Central African Journal of Medicine* 31(9):166-170.

United States Embassy. 2003. [Online]. Available: http://usembassy.state.gov/Cambodia [accessed 2003].

WHO (World Health Organization). 2003. More equitable pricing for essential drugs: What do we mean and what are the issues? In: *WHO Commission on Macroeconomics and Health, Norway.* Background paper for the WHO-WTO secretariat workshop on differential pricing and financing of essential drugs, Høsbjør, Norway, April 8-11, 2001. World Health Organization. [Online]. Available: www.who.int/medicines/library/edm_general/who-wto-hosbjor/equitable_pricing.doc.

WHO Regional Office for South-East Asia. *Malaria: Issues and Challenges.* [Online]. Available: http://w3.whosea.org/mal/issues.htm [accessed April 7, 2004].

WHO/UNICEF. 2003. *The Africa Malaria Report 2003.* Geneva: World Health Organization.

Wilkinson D, Holloway J, Fallavier P. 2000. *Findings from the Evaluation of User Fees, Categorized by Evaluation Objectives.* Draft study to evaluate the impact of user fees on access, equity and health providers' practices. Phnom Penh, November 2000.

Winch PJ, Makemba AM, Kamazima SR, Lurie M, Lwihula GK, Premji Z, Minjas JN, Shiff CJ. 1996. Local terminology for febrile illnesses in Bagamoyo district, Tanzania and its impact on the design of a community-based malaria control programme. *Social Science and Medicine* 42(7):1057-1067.

World Bank. 1999. *Volume Two: Main Report. Poverty Reduction and Economic Management Sector Unit, East Asia and Pacific Region. Cambodia: Public Expenditure Review.* Washington, DC: The World Bank.

World Bank. 2002. *World Development Indicators.* Washington, DC: The World Bank.

World Bank. 2003. *World Development Indicators.* Washington, DC: The World Bank.

APPENDIX 1A
THE TEHIP STUDY

Why Do They Die?
An Inquiry into Treatments Preceding Deaths from Malaria[5]

A child in rural Tanzania dies from malaria. One can hardly help but envision the cascade of events—what might have happened or not happened—that led to such a sorrowful ending. But guesswork is not an adequate substitute for knowing. The solutions that will keep such children alive and malaria-free depend on understanding why and where the fatal failures of social transactions occurred.

The Research Area

TEHIP studied the circumstances leading to deaths from malaria in the stable, perennial malaria-transmission belt that runs along the coast of Tanzania and up the Rufiji and Kilombero River basins. The transmission risk there is typical of the majority (75 percent) of Tanzania and of sub-Saharan Africa in general (MARA Collaboration, 2003). The population of Rufiji District is 203,000, divided among several ethnic groups. The district occupies 14,500 km² and is entirely rural, with 94 registered villages.

There are 57 formal health facilities: two hospitals (one government and one NGO), five health centers with inpatient facilities (all government), and 50 dispensaries (46 government). Over-the-counter drugs are available from many private shops and kiosks in the villages. People also consult traditional healers and traditional birth attendants.

Integrated management of childhood illness (IMCI) services, intermittent presumptive treatment (IPT) of malaria in pregnancy, and 1st, 2nd, and 3rd line antimalarial services are available at all formal health services. Within the District, insecticide treated nets (ITNs) are distributed through social marketing.

The Rufiji Demographic Surveillance Site (DSS) covers part of Rufiji District, including 1,800 km² north of the Rufiji River and west of the Rufiji Delta, with a population of 85,000 in 17,000 households in 31 villages. The DSS registers all births, deaths, in-migrations, out-migrations, pregnancies, and other vital events. Events are detected by 150 village "key informants," and verified by DSS staff. Twenty-eight full-time enumerators update the population register every 4 months, based on household surveys.

---

[5]Based on an analysis prepared for this study (de Savigny et al., 2003).

Verbal Autopsies

The information available for each death is gathered during the process of "verbal autopsy" (VA). Once a key informant documents a death in the study area, a DSS VA supervisor, who is also a trained clinical officer or health officer, conducts the VA interview using standard questionnaires that are designed specifically for deaths of: a) children under 31 days of age; b) children under 5 years but 31 days and older; and c) population aged 5 years and above. The questionnaires and responses are in Kiswahili, the common language of the area. Open-ended and closed questions are asked on the history of events leading to death, as well as about previously diagnosed medical conditions, and signs and symptoms before death. Use of health facilities prior to death, reasons for using or not using a particular health facility, and confirmatory evidence of cause of death (if available) are asked about and recorded. A typical bereavement interview for a VA takes 45 to 60 minutes.

The VA supervisor establishes a tentative cause of death from signs, symptoms, sequence, and severity, as well as any confirmatory evidence. A physician reviews the material and makes the final determination of cause of death that is subsequently entered in the database.

Malaria-Related Deaths

This study covered the period January 1999 through the end of December 2001, during which 3,023 deaths occurred and 2,953 (97.7 percent) verbal autopsies were conducted in the DSS. Of these deaths, 722 which fell under the following codings were suspected to be directly or indirectly due to malaria:

- acute febrile illness 1-4 weeks
- acute febrile illness ≤7days
- acute febrile illness including malaria
- acute febrile illness with seizures
- acute febrile illness with anemia
- cerebral malaria
- fever plus malnutrition
- malaria
- malaria confirmed
- unspecified acute febrile illness

Among these 722, 45.8 percent were male, 54.2 percent female; 44.3 percent were under 5 years of age, 55.7 percent were 5 years or older; 39 (5.4 percent) had convulsions and possible cerebral malaria, while 94.6 percent reported no convulsions.

As a cautionary note, VA methods have distinct limitations. Specifically, not all the cases identified as "malaria" in this series truly represent malaria, especially those with unspecified acute febrile illness at an older age. And undoubtedly, some malaria deaths were coded as nonmalaria. For example, life-threatening anemia, likely due to malaria, is prevalent in young children over 6 months of age in the study area, yet VA coded deaths due to anemia with malaria are infrequent among recorded malaria deaths.

Types of Care Sought

The term *modern care* describes what conventionally includes biomedical, Western, pharmaceutical, professional, official, or formal health care. *Traditional care* describes what conventionally includes traditional medicine, traditional healers, traditional providers, lay providers, traditional practices, or folk care. From the VAs, 13 possible sources of treatment were collapsed into six subcategories of provider type:

1. Government
2. Home/Shops
3. Non-Government
4. Traditional Medicine at Home
5. Traditional Medicine at Practitioner
6. No Care

and into three broader subcategories:

1. Modern Care
2. Traditional Care
3. No Care

Of the 722 individuals whose deaths were ascribed to malaria, 626 (87 percent) sought care at least once before death, while 96 (13 percent) did not, or could not, seek care. Treatment usually starts at home using antipyretics and antimalarials from local shops or left over from previous episodes. Malaria is perceived by adult caregivers as a mild disease, and if it becomes serious or life threatening, the presumptive diagnosis changes from malaria to something that is more often treated with traditional medicine or practices. Yet these beliefs are not rigid. Every case is subject to a process of continuing debate and reevaluation within the family. As a result, modern pharmaceuticals also are sought, albeit with delay, when convulsions fail to resolve, or recur after traditional medicine (Oberlander and Elverdan, 2000). Significant switching from one provider to another occurs over time; this phenomenon is most apparent when comparing treatment of malaria without convulsions to malaria with convulsions.

Key Observations

- Cases with convulsions were significantly (p<0.05) more likely to receive care.
- Of the group that did *not* have convulsions, 91 percent used modern care first, and by the second treatment, more than 99 percent used modern care. Hence traditional care delayed modern care for 9 percent of cases.
- Of the group that had convulsions, 90 percent used modern care first, but only 63 percent continued with modern care for a second treatment.
- Government health facilities and shopkeepers were the main source of antimalarial drugs. This pattern held up over broad age groups, sex, and socioeconomic status. (At the time of the study, all government providers had adequate drug supplies, which could be a factor in their popularity. The first-line drug was chloroquine, however, at a time when drug resistance was already widespread in this area.)

Other Relevant Factors

In this study, modern care was more popular than previous reports would suggest. But some part of that modern care involved self-treatment and a variety of private providers. Knowledge of appropriate treatment regimens is lacking on the part of the public as well as the private providers (Brugha et al., 1999; Marsh et al., 1999), and under-dosing in home-based care is common. These may account for at least some treatment failures.

The only other study of health-seeking patterns in a large series of VAs is from the mid-1980s from the Bagamoyo District of Tanzania, another district in the Coast Region (Mtango et al., 1992). In that series, malaria deaths were not analyzed separately, but government providers were the choice in only 45 percent of all deaths. A preference for traditional healers was cited by 41 percent of mothers as the reason for not using government services. At that time, it was also true that government providers were often without adequate drug supply.

Why Did They Die?

The study results to date cannot answer that question, but they begin to narrow the possibilities. Some form of care was sought in the majority of malaria deaths (88 percent). No care was sought for 12 percent of child deaths. Included among these were sudden deaths following apparently mild illness, which may have been impossible to prevent under the circumstances. This pattern is considerably better than was seen in the mid-1980s in Bagamoyo, when 55 percent of children who died had not utilized any modern care (Mtango et al., 1992), and better than for all deaths in the same area during the same period when 20 percent of all-cause deaths had no prior health-seeking events (Tanzania Essential Health Interventions Project and Ministry of Health of Tanzania, 2002).

With belief systems for malaria treatment-seeking now firmly on the side of modern care, there is obviously something still failing in the transaction to obtain this care, or in the quality of the care and referral once it is accessed. TEHIP is continuing to refine the information from this study, and will be analyzing the narrative portion of the verbal autopsy questionnaires to look at some specific aspects of the health care received, including:

• delay in seeking modern care (e.g., tried to treat at home without antimalarials, no transport, beliefs, poor recognition of severity, lack of confidence in modern care, no power to decide, insufficient finances);
• delay in receiving modern care (e.g., after working hours, weekends, long queues, satisfaction); and
• ineffective modern care (e.g., poor communication, no referral, drugs not available, abusive health worker, non-compliant providers, poor adherence of patients).

All of these factors could have contributed to failed treatment. The study, as yet, can provide no direct information on the possible contribution of drug resistant malaria to these deaths.

The current results suggest that policies and efforts aimed at improving early recognition of symptoms and danger signs at home, prompt treatment or treatment-seeking, compliance with the full course of treatment, and the quality of the antimalarial available are highly justified.

REFERENCES

De Savigny D, Mwageni E, Mayombana C, Masanja H, Minhaj A, Momburi D, Mkilindi Y, Mbuya C, Kasale H, and Reid G. 2003. Care seeking patterns in fatal malaria: Evidence from Tanzania. Paper commissioned by the Institute of Medicine.
MARA Collaboration. 2003. *MARA LITe for Africa CD version 3.0.0.* South Africa: Medical Research Council of South Africa.
Mtango FDE, Neuvians D, Broome CV, Hightower AW, Pio A. 1992. Risk factors for deaths in children under 5 years old in Bagamoyo District, Tanzania. *Tropical Medicine and Parasitology* 43(4):229-233.
Oberlander L, Elverdan B. 2000. Malaria in the United Republic of Tanzania: Cultural considerations and health-seeking behaviour. *Bulletin of the World Health Organization* 78(11):1352-1357.
Tanzania Essential Health Interventions Project, Ministry of Health of Tanzania. 2002. *Burden of Disease Profile 2001—Coastal Zone.* Dar es Salaam: Ministry of Health of Tanzania.

2

The Cost and Cost-Effectiveness of Antimalarial Drugs

In one sense, the economics of antimalarial drugs are simple: currently effective drugs—those recommended by the global community for most of Africa and Asia—are not affordable by the endemic countries, so few people are getting them. This is in contrast to the previous generation of effective drugs, which were exceedingly cheap by any standards, but which no longer work because drug resistance is so widespread. As a result, malaria mortality rates are rising in Africa, and more cases are inadequately treated.

The Immediate Problem of ACT Affordability

Chloroquine—the standard, effective drug for decades—costs about 10 U.S. cents per course of treatment for an adult. The new effective drugs—artemisinin combination therapy (ACT)[1]—today cost US$2.40 per course wholesale, and can be marked up to five times that amount in pharmacies in Africa. There are limited alternatives to ACTs for effectiveness and safety for widespread use, and their adoption is recommended by WHO and virtually all other expert bodies. Even 10 cents is too much for the poorest of the poor in every endemic country (which equals substantial numbers of

---

[1]The rationale for combining two or more drugs is that doing so dramatically reduces the odds that malaria strains resistant to any of the drugs in the combination would survive to be transmitted. In this report, ACT is used mainly to describe a drug "coformulation" (i.e., two drugs in one pill), and not just two separate drugs taken at the same time.

people), but it is affordable for many, and governments generally have been able to afford that price (or find external financing) for their public-sector needs. Multiply the per-dose difference in price by the millions or tens of million courses used per year in each country in Africa, and the money adds up. Continent-wide, an estimated 200-400 million courses of treatment are used per year, and an additional 100 million courses in the rest of the world. Realistically, the endemic countries are able to contribute very little of the incremental cost, and that is not likely to change for many years, given the pace of economic development in Africa and in poor nations elsewhere. One positive change that is almost certain, however, is that several different ACTs will become available,[2] and their price will come down by more than half, to about 10 times the current price of chloroquine, or about US$1 per adult course and US$0.60 for an average child's course.

The Cost of Producing ACTs and Future Prices

Why are ACTs so much more expensive than chloroquine? Even at prices anticipated after the massive scale-up that would be necessary to supply the African market—should funding become available for large-scale purchase—the price as sold by the producer will likely remain at about 10 times the price of chloroquine (Table 2-1 lists prices offered by major producers to Médecins Sans Frontières [MSF] in 2003). These prices reflect the production costs of artemisinins without a premium for any exclusivity related to patents.[3] They are high because the process involves growing the source plant, *Artemisia annua*, extracting the active moiety, and creating the desired artemisinin derivative (artesunate, artemether, etc.). Coformulation with the companion drug follows. The price of the finished product is driven mainly by the cost of the artemisinin derivative, but also is affected by the companion drug (e.g., lumefantrine, the companion drug in Coartem, is a relatively expensive drug on its own, which contributes to the high price of the coformulation).

There is something of a chicken-and-egg quality about the current price of artemisinins, and the prospect for significantly lower prices. Lower prices can be expected in response to large-scale demand, which, in turn, will induce competition among producers. However, without assurances from the global community that there will be a market for large quantities of

---

[2]There are several companion drugs with which the artemisinin may be combined, and the development work on these new combinations is due to be completed within the next 2 years.

[3]Coartem has some patent protection, but Novartis is selling it in developing countries for less than production costs, i.e., at a loss.

TABLE 2-1 Wholesale Prices (Offers) for Artesunate and ACTs in 2003 (US$)

Drug	Range of prices for standard adult course
Artesunate	*Asian suppliers:* • US$0.50 (not yet in production); less for greater quantities • US$0.63; 15% discount for greater than 1 million treatments • US$1.25 (not yet in production) • US$1.26; decreasing to US$1.01 at 3 million treatments • US$1.35 *European suppliers:* • US$2.68 (2.10 Euros) • US$2.42 (1.90 Euros) *African supplier:* • US$5.36
Coartem	US$2.40 for public services of developing countries (tiered pricing; higher for all other buyers)
CV8 (8 tablets)	US$1.21 for <1 million treatments; US$0.97 for > 1 million treatments
Artekin II	US$1.00 at retail
AS + AQ blister	*Asian suppliers:* • US$1.50 (not yet in production) • <US$1.91 (1.50 Euros) (not yet in production) *European suppliers:* • US$1.53 (1.2 Euros) • US$1.91 (1.5 Euros) • US$2.68 (2.10 Euros) for <500,000 treatments; US$1.39 (1.09 Euros) for >500,000 treatments
AS + SP blister (6 tablets)	*European supplier:* • US$2.42 (1.90 Euros) for <500,000 treatments; US$1.24 (0.97 Euros) for >500,000 treatments

AQ=amodiaquine
AS=artesunate
SP=sulfadoxine-pyrimethamine
CV8=a new combination of dihydroartemisinin, piperaquine, trimethoprim, and primaquine

SOURCE: J.M. Kindermans, Médecins Sans Frontières, 2003.

ACTs, manufacturers will not have the incentive to scale up production, and prices will not drop. In addition to competition driving prices down (i.e., companies being willing to accept lower profits per dose with higher volumes), technological improvements in the process could bring down the actual production costs, which would be passed along to purchasers in a competitive environment.

The real price breakthrough will likely occur only when a fully synthetic artemisinin is developed, eliminating the growing and extraction process. The Medicines for Malaria Venture (MMV) has such a compound under development, which they predict could be available in 5-6 years. The ultimate price is not known, but it should be significantly less expensive than current artemisinins (assuming no premium for exclusivity). If the synthetic product is better than, or at least as effective as the extracted ones, the market would change dramatically. A global subsidy might still be needed, but it could be less than what is needed now.

The Global Cost of ACTs and Future Antimalarials

A per-course price of US$1 can be taken as a reasonable upper limit for the wholesale cost of ACTs purchased in large quantities (e.g., 1 million or more courses) within 1 to 2 years. Prices of US$1 and less have already been offered to MSF by several companies, assuming that no major problems are encountered in scaling up, and producers can meet quality standards (no major problems are foreseen for either issue).[4] Using our estimate of 300-500 million episodes treated each year, the math is simple: US$300-500 million per year. This quantum jump in the global cost of antimalarials is, in all likelihood, a one-time phenomenon, for the following two key reasons.

First, the *volume* of antimalarials needed is not expected to increase significantly—assuming that treatment and other control measures remain at least at current levels. If treatment coverage could be expanded, more treatments might be required, but such changes are likely to be incremental and small in relation to the current treatment volume. Currently, treatment failures account for some number of treatments, and these should be reduced with effective drugs, balancing out some of the incremental increases. In the lower transmission areas at least, if used optimally, ACTs have the potential to decrease malaria transmission, and therefore the volume of drugs required, as has occurred in KwaZulu Natal, South Africa, as part of an integrated control program.

The second reason is, as already stated, future drugs are likely to be

---

[4]According to MSF, these are not preferential prices for that organization, but prices that any major buyer would be offered.

cheaper to produce than artemisinins (although probably not as cheap as chloroquine). And because, realistically, any new antimalarial with global promise is likely to emerge from MMV or another publicly funded source (e.g., the U.S. military), the need to recoup R&D costs through sales will be minimal. The day of the ten cent course of antimalarials may be gone, but newer, effective combination treatments still will be a relative bargain.

Another thing that is not likely to change quickly, however, is the inability of the endemic countries to absorb the higher costs. This means that without a global subsidy that is assured at least in the medium term, governments (through the public sector), and families (through their largely private-sector purchases) could be left without financial access to ACTs, or newer antimalarials, as they are introduced.

Inability to Rely on Tiered Pricing

Malaria affects only poor nations, those with highly restricted purchasing power. As is well known, the R&D costs of new drugs, together with the profits, are recovered in a markup of price over the costs of producing the drug. For those medicines with worldwide demand, it is possible to recover the fixed costs and make the bulk of the profits from sales in the richer countries, while selling at much lower prices in poorer countries. Price discrimination—tiered pricing—is clearly emerging as the pattern for antiretroviral drugs for people with HIV, for the panoply of drugs needed for tuberculosis, for childhood vaccines, and others.

In the case of malaria, the market is very small outside of endemic nations, nearly all of which are in the low-income category: within these countries, there is no room to charge anyone substantially above the marginal cost of production in order to create incentives for R&D. The exception to this generalization is that antimalarials are needed by travelers, and by the military of high-income countries. These groups, however, need antimalarial *prophylactic* drugs, and to a much lesser extent, *treatments* for clinical disease. In the past, chloroquine filled both roles, but just as with treatment, because of widespread resistance, chloroquine can no longer be used for prophylaxis. Some other drugs still can be used for both purposes. Mefloquine and Malarone fall into this category; both are quite expensive when bought in the United States or Europe. However, artemisinins are not good candidates for preventing malaria because they have extremely short half-lives, a characteristic that may prevent the easy emergence of resistant parasites. A good prophylactic drug needs to remain in the body between doses, and the longer the interval between dosing, the better people's adherence to the regim.

COST-EFFECTIVENESS OF ACTs AND
OTHER ANTIMALARIAL DRUGS

Antimalarial drugs are not the only pressing health care need in sub-Saharan Africa, where AIDS, tuberculosis, and a host of other infectious and other diseases also claim lives prematurely. And resources allocated to malaria can be spent on bednets, indoor spraying, or other measures, and not necessarily on antimalarial drugs. Thus drugs must compete for both public and private funds on grounds of their value for the dollars spent: their cost-effectiveness.

The question most relevant to this study is the cost-effectiveness of treating versus not treating acute episodes of malaria (the latter includes using an ineffective drug as well as no treatment). In the short term (possibly the next 5 years), it also is relevant to ask whether it would be beneficial to switch from failing but affordable chloroquine, to an intermediate drug that is as inexpensive as chloroquine, but which can only last a few years because of rapidly evolving resistance. In this scenario, a switch to more expensive ACTs would be expected within a few years, but in the meantime, considerable funds might be saved. The only drug that currently meets the conditions for such an intermediate is SP, but the analysis might apply in the future to other drugs. We look at both the cost-effectiveness of treatment versus no treatment, and of switching to a stopgap drug and then to ACTs.

Benchmarks for Cost-Effectiveness

There are no firm benchmarks or cutoff points to separate interventions that are deemed worth the cost ("cost-effective") and those that are not, but there are some guidelines.[5] At one end, a 1996 WHO Ad Hoc Committee recommended that, for low-income countries with a GDP per capita of less than $765, interventions that cost $25 or less per disability-adjusted life-year (DALY)[6] were "highly attractive," and those costing $150 or less per DALY were "attractive" (all figures in 1996 dollars) (World Health Organization, 1996).

More recently, the Commission on Macroeconomics and Health suggested that interventions costing less than three times GDP per capita for

---

[5]All link cost-effectiveness judgments to some measure of national wealth. Cost-effectiveness is a relative concept: what is considered a bargain in a high-income country may be completely out of range for a low-income country.

[6]The DALY is a summary measure of disease burden that incorporates years lost by premature death with years of life lived with disability. It allows comparison of the influence of different diseases whose effects on mortality, morbidity, and disability differ. One DALY can be considered as one year of "healthy" life.

each DALY averted represent good value for money (Commission on Macroeconomics and Health, 2001). WHO's World Health Report for 2002 built on this principle, defining "very cost-effective" interventions as those that cost less than GDP per capita to avert each additional DALY, and "cost-effective" interventions as those where each DALY averted costs between one and three times GDP per capita (World Health Organization, 2002).

It bears noting that cost-effectiveness analysis is an inexact science, more so in cases, such as this one, where many assumptions must be made on scant data. Uncertainty bounds are very wide. At its best, cost-effectiveness can help to define the relative positions of interventions by grouping them according to reasonably similar cost-effectiveness. Then, broad policy questions related to health care spending can be addressed, e.g., why are some interventions supported that cost more than three times GDP per capita, while others that appear to be better buys are not? One important aspect, relevant to ACTs, is that cost-effectiveness analysis does not address the total cost of an intervention for a country. Something that is very cost-effective—because it costs little and works well—could be very expensive per capita if a large proportion of the population needs it, which is the case for malaria treatment. It may not be affordable without additional resources, even though it is desirable and relatively cost-effective.

Two Models

We present two simplified models to examine the consequences of treating versus not treating (i.e., treating with a wholly ineffective antimalarial): switching drugs once—directly to ACTs—versus twice—to a less expensive but less durable alternative first, thence to ACTs. In the analysis of treating versus not treating, the evolution of resistance is not introduced (although the model from which this was adapted does include resistance), the aim being to define a basic level of benefit from effective treatment. The second analysis (one change versus two) is based on a different model, which does, of necessity, take into account the evolution of resistance. It also incorporates the effects of partial coverage within a population. Neither analysis attempts to model large-scale spatial effects if certain countries adopted effective antimalarials but others did not.

Treatment versus No Treatment

The model used to generate cost-effectiveness estimates for malaria treatment with ACTs was adapted from an earlier model looking at other aspects of malaria treatment (Box 2-1). Here, we compare ACT treatment with no treatment under two sets of treatment conditions. Treatment is either presumptive (i.e., everyone with fever suspected to be malaria is treated) or only after diagnosis of symptomatic individuals with a "hypothetical rapid diagnostic test" (RDT).[7] Under the assumptions of this model, treatment with ACTs saves lives, and at a cost that is well under even the low cutoff for a "highly attractive" or "very cost-effective" intervention for children under 5, at less than US$8 per DALY with presumptive treatment, and US$6.23 with an RDT. A life saved for US$209 or US$171 (without and with RDT) is also considered a bargain. For the over-5s, the answer from this model is not as clear-cut, though the point estimate of the cost-effectiveness ratio still falls within the "attractive" or "very cost-effective" range, at US$112 per DALY with presumptive treatment, and US$81.61 with RDT. Saving the life of someone over 5 (the model uses "adult" assumptions for this whole group, so this really applies to the adult population) costs about US$2,800 with presumptive treatment, and US$2,027 with RDT. It is important to note that these benefits apply only to reduced mortality, except for a very small portion for permanent disability caused by severe malaria. The model does not give any value to reduced morbidity; while the benefit per case may be small, for adults, the loss of a few days to 2 weeks of work are not trivial financially, and in the aggregate, can be very large.

Most of the variables in the model are subject to greater and lesser degrees of uncertainty, to which the authors have assigned ranges of values. Here we present single values based on the best (or central) estimate for each variable.

The analyses based on presumptive treatment should be closer to the current and near-term reality in Africa, where RDTs are seldom used. RDTs are used routinely in at least some parts of Asia, but the variables in this model (e.g., the proportion with fever who have malaria and the probabilities of death at different ages) are not applicable to most of Asia without significant modification.

Another way the model has been simplified is to assume that ACT resistance does not exist, thus the costs and benefits would remain perpetually the same. The model from which this was adapted does build in the spread of drug resistant malaria. As time goes on, costs increase (because of the cost of re-treating initial failures) and benefits decrease. It is reasonable to assume that, even if ACTs are used well, malaria strains resistant to ACTs will eventually develop and spread (as discussed elsewhere in this report), but it also is reasonable to anticipate that ACTs could remain

---

[7]The hypothetical RDT is 100% accurate, which does not exist in reality. There are places where RDTs are in use, but in most African settings, they would not be appropriate for a variety of reasons. This analysis is included as a window on a possible future scenario.

BOX 2-1
ACTs versus No Treatment: Key Points in the Cost-Effectiveness Analysis

This cost-effectiveness analysis is adapted by Shillcutt and Mills from a model[a] (Coleman et al., forthcoming) that describes clinic-based treatment for malaria, specifically where malaria is highly endemic. Most of the assumptions were taken from a cost-effectiveness analysis of a range of malaria control methods (Goodman et al., 2000).[b] Cost figures (in US$) were inflated to 2003 levels.

The results of this simplified model are for a single year, both for children under 5 years of age, and for everyone over 5 years.

The analysis was carried out two ways: 1) giving ACTs to all patients who come to the clinic with fever (presumptive treatment), and 2) using a rapid diagnostic test (RDT; a "dipstick") for all fever patients, but treating only those with a positive test.

Assumptions

Patients

- 45% of people coming to the clinic with fever have malaria.
- The average age of patients under 5 years is 2 years.
- The average age of patients over 5 years is 27 years.

Natural History of Malaria

- Without treatment, 5% (3-7%) of malaria cases in under-5s, and 1% (0.5-1.5%) in over-5s progress to severe malaria.
- 50% of under-5s (40-60%), and 25% (20-30%) of over-5s with severe malaria die from the episode.
- 1.3% of under-5s (0.4-2.2%), and 0.5% (0.25-0.75%) of over-5s with severe malaria develop neurological sequelae.

Effectiveness of RDTs and ACTs

- RDT has perfect accuracy (no cases missed or misdiagnosed).
- ACT is 100% effective if a full course is taken—no resistance has yet developed.
- 70% (the midpoint of the estimated range of 60-80%) of patients take the full course.
- If less than the full course is taken, the patient will be "cured" (an "adequate clinical response") 20% (10-30%) of the time; 80% (70-90%) of the time the patient will not be cured and will either have fever >37.5°C or detectable malaria in the blood 14 days after treatment.

---

[a]This adaptation differs from the original model in having a no-treatment comparison.
[b]The costs of ACTs and RDTs were estimated from data available to the committee.

continued

BOX 2-1 Continued

Costs

- International wholesale cost of a course of ACTs: US$0.50 for a child, US$1 for an adult.
- Cost of transporting the drug from producer to clinic: 20% of drug cost (US$0.10 for a child course; US$0.20 for an adult course).
- Clinic cost (staff, equipment, capital): US$1.14 per patient.
- Cost of one RDT: US$0.50

Effects of ACTs

- Disability-adjusted life-years (DALYs) averted for each death avoided by treatment. This is roughly the difference between dying from the episode and living out an average lifespan, plus a small number of years lived with a disability for those who would have had long-term neurological effects from severe malaria. Separate calculations were done for under-5s and over-5s. A discount rate of 3% was applied (so future "years" are considered less important and add progressively smaller increments to the total).

— DALYs averted for each under-5 death avoided: 27.5
— DALYs averted for each over-5 death avoided: 24.9

Key Results

Presumptive Treatment

Under 5 years of age

Effect per person (DALYs)	0.262
Costs per person ($US2003)	US$2
Cost-effectiveness ratio (CER) per DALY	US$7.62
CER per death averted	US$209.23

Over 5 years of age

Effect per person (DALYs)	0.023
Costs per person ($US2003)	US$2.60
CER per DALY	US$112.11
CER per death averted	US$2,784.16

With Diagnosis by RDT

Under 5 years of age

Effect per person (DALYs)	0.262
Costs per person ($US2003)	US$1.64
CER per DALY	US$6.23
CER per death averted	US$171.21

Over 5 years of age

Effect per person (DALYs)	0.023
Costs per person ($US2003)	US$1.90
CER per DALY	US$81.61
CER per death averted	US$2,026.72

Notes on Results

- Level of effect for adults is much lower than for children because adults are much less likely to die.
- Costs for adults are higher because drug costs are higher.
- Comparing presumptive diagnosis with use of the RDT, the effects are the same because, in both cases, everyone with malaria is treated. Average costs are lower because the RDT costs less than the drug and 55% of "fever" patients do not have malaria in this model.

Not Included in This Model

Certain aspects of how malaria is treated and its effects are not captured in this model. The most significant are:

- A large (but variable, geographically and by age) proportion of antimalarials are acquired outside of clinics after self-diagnosis, from pharmacies, drug sellers, and other outlets, with the following consequences. Costs will vary from the model (e.g., the drug cost may be higher than in the clinic, but no clinic fee would be charged; if only a partial course is purchased, it could be less expensive than the clinic, however). Benefits also will vary (e.g., fewer people are likely to take a full course, resulting in more treatment failures). There is insufficient information to make useful estimates of this scenario.
- Curing an episode of malaria in itself does not count in the benefits: only deaths and long-term disability averted are included. However, both children and adults benefit from fewer days of illness (children can attend school, adults can work). The benefit of early cure is not easily captured in this type of model, but does figure in microeconomic analyses of the costs of malaria. In this sense, the analysis understates the benefits, hence the cost-effectiveness, of ACTs.
- Only the direct costs of treatment at the clinic are included. Other direct costs to the patient (or family), including transportation, and indirect costs (lost wages) are not counted. Including these would tend to increase the costs but not the benefits, hence reducing the apparent cost-effectiveness of ACTs.
- Taking the whole population over age 5 in one analysis may mask differences among the younger and older members of the group.

effective for a relatively long period. In fact, they could well be superseded by newer, less expensive drugs before they lost effectiveness. Leaving resistance out of the model means possibly overestimating the cost-effectiveness of ACTs *in the long term*, but it may still be realistic in the short and medium term.

One Change versus Two: Chloroquine → ACTs versus Chloroquine → "Intermediate" → ACTs

ACTs are recommended by WHO as the drug of choice for policy change in countries with significant chloroquine resistance. Within a few years, this will include every country in sub-Saharan Africa. But if these countries were to switch to an inexpensive intermediate drug or an inexpensive combination that does not include an artemisinin (e.g., chloroquine + SP) as an interim measure, this would delay the higher treatment cost of ACTs. As recently as a year ago, changing to SP was a potentially viable option, with the understanding that resistance was likely to develop within a few years. A model was developed by a member of the IOM committee (Laxminarayan, forthcoming) to compare the costs and effects of a direct change to ACTs versus changing first to SP and then to ACTs. The model incorporates aspects of malaria transmission, levels of immunity, and drug resistance, and the costs of a malaria episode (including the cost of the drug, but no dispensing costs; and the costs of morbidity and mortality, set at US$0.50 per patient per day with malaria). Although based on SP as the intermediate, the model is indicative of a change to any relatively cheap alternative antimalarial with the potential for rapid development of resistance.

Characteristics that affect both the costs and effects of the two strategies are the level of coverage (i.e., the number and proportion of the population who get treatment for malaria when needed); the level of immunity to malaria in the population, which is related directly to the intensity of malaria transmission; and how quickly patients are treated after becoming symptomatic (this is dependent on access).

The level of coverage has an obvious influence on both costs and effects, which would be proportional to the number treated, but it has a second, less obvious, but extremely important, effect. The level of coverage is the most important factor in determining the level of "drug pressure," which determines the rate at which drug resistance spreads (see Chapter 9 for more detail on drug pressure and drug resistance). In the medium to long term, this effect dominates the results.

For the individual, immunity to malaria reflects exposure through the bites of infective mosquitoes. At the community level, immunity increases with the intensity of transmission and decreases with the extent of treatment coverage with an effective drug (Pringle and Avery-Jones 1966; Cornille-Brogger et al., 1978).

Where transmission is most intense, the level of immunity is highest and becomes evident at the earliest ages. Where infective bites are rare (e.g., in much of Asia), very little immunity develops. Immunity to malaria is a temporary phenomenon, waxing and waning with exposure.

For the purposes of this model, an initial frequency of drug-resistant parasites of 10^{-12} (a number very close to 0) was arbitrarily chosen for the artemisinin-based combinations, and for SP, 10^{-3} (one in one thousand) (Laxminarayan, forthcoming). Over time, treatment selection pressure leads to a greater prevalence of infected individuals who carry the drug-resistant strain relative to those carrying a drug-sensitive strain. The model was used to compare the economic consequences of two strategies: 1) replacing chloroquine (CQ) with ACTs and 2) replacing CQ with SP and waiting for resistance (to a level of 20 percent) to develop before introducing ACTs. A 3 percent discount rate is used for all relevant aspects of the model.

Using either strategy, the total costs of infection decrease with increasing levels of coverage with either strategy. This is attributable to faster cure rates, lower morbidity, and less need for re-treatment because of initial failures. At very low levels of treatment coverage (and low drug pressure), resistance to the intermediate drug is not a problem, so the least expensive drug gives good results for less money. At high levels of treatment coverage (and high drug pressure), resistance evolves so rapidly regardless of which strategy is followed that the faster acquisition of immunity with a less effective drug plays a critical role in determining the superior strategy.

The bottom line is that if one were interested in only the short term, using the less expensive drug makes better economic sense since the costs of resistance-related morbidity do not enter into the considerations. However, for longer planning horizons, a direct switch to ACTs is advantageous, given the costs of higher morbidity associated with increasing resistance to the intermediate drug. In theory, with higher intensity of disease transmission, the benefit of switching to ACTs directly may be diminished because of greater immunity associated with higher transmission, and hence a lower risk of resistance developing to the intermediate drug, whatever it is. Resistance to the intermediate would be expected to take longer to develop and, therefore, the benefits of switching to using it first, then switching to ACTs, increase.

One factor that is not taken account of in this model is the likelihood that, during a period of use of an intermediate drug, artemisinin monotherapy might gain in popularity, and during that time, some of the ACT companion drugs would continue to be used as monotherapy. This could result in higher levels of resistance to ACTs before they are introduced formally as first-line treatment. In general, the greater the coverage with

ACTs, and the sooner their use begins, the lower the likelihood of widespread monotherapy use, which could lower the likelihood of resistance to ACTs.

If it were easy for countries to switch drugs, it might make sense to introduce the cheaper drug first, and then move to ACTs before resistance has had much effect on malaria morbidity. However, this is not likely to happen for two reasons. First, malaria-endemic countries have found it difficult to modify their malaria treatment policies proactively in response to impending resistance-related morbidity. The fact that CQ is being used even with high treatment failure rates when an alternative drug is available is emblematic of these difficulties. Second, each change in treatment policy incurs costs associated with retraining health workers, printing material that explains new dosing regimes, restocking new drugs, and so forth, which can be significant in the short term. In the case of a switch to an intermediate that lasts only a few years, these policy change costs would have to be amortized over a much shorter life of the drug than in the case of a switch to ACTs. At a human level, knowledge of which antimalarial is recommended, and how it should be used must penetrate deep into society not only through the formal sector but through the many-layered informal sector. People must gain collective experience with a new drug, and observe its effects consistently to make the change complete, which can take years. This model does not incorporate policy change costs or other difficulties, so it may mask a portion of the true costs of switching first to an intermediate antimalarial and then to ACTs, versus a single switch to ACTs.

Antimalarial R&D: Effects of Lack of Global Purchasing Power

Malaria has never been an attractive target for the research-based pharmaceutical industry for the very reason the current crisis exists: lack of funds to pay for even modestly priced drugs. Most of the antimalarial drugs developed in the past half century are the products of publicly financed R&D. Up to now, the largest number of new products has come from R&D conducted by the Chinese government and the U.S. military. Most recently, the early development of the artemisinins was launched by Chinese government scientists, in response to concerns of the North Vietnamese government over the toll of chloroquine-resistant malaria on its soldiers during the conflict with the United States. The U.S. military continues its research program (though at a considerably lower level than its peak, during the Vietnam War), but in the past 5 years, has been upstaged—in a positive way—by the Medicines for Malaria Venture (MMV), an international "public-private partnership" with the sole mission of developing new antimalarial drugs. MMV today has the most active pipeline of research and products in various stages of development that has ever existed (see chapter 10 for a more detailed discussion of antimalarial drug R&D).

The current inaction over funding ACTs could call into question the sense of continuing to allocate public funding and solicit private contributions toward R&D for new antimalarials. The unstated implication of the failure to purchase ACTs is that only drugs that are about as inexpensive to produce as chloroquine are worth developing for first-line treatment. There may well be new drugs, cheaper than ACTs, in another 10 years, but they may still be unaffordable to most users. Rationalizing current R&D expenditures is not a reason to establish a global subsidy for ACTs, but the failure to do so may well have consequences for the R&D process that are detrimental and difficult to reverse.

CURRENT LEVELS OF GLOBAL FINANCING FOR MALARIA CONTROL

Families bear much of the financial burden of malaria treatment in sub-Saharan African and elsewhere. Funds deployed by governments come from internal country resources as well as from the major donors of development assistance, including support from individual countries (bilateral aid), and from international organizations, most importantly, the International Development Association of the World Bank, and other United Nations agencies. Nongovernmental organizations (particularly church-run medical services and groups like MSF) have for decades directly provided significant amounts of medical care, including drugs, in some cases (e.g., Zambia) acting as part of the public medical care system. Newer foundations—in particular, the Bill and Melinda Gates Foundation—and the beginning of operations by the Global Fund have provided significant increments of new funding, but also have highlighted the very low levels available in comparison to stated needs.

Although difficult to track accurately, the level of external support for malaria control from the key bilateral and multilateral agencies appears to have remained relatively static in recent years. The Commission on Macroeconomics and Health (Commission on Macroeconomics and Health, 2001) reported on contributions to health development assistance by bilateral and multilateral donors in the late 1990s, which totaled about US$1.7 billion for all diseases and programs. The biggest share—about US$287 million per year—went to HIV/AIDS. Malaria-specific funding was US$87 million, and for tuberculosis, US$81 million. These are the funds earmarked for specific diseases, but it is likely that other general funds were also used for them. A more recent estimate for international funding of malaria control, including bilateral aid and low-cost loan assistance from multilateral organizations for the years 2000 and 2002, totals about US$100 million per year (Narasimhan and Attaran, 2003). This figure is for all aspects of control (insecticide-treated nets, household spraying, and other preventive measures), and not just treatment. The amount that would have gone toward the cost of antimalarial drugs would be some fraction of the total.

Foundations have, for many years, contributed to global public health initiatives. In recent years, the Bill and Melinda Gates Foundation has entered at a level surpassing any other such efforts, spending close to US$1 billion per year on a variety of programs, some funded independently, and some through existing programs (e.g., the Gates Foundation is a major donor to the Global Fund, MMV, GAVI, and a number of other initiatives). This single entity is spending well over half of the amount spent by all governments and multilateral institutions together.

The advent of the Global Fund to Fight AIDS, Tuberculosis and Malaria represents the other big change in the funding landscape for global health. In their first three rounds of grants (from mid-2002 through the end of 2003), the Global Fund approved US$2 billion in 2-year grants to about 100 of the world's poorest countries. About one-quarter—US$475 million—was allocated to malaria projects, although very little so far involves funding the purchase of ACTs.

PROJECTED FINANCING NEEDS FOR
GLOBAL MALARIA CONTROL

In April 2000, more than 20 African heads of state met in Abuja, Nigeria for the first-of-a-kind political summit on malaria. It was one of the seminal events of the Roll Back Malaria (RBM) partnership. The African leaders called on the world community to allocate substantial new resources—at least US$1 billion per year—toward reaching the RBM goal of halving malaria deaths by the year 2010. Development partners also were called upon to cancel the debt of poor and heavily indebted nations so that more resources could be released to address malaria and otherwise alleviate poverty. In addition, the Abuja summit sought resources to support R&D for the whole range of malaria control measures.

The derivation of the US$1 billion was not stated explicitly, but this amount does not seem to overstate how much is needed. In the following year, 2001, the Commission on Macroeconomics and Health published a comprehensive and systematic analysis of how much it would cost to "scale up" a set of "priority" interventions for the world's poor ("priority" being defined by acceptable effectiveness, cost-effectiveness, and overall cost, with costs representing incremental costs over existing expenditures).

Malaria was singled out for individual analysis as one of the most important illnesses (in terms of both the burden of disease and its costs to society) to be addressed by increased resources for worthwhile interven-

TABLE 2-2 Annual Incremental Cost of Scaling Up Priority Interventions

TOTAL DOLLARS (BILLIONS OF U.S. DOLLARS)

	2007 Average Estimate	2015 Average Estimate
All interventions	26	46
TB treatment	0.5	1
Malaria prevention	2	3
Malaria treatment	*0.5*	*1*
HIV prevention	6	8
HIV care	3	6
HIV treatment (HAART)	5	8
Childhood-related illness—treatment	4	11
Childhood-related illnesses—immunization	1	1
Maternity-related illnesses	4	5

SOURCE: Commission on Macroeconomics and Health (2001).

tions (Table 2-2). What do these figures say about the costs of scaling up malaria treatment interventions? First, US$0.5 billion for malaria treatment in 2007 (US$1 billion in 2015) does not include treating children under 3 years old, because treatment of childhood-related illness (a few lines down) is linked to a specific mechanism for delivering care (Integrated Management of Childhood Illness, IMCI). Likewise, intermittent preventive therapy (IPT) for pregnant women is included in the estimate for "maternity-related illnesses." Malaria features large in the childhood burden of illness, in particular, so some substantial amount of the IMCI figure could be directly attributable to malaria (but the figures cannot be broken out in that way). The costs included in these estimates are basically the local cost of the interventions, their delivery, and local management support, but not of broader health sector improvements that would be needed to make them possible. Taking those higher-level costs into account roughly doubles the disease-specific estimates (Commission on Macroeconomics and Health, 2001).

If we take current external annual funding to be about US$100 million from bilateral and multilateral sources, plus another US$250 million from the Global Fund, and generously, $100 million from other sources, the total is still less than half of the US$1 billion suggested by the African leaders, and an even smaller fraction of the amount the Commission on Macroeconomics and Health projected. Both estimates of global need include some provision for incremental spending on ACTs, although not at the level of subsidy suggested in this report, which means that some portion of the estimated US$300-500 million for a global antimalarial drug subsidy should be added to the total.

REFERENCES

Coleman PG, Morel CM, Shillcutt SD, Goodman CA, Mills AJ. Forthcoming. A threshold analysis of the cost-effectiveness of artemisinin-based combination therapies in sub-Saharan Africa. *American Journal of Tropical Medicine and Hygiene.*

Commission on Macroeconomics and Health. 2001. *Macroeconomics and Health: Investing in Health for Economic Development.* Geneva: World Health Organization.

Cornille-Brogger R, Mathews HM, Storey J, Ashkar TS, Brogger S, Molineaux L. 1978. Changing patterns in the humoral immune response to malaria before, during, and after the application of control measures: A longitudinal study in the West African savanna. *Bulletin of the World Health Organization* 56(4):579-600.

Goodman CA, Coleman PG, Mills AJ. 2000. *Economic Analysis of Malaria Control in Sub-Saharan Africa.* Geneva: Global Forum for Health Research.

Laxminarayan R. Forthcoming. ACT now or later: Economics of malaria resistance. *American Journal of Tropical Medicine and Hygiene.*

Narasimhan V, Attaran A. 2003. Roll Back Malaria? The scarcity of international aid for malaria control. *Malaria Journal* 2(1):8.

Pringle G, Avery-Jones S. 1966. Observations on the early course of untreated falciparum malaria in semi-immune African children following a short period of protection. *Bulletin of the World Health Organization* 34(2):269-272.

WHO. 1996. *Investing in Health Research and Development: Report of the Ad Hoc Committee on Health Research Relating to Future Intervention Options. TDR/Gen/96.1.* Geneva: World Health Organization.

WHO. 2002. *World Health Report 2002.* Geneva: World Health Organization.

3

The Case for a Global Subsidy of Antimalarial Drugs

INTRODUCTION

Subsidies of public money increase access to goods or services that, from a societal perspective, are necessary or highly desirable but would not otherwise reach intended users because of cost. In cases where the item being subsidized also produces "positive externalities" that benefit everyone, the rationale for subsidizing individual access is strengthened. Artemisinin combination therapies (ACTs) have proven effective at the indivdual level in every setting where they have been tried. Used in combination with another effective antimalarial—as opposed to an artemisinin alone—a "global public good" results from the reduced risk of early development of resistance to this class of drug. A global subsidy, therefore, benefits not only those using the drugs directly but the global community.

Without subsidies, a large proportion (in some countries, a majority) of residents of sub-Saharan Africa and the poorer malaria-endemic countries of Asia will not be able to afford appropriate courses of ACTs. Moreover, evolving patterns of use are likely to create a negative externality—an increased chance that artemisinin-resistant strains will develop and spread, to the detriment of all. To round out the arguments for a global subsidy, ACTs are cost effective by global standards, and the full subsidy has a reasonable global price tag when held against the human and economic burden of malaria.

This chapter presents the pros and cons for a global antimalarial drug subsidy, using the specific case of ACTs, the only family of drugs that would currently meet worldwide needs. It ends with a discussion of how such a subsidy might be financed.

The Case for an Antimalarial Subsidy of Any Kind

The Humanitarian Case: Saving Lives

The primary reason for subsidizing antimalarials is to increase access to ACTs (and other drugs in the future) with the aim of reversing the recent upward trend in deaths and illness from drug-resistant falciparum malaria. Despite WHO's recommendation that ACTs be adopted as the first-line treatment for uncomplicated falciparum malaria where drug resistance has already reached significant levels (defined as greater than 15-25 percent failure to cure in standard clinical tests), few countries of sub-Saharan Africa that meet this definition of drug failure have named ACTs as their first-line malaria treatment. The few that have made the change have done so only after securing means to finance at least the public portion of the cost for a few years (i.e., drugs sold through the private retail sector are not subsidized). Other countries have made other decisions, e.g., switching to sulfadoxine-pyrimethamine (SP), or chloroquine plus SP, as first-line treatments (both regimens are in the same price range as chloroquine), merely postponing the inevitable change to ACTs for the time being.

Informally, knowledgeable individuals from endemic countries readily disclose that cost is the main factor preventing governments from switching to ACTs. Even if the prospect of funding exists, e.g., through the Global Fund, governments are wary about changing because of the uncertain sustainability of financing in the longer term. This has led to the continuing spread of chloroquine resistance to current high levels in many countries. The current dilemma clearly supports a subsidy of some type that would make the choice of adopting ACTs as first-line antimalarials a financially feasible option for countries unable to do so under existing circumstances. The fact that no country in Africa has adopted ACTs as first-line treatment without external funding indicates that widespread coverage will not be achieved across the continent without a global plan and a subsidy available to all countries. Currently, not enough money is available through the Global Fund or bilateral agencies to accomplish this.

Creating a "Public Good:" Buying Time against Drug Resistance

In addition to the humanitarian rationale, there is an economic rationale for international subsidies of ACTs. Treating any contagious disease creates a "positive externality" by reducing the chances that other people nearby will contract the disease. In the case of malaria, this argument for public financing would justify making transfers only to governments. There is, however, an international externality: if a country does not use ACTs— in particular, if it uses artemisinins as monotherapy—the possibility that resistance will develop is much greater. The subsequent spread of artemisinin resistance—first directly to neighboring countries and then to more distant ones via migrants and travelers—is inevitable. It is therefore in the interest of the global community to maintain the efficacy of artemisinins through "universal" adoption of ACTs and to discourage monotherapies that would compromise either the artemisinins directly, or the ability of companion drugs to protect artemisinins in a combination. It is impossible to assign a dollar value to this international public good, but it must include both the ability to treat hundreds of millions of cases of malaria with these drugs (over the number of years of extra effective life produced), and potential moderation of future R&D costs for first-line antimalarials.

Stimulating the ACT Market

An additional rationale for a substantial international ACT subsidy is to provide the impetus needed for more generic drug manufacturers to enter ACT production, and for those already producing artemisinins to increase output. Companies have not invested in producing ACTs on the scale needed to supply Africa because there has been no assured market. Starting with cultivation of *Artemisia annua*, it takes about 18 months to produce a finished ACT, which currently has a 2-year shelf life. A visible, global subsidy would provide the security needed for private concerns to ramp up for African demand.

Maintaining the Impetus to Develop New Antimalarial Drugs

The push to develop new and better antimalarial drugs is not driven by profitability but largely by a sense of public and private sector responsibility to address a major health need that otherwise would likely be neglected. (Chapter 10 describes the recently revitalized R&D pipeline for antimalarials, largely through the Medicines for Malaria Venture [MMV], a public-private partnership.) The need is great, but demand is weak because the potential customers are among the world's poorest people. The current situation with ACTs is just the consequence that would be expected. Without a system in place to pay for new drugs emerging from MMV (and possibly other sources), it is likely to become increasingly difficult to maintain support for R&D programs.

Goals of a Subsidy for ACTs

The broad goals of a subsidy for ACTs correspond one-to-one with the goals of this study:

- To ensure access to ACTs for the greatest number of patients, aiming to at least match historic access to chloroquine, which would require access in both the public and private sectors in most, if not all, countries
- To delay for as long as possible the development and spread of resistance to artemisinins and currently-effective partner drugs by:
   — discouraging the use of artemisinin (and other) monotherapy for uncomplicated malaria, and
   — encouraging use of ACTs in recommended courses.

The following discussion proceeds through the arguments that lead to this report's central recommendation: a supranational, broad subsidy of ACTs (a "global subsidy") near the top of the distribution chain.

The Case for a Global Subsidy of ACTs

Under ideal circumstances, the following conditions would be met when ACTs are introduced into Africa and Asia on a widespread basis. Within a relatively short time (i.e., a few years):

- Full courses (i.e., doses taken once or twice a day for a total of 3 days, depending on formulation) will be taken to ensure that an individual's current malaria infection is cured, since partial courses typically produce incomplete cure, and also increase the possibility of recurrence with drug-resistant malaria parasites.
- Monotherapy with either the artemisinin or the companion drug will be avoided (except in special circumstances that demand customized monotherapy treatment). (One practical benefit to individuals taking ACTs as opposed to artemisinin monotherapy is a shorter course: 3 days vs. 7 days, respectively. The main benefit to the global community is a greatly reduced probability of resistance.)
- ACT coverage of people with clinical malaria will be as high as possible to achieve the greatest benefit in terms of reduced morbidity and mortality. High coverage also could result in reduced transmission, at least in areas of low and moderate transmission. Whether transmission will be affected in areas of intense transmission is not yet known. A high degree of coverage will require that ACTs be made available through both public and private outlets.

There is one other condition that ideally should be met, but which is less time-sensitive:

• ACTs will not be used by people whose clinical illness is not due to malaria. Use by nonaffected people has several consequences: 1) for the individual, the true cause of illness goes untreated, with whatever consequences that may entail (including also loss of confidence in ACTs); 2) in people with low level, asymptomatic malaria infections, unwarranted ACT use (particularly in partial doses) may actually enhance the development of drug resistant parasites, although this risk is probably very low;[1] 3) the ACT (and associated subsidy) is essentially wasted.

These are the ideal conditions, but they must be approached with current conditions as a starting point. Given the existing deficiencies of health care systems and the treatment of malaria in particular, the goals are only partially achievable in the short-to-medium term. Nonetheless, the introduction of ACTs will provide immediate, major benefits in all endemic countries.

A key question for this study is whether countries acting on their own could create the conditions set out above that would sustain the benefits of ACTs within their national borders. If not country-by-country, would it be possible to maintain drug efficacy regionally? But these turn out to be merely rhetorical questions, because national borders have little effect on the spread of disease or resistant strains, generally. Furthermore, the spread of malaria resistant to chloroquine and other widely used antimalarials has already occurred. Even when disease agents are not spreading, drugs move readily across borders wherever a sufficient disparity exists in availability or price. If subsidies for antimalarials were available in some countries and not others, the result could be inexpensive, nationally subsidized ACTs moving into countries that lack subsidies, or inexpensive monotherapies moving from one country in which they are available to a neighboring one where they are not. Regulatory systems and surveillance may be better in some countries than others, but weak links are bound to exist that will facilitate such transfers. Practical market realities suggest that similar access and similar prices should prevail everywhere if ACTs are to become a reliable medical staple and be reasonably protected from the premature development of artemisinin-resistant malaria.

---

[1]Inappropriate treatment of a person with another cause of fever, who happens to have coincident asymptomatic malaria, does not encourage resistance. Even what are considered inadequate doses may be sufficient to eradicate asymptomatic parasitemias, and will contribute little or nothing to drug pressure. If the person does not have malaria at all, treatment would have no relevance to the development of resistance.

Avoidance of Macroeconomic Distortions in Endemic Countries

An issue that surfaces in discussions of a significant expansion of over-seas development assistance flowing into countries is that it can lead to unintended and often detrimental macroeconomic effects. These include unfavorable effects on the currency exchange rate, imbalances among sectors in the wage structure, and the diversion of resources from intended uses to other sectors. The nature and consequences of such effects was reviewed by the Commission on Macroeconomics and Health in relation to their recommendation for a large increase in external funding for core health services (Commission on Macroeconomics and Health Working Group 3, 2002).

The design of the subsidy recommended in this report should avoid these effects, to the greatest extent possible. The subsidy arrives in each country in the form of lower prices for antimalarial drugs (prices that should be similar to prices for chloroquine and SP in recent years), not as currency. No other method of subsidization would appear to be as neutral in this respect.

Potential Difficulties with a Global Subsidy for Antimalarials

A global subsidy for ACTs does pose some difficulties, in terms of both how ACTs are used and the way in which bilateral and multilateral aid programs are structured.

Potential Negative Impacts of ACT Use

If ACTs become as inexpensive to consumers as chloroquine is now, chances are they will be used as frequently as chloroquine, including over-use for febrile illnesses due to causes other than malaria. All overuse increases the probability that artemisinin-resistant parasites will arise and spread. Experience with other antimalarials suggests that resistance is less likely to develop in high-transmission areas than in low-transmission areas where people develop high parasite loads accompanied by clinical symptoms of malaria (see Chapter 9). This is not guaranteed, however.

Low-priced ACTs also could dampen incentives to expand the use of diagnostic tests (traditional microscopy or rapid dipsticks) for malaria. Currently, most antimalarial use in sub-Saharan Africa follows self-diagnosis (or parental diagnosis, in the case of children) and purchase of drugs through the private sector. Even in formal health facilities, diagnosis is often based on clinical symptoms. One confounding issue is that the currently available diagnostic tests have drawbacks. Microscopy is time-consuming, and technically demanding. Present-day dipsticks are relatively expensive and do not discriminate between a true clinical case of malaria and illness of another cause in someone with a chronic but asymptomatic malaria infection, which is common in high-transmission areas. Work is progressing toward appropriate rapid diagnostics for such areas, but validated tests are not yet available.

Difficulties Related to International Aid Programs

The main purpose of bilateral and multilateral aid is to provide benefits to nations (or groups within them) who have been identified as appropriate beneficiaries of the particular type of assistance given. A global subsidy takes away the opportunity to select beneficiaries. In the case of ACTs, this means that some nations as well as certain individuals within virtually every nation will benefit when they could afford to pay the full price or something between the fully subsidized and nonsubsidized price.

Concern over Setting Precedents

Concerns may arise that a global subsidy for ACTs sets a precedent for other drugs or health interventions. The main precedent would be to subsidize other antimalarials which international consensus deems should either supplant ACTs or serve as another first-line therapy. If economic conditions in endemic countries are substantially unchanged when that time comes and the new product meets appropriate cost and cost-effectiveness criteria, it would be difficult to exclude it from subsidies.

On the other hand, the possibility that a global subsidy for ACTs would lead to pressure to subsidize drugs for treatment of other diseases should be a lesser concern. A few key factors related to malaria and its treatment, taken together, are unique among the major diseases. These factors are:

- Predominance of self-diagnosis and treatment of a life-threatening disease, with private sector drug purchasing, for an unpredictable need at the level of the individual or family
- Negligible market for drug in wealthier countries, so minimal opportunity for tiered pricing (particularly because ACTs are not appropriate for prophylaxis for travelers)
- Lack of a viable replacement for artemisinins as first-line drug
- Need for drug change because the historically effective drug has failed rather than extending a new medical benefit (as with the provision of long-term treatment for HIV-infected individuals); the major aim of replacing current antimalarials is to prevent further deterioration of clinical management

The first two points are particularly important. Taking tuberculosis and HIV as the two most important global comparator diseases, there are significant differences. Neither is commonly self-treated, and for both, the courses of treatment are long-term and predictable. The market for drugs to treat both TB and HIV are global, although the TB market is heavily weighted toward poor countries. Thus, no current disease is analogous, but one could arise in the future that has characteristics akin to malaria and ACT treatment. In such a case, the experience gained with ACTs will undoubtedly provide guidance.

How Can a Subsidy Be Structured to Achieve the Goals of ACT Use?

Subsidies can be structured in many ways. A major division is between "broad" and "targeted" subsidies. *Broad subsidies* apply equally to all members of society. In the case of ACTs, a lower (subsidized) price would be available to everyone, regardless of their income. In theory, broad subsidies can reach into the private sector; however, they often are made available only through the public sector, which deters some people from taking advantage of them. *Targeted subsidies* are designed to benefit particular groups within society. The main reasons for choosing to target a subsidy often relate to equity, efficiency, sustainability, and meeting community needs (Worrall et al., 2003). However, there are no standard formulas and each situation must be assessed based on the specific goals of the subsidy, the feasibility of delivering it in different ways, and the potential for unwanted effects.

Whether broad or targeted, *levels* of subsidy can vary, with effects on consumer price that range from lowering the price by a small decrement to a full subsidy that makes the item free. The overall cost of subsidies is determined both by how broad or targeted they are and the level of the subsidy.

The point at which the subsidy is applied also affects how it operates, and its costs. In the case of ACTs, the point of subsidy could be anywhere along the distribution chain, from the top (somewhere close to where the drugs are produced and first sold as finished products) to the bottom, i.e., the consumer. A consumer might receive a drug voucher for redemption at various outlets, or obtain free drugs from a public clinic or other specified outlet, with the cost differential directly channeled to the providing facility.

The advantages and disadvantages of broad and targeted subsidies, and considerations specific to ACTs, are summarized in Table 3-1 (Derriennic and Mensah, 2003) and discussed below.

Broad versus Targeted Subsidy for ACTs

Wealthier individuals in every endemic country are able to afford ACTs for malaria treatment at the current retail price, which ranges between US$5 and US$20 in private pharmacies throughout Africa. The price is likely to fall over the next few years (for newer ACTs), which will expand the numbers of people with financial access. Consequently, a broad subsidy that reduces the price of the entire ACT supply will benefit some people who do not need it. This could be the basis for arguing for a targeted subsidy over a broad one on grounds of equity, efficiency, or both.

Improving equity is a common objective of targeted subsidies, with the aim of redressing imbalances in access to vital goods or services, particularly for health care and food, but also in areas such as education for women (Worrall et al., 2003). If targeting is feasible, it can reduce the cost of the subsidy while at the same time concentrating it on those who would benefit most. In the case of ACTs, in areas of high transmission, young children and pregnant women are at greatest risk of death or serious consequences of malaria; in low-transmission areas, everyone who contracts malaria is at some risk of serious illness and death, including healthy adults. Considering only short-term gains in morbidity and mortality, the greatest benefits could therefore be achieved by targeting young children and pregnant women in high-transmission areas, and patients of all ages with confirmed falciparum malaria in low-transmission areas.

Another important factor in deciding between broad and targeted subsidies is the proportion of the population who would be eligible for a subsidy. In the case of ACTs, we would want to know: 1) the proportion of the population who would be unable to buy the drugs without a subsidy, and 2) something about the price elasticity of demand (i.e., how demand changes with changes in prices), to determine the level of subsidy needed per dose to reach the target population. The larger the proportion of the population who would be eligible, and the larger the subsidy per dose, the closer we come to a broad subsidy covering a substantial proportion of the drug's purchase price. If there were no administrative costs to delivering subsidies and/or negative effects of targeted subsidies, it would always make sense to target, but this is not the case.

Not surprisingly, it is difficult to estimate the proportion of the population in endemic countries that would find ACTs financially inaccessible, either at current prices or at the somewhat lower prices projected over the next few years, because information is limited. However, we have estimated that in many countries in sub-Saharan Africa and some in Asia, where per capita incomes are very low, well over half of the population would be unable to afford ACTs without a subsidy, and the proportion may be substantially higher in some countries.

TABLE 3-1 Types of Subsidy That Could Be Applied to ACTs

Population to Be Reached	Channel and Method	Advantages
BROAD SUBSIDIES		
Broad subsidies would have the highest total drug costs, but administrative costs are likely to be substantially lower, and coverage substantially higher, than with targeted subsidies.		
All endemic countries, total population ("global")	Public and private (including NGO) sectors	Widest possible access created (depending on level of subsidy)
	Global (supranational) level purchase or other high-level subsidy in ACT production chain	Maintains existing drug flows with minimal market distortion
	Supplies to public and private sectors through existing channels (with acceptance of each government for private sector access)	Administrative simplicity within countries
Country-specific, but covering total population within subsidized countries (national)	Direct subsidy of public sector from central government to reduce drug costs in clinics and other facilities	Same as above
	Sale of ACTs at highest levels of private sector, including NGOs (by government?)	

Disadvantages	ACT-Specific Issues
Higher drug costs than other subsidies	To meet the goal of access equal to historic levels of chloroquine access, end-user price would have to be no more than chloroquine.
Requires international financing mechanisms outside the current norm	To meet the goal of discouraging the use of monotherapies, the price would have to be no higher than the least expensive of the two components (the artemisinin and the companion drug).
Poorest of the poor still would be excluded by cost; additional coverage would require additional targeted programs	
Greatest potential for overuse of drug and increased drug selection pressure for resistance	
Same as above, and:	Same as above
Potential for diversion to neighboring countries without subsidized ACTs	

Continued

TABLE 3-1 Continued

Population to Be Reached	Channel and Method	Advantages

TARGETED SUBSIDIES

Under any targeted approach, the potential for controlling the use of artemisinin (and companion drug) monotherapy is very limited. Market conditions may make monotherapy the rational choice for consumers, and the global community will have little leverage over production practices of manufacturers.

Population to Be Reached	Channel and Method	Advantages
Age under 5 years and pregnant women (at-risk targets)	Public or public and private sectors Public sector through clinics and other public facilities If private sector is included, through vouchers	Focuses on most at risk of serious outcome (in highest-transmission areas only) Relatively easy to identify target population Lower drug selection pressure for resistance
All those unable to afford market price of ACTs (economic target)	Public or public and private sectors Public sector through clinics and other public facilities If private sector is included, through vouchers	Focuses on poor Lower drug selection pressure for resistance
Age under 5 years and pregnant women AND unable to afford market price of ACTs (at risk and economic targets)	Public or public and private sectors Public sector through clinics and other public facilities If private sector is included, through vouchers	Targets those most likely to gain access and benefit Lowest drug costs of all options Lower drug selection pressure for resistance

SOURCE: Based in part on Derriennic and Mensah, 2003.

Disadvantages	ACT-Specific Issues

High administrative burden and costs to develop and monitor program, particularly private sector involvement

If public sector only, poor coverage in many countries and public sector could be overwhelmed with demand

High risk of leakage to adult population

Misses adults at risk in lower-transmission or epidemic-prone areas

Subsidizes some who could afford ACTs without subsidy

High administrative burden and costs to develop and monitor program, particularly private sector involvement

Depending on how the target group is defined, it could be a very large proportion of the population—possibly greater than half in many sub-Saharan African countries. The number will be large if the target is to achieve access at least equivalent to historic access to chloroquine.

If public sector only, poor coverage in many countries and public sector could be overwhelmed with demand

High risk of leakage to private sector for those not eligible for subsidy

Unclear how the overall cost of this approach would compare with other subsidies

Same as above

What the optimal price or prices should be to the end user also is difficult to answer, but research indicates that even chloroquine—at around 10 U.S. cents per dose—is too expensive for the very poor. If we accept that ACTs should achieve access at least as widespread as that of chloroquine, the subsidized price could be no higher than chloroquine's.

All forms of subsidy incur administrative costs as well as direct costs (i.e., the amount of subsidy per drug course), but these vary depending on how the program is organized. As a general rule, broad subsidies should require less administration than targeted subsidies, since the latter involve either delivering the subsidy (in the form of a voucher, or the commodity itself) or setting up a system to identify those eligible for the subsidy, maintaining records, reimbursing the implementing sites, auditing to ensure that the subsidies reach their intended target group and are not diverted, and other record keeping. A broad subsidy, because it is available to everyone, requires less effort, although record-keeping for accountability still is needed. With all subsidies, methods should be built in to evaluate the effect on stated goals (which could include both process—e.g., how many courses of subsidized ACTs are delivered to patients—and outcome measures—the effect on a key health measure).

Placement of the Subsidy in the Path from Production to End User

Where the subsidy is placed in the chain from drug manufacturer to consumer will affect the accessibility of ACTs by consumers in several ways. Subsidizing drugs high up in the chain, near the producer level and above the level of individual country procurement (what will be referred to here as "supranational" subsidy), will almost certainly make them available in more *countries* than would be the case if the subsidy worked through procurement mechanisms on a country by country basis. Precedents for supranational subsidies include the historic smallpox eradication campaign and current program to eradicate polio.

A key argument for a high-level global subsidy is to avoid undermining the private distribution systems that currently supply most of the antimalarials purchased in Africa and elsewhere. It is difficult to imagine how to subsidize at a local level and maintain the reach of the private distribution system. Subsidy at the highest levels will permit resale to the private sector, at a subsidized price. At the same time, it does not preclude national decisions about how subsidized antimalarials will be made available through the public sector. A country could, for instance provide antimalarials free in public sector facilities (with an additional subsidy), while at the same time ensuring that they are available for sale at a reasonable price in pharmacies and other private sector outlets.

There also are disadvantages to a supranational subsidy. One is that it minimizes influence over end-user prices. Drugs gather costs as they move along the distribution chain to consumers. Overall mark-ups can be considerable, as seen in the three countries for which information on drug flows was discussed in Chapter 1 (Senegal, Zambia, and Cambodia). A recent detailed study of the retail sector in Tanzania confirms some lack of price competition in the private sector (Goodman et al., 2004) (Box 3-1).

We have assumed that as long as there is a sufficient supply of ACTs, the end-user price should be at least as low as chloroquine if the drugs were subsidized to the full cost of original purchase from the manufacturer. We also know, however, that even chloroquine is still out of economic reach for many people, both because even the lowest price is unaffordable, but also because price competition does not function everywhere. A subsidy lower down in the chain could allow drugs to reach the end users at lower prices (or free, if a voucher or targeting program is employed). A program that would address this problem can still be put in place within countries, even in the presence of the supranational subsidy. In fact, countries might find this more feasible in the presence of a global subsidy, because it would require less country-level funding.

Both an advantage and a disadvantage of a supranational subsidy is that it perpetuates both the best and worst elements of an existing distribution system. We have already seen that the quality of drugs obtained from drug peddlers and small shops can be low—sellers are willing to sell partial doses, and drugs may be poor quality. These conditions are conducive to the development of drug resistant malaria strains, and most important, lack of cure for those who use these services. On the other hand, problems of substandard drugs are not limited to the private sector. In Cambodia, counterfeit and poor quality drugs were found more frequently in public outlets.

What would be the alternative if ACTs at subsidized prices were not available to private sellers in these small outlets? They might well be selling artemisinin (and other) monotherapies, also in partial doses, in which case the drug pressure would be even greater. Whether involving ACTs or other drugs, these are the very conditions that must be addressed by initiatives to improve the use of antimalarials (see Chapter 11). The point we make here is that it is not feasible to reform and improve the "system" *before* the widespread introduction of ACTs. On the positive side, one aim of the centralized management of ACT procurement will be to encourage packaging of ACTs in ways that will improve adherence and reduce the likelihood of partial dosing. At the same time, attention still will be needed at the local level to minimize the misuse of ACTs.

It is the second goal—achieving high overall coverage with ACTs and, to the extent possible, eliminating use of monotherapies—that will be difficult or close to impossible to achieve with any approach other than a global subsidy. As long as ACT prices are low enough (in particular, lower than

BOX 3-1
Investigating Competition and Regulation in the Retail Market
for Malaria Treatment in Rural Tanzania

Goodman and her colleagues (Goodman et al., 2004) studied the functioning of the retail market for antimalarials in rural areas of Tanzania (parts of the Kilombero, Ulanga, and Rufiji districts) in 2001/2002. As in much of sub-Saharan Africa, most antimalarials in the study sites are acquired directly through a retail shop. In this case, 54 percent of people seeking treatment for fever went to a shop, compared with the 38 percent who went to a health facility. There were no pharmacies in these areas, only drug stores and general shops or stalls where drugs are sold. General shops (one for every 273 people) far out numbered drug stores (one for every 4570 people), but the proportion of general stores that stocked antimalarials was low and falling, with the result that 85 percent of retail antimalarial sales were through drug stores.

Drug stores were competing with the public sector on drug availability, stocking effective antimalarials when government facilities had only chloroquine (when it was no longer effective), or had run out of antimalarials. However, price competition among private retailers was weak, with drug store markups for antimalarials ranging from two to more than six times in relation to an international reference price (although there is no firm rule about what price ratio is appropriate, a ratio greater than two is often taken as excessive). The reasons are most likely the obvious ones: there are few outlets, so little reason to keep prices low, and people tend to seek care close to home, further reducing competition. There also may be some implicit collusion to avoid antagonizing fellow traders.

The high prices (and other factors) contributed to poor quality care for people seeking treatment for malaria through the private sector. People often bought only partial courses of antimalarials, or bought only antipyretics, which are cheaper.

Unless preemptive steps are taken, the same problems of high retail markups and poor quality treatment are likely to occur when ACTs subsidized high in the distribution chain flow through the system. In the absence of major system changes, Goodman and her colleagues identified other measures that could be used to improve access, including:

• Encouraging over-the-counter sale of prepackaged ACTs with clear labelling and locally tested instructions
• Widespread distribution of a single branded product, or a limited number of quality-marked brands
• Retail price maintenance by price labelling and consumer education campaigns
• Encouraging sale of products in a wide range of outlets, including drug shops and general stores in remote areas
• A positive role for regulators in improving knowledge and encouraging regular stocking

It will be important, as well, to monitor prices and their effects on access to ACTs, once a subsidy is in place.

artemisinin and companion drug monotherapies), market mechanisms of supply and demand should ensure that they become the most widely used drugs for malaria with relatively minimal government actions. All other antimalarial drugs (excluding chloroquine and SP) would be more expensive and (most likely) less effective. Chloroquine and SP would certainly be less effective overall for true malaria cases. Soon, African consumers would appreciate that ACTs are far more desirable than alternative treatment options, as have Asian consumers.

Artemisinin monotherapies and monotherapy formulations of companion drugs could be excluded from the market in each country by legal and regulatory mechanisms (with some provision for special cases that require monotherapies). Even if those laws and regulations were less than fully effective, the monotherapies would probably gain a very low market share because they would be more expensive than subsidized ACTs. If subsidies were targeted, in contrast, most people would have to pay full market costs for ACTs, and it would be extremely difficult for countries to control the flow of monotherapies (which could be less expensive than ACTs), particularly in the private sector.

Anticipated Benefits of a High-Level Global Subsidy

A global subsidy of ACTs near the top of the distribution chain accomplishes several things that are consistent with the optimal use of ACTs, which targeted subsidies, or subsidies at points lower in the distribution chain, cannot accomplish:

• With the assent of individual countries (but without the need to set up new programs, should countries choose not to), it would allow ACTs to flow through both public- and private-sector channels that already exist to deliver antimalarials to consumers, even in remote places.
• It would allow all countries to adopt the malaria treatment policies best for their populations, including ACTs as first-line treatment, without concern about the sustainability of country-level external funding for purchase.
• It would not force countries to choose between effective antimalarials and spending on other measures to enhance malaria control.
• It would provide equitable access to inhabitants of all endemic countries, including those that, for a variety of reasons, may not be applying for funds specifically earmarked for purchasing ACTs.
• It gives the global community leverage with artemisinin manufacturers who wish to sell through the subsidized system not to produce artemisinin monotherapies.

- It minimizes the administrative costs of applying the subsidy.
- It minimizes the incentives for counterfeit ACT production.
- It minimizes incentives for diversion and smuggling of ACTs.

FINANCING A GLOBAL SUBSIDY OF ACTS

If the added expense of ACTs were affordable within the budgets of governments and families of endemic countries, the current crisis would not exist. The fact that not even one country in sub-Saharan Africa adopted ACTs as first-line treatment without first having secured funding from the Global Fund suggests a problem of considerable breadth and depth. Even in countries with funding, thus far, ACTs will be distributed only through the public sector (and possibly NGOs); no subsidized ACTs will appear in the private retail market, at least through legal channels. This chapter has already made the case that the goals of a subsidy for ACTs would be best met through a centralized, global system, where all potential consumers have access to subsidized drugs, regardless of where they get them. Where will the funding for such a subsidy come from and how will it be handled?

Funds for ACTs will have to come from a mix of internal financing from endemic countries, and external funding from the range of sources available for health programs generally.

Ability to Mobilize Additional Domestic Resources in Africa to Fund ACTs

Current Spending on Health

Spending for malaria treatment and prevention is a subset of health spending in general. In Africa, only seven countries spend more than US$100 per person each year on health, including both public and private spending, whereas 27 spend less than US$50 and another seven, less than US$20. Government spending on health can be as high as US$364 per person in South Africa or US$223 in Namibia, but in most countries it is below US$40, and in 17 countries, below US$20 (Table 3-2).

Out-of-pocket spending represents a high proportion of total spending on health in those countries that spend the least on health. Of the seven countries that spent a total of less than US$20 per head on health, in two (Madagascar and Niger) more than one-third was represented by out-of-pocket spending, and in three (Burundi, Nigeria, and Sierra Leone) more than half.

By any standards, spending levels in most sub-Saharan countries are so low that there is little hope for improving the principal measures of the population's health as long as spending on health in general remains at such levels. Estimates suggest that US$80 per person per year (in PPP dollars) are needed for effective health services (Commission on Macroeconomics and Health Working Group 3, 2002). This is equivalent to about US$33-40 in current (and not PPP) dollars.

In most of Africa, US$30 to US$40 per capita health spending translates into more than 10 percent of GNP, a figure far in excess of what such low-income countries attain in practice, and far beyond what most countries can reasonably be expected to generate. Most African countries spend less than 5 percent of GDP on health, and some, less than 3 percent. Spending on health in Africa is probably below the amounts needed to maintain health at present levels, much less improve it.

Those countries where out-of-pocket expenditures represent a large proportion of the total spent on health would seem to have the least hope for improvement unless substantial increases can be made in resources for health flowing through the health system as a whole. The sacrifices already being made to spend household moneys on medicines and health care, often for catastrophic illnesses, suggest that the availability of additional funds for even more expensive treatments must be slight. To raise health spending, including spending on antimalarial drugs, in those poorer countries will require an increase in public health spending that, in turn, will demand either increased government revenues, a marked reordering of government spending priorities, or an increase in external aid designed to reach the ultimate consumer.

Potential for Increased Tax Revenues

In Africa, tax revenue as a proportion of GDP can range from below 10 percent (Burkina Faso, Cameroon, the Democratic Republic of the Congo, the Republic of the Congo, Madagascar, Rwanda, and Sierra Leone) to much higher figures, such as 25 percent for the Gambia, 23 percent for Kenya, and 29 percent for Namibia. The unweighted average is 17.7 percent. Notwithstanding the considerable problems with international comparisons of taxation, the large differences in the tax-to-GDP ratio among countries in Africa suggest that scope exists for many to increase revenue through higher tax rates, better compliance, and improved tax administration. However, the structure of tax rates in any country reflects a complex mix of judgments as to what the government considers politically tenable, what the population perceives as fair, the margin beyond which evasion defeats rate increases, and the capacity of officials to administer the tax system.

If the argument that more government funds should be spent on health was persuasive, could those funds come from taxation? Almost certainly

TABLE 3-2 Annual Per Capita Health Expenditures in Sub-Saharan Africa (purchasing power parity, US$)

	Total	Public Sector	Out of Pocket	Total Health Spending % Share of GDP
Angola	62	30	32	4.1
Benin	27	13	14	3.1
Botswana	220	155	24	3.4
Burkina Faso	32	22	10	4.0
Burundi	12	5	7	2.1
Cameroon	44	15	23	3.0
Cape Verde	87	62	24	2.6
CAR	25	13	9	2.4
Chad	25	20	5	3.1
Comoros	53	36	17	4.5
Congo, Rep. (Brazz)	28	18	10	2.8
Cote d'Ivoire	46	21	21	3.0
Dem. Rep. Of Congo	15	11	4	1.6
Equatorial Guinea	59	33	26	3.6
Eritrea	42	28	14	4.4
Ethiopia	29	12	15	4.7
Gabon	197	131	66	3.1
Gambia	45	36	10	3.0
Ghana	63	35	28	3.6
Guinea	58	33	25	3.6
Guinea Bissau	34	22	12	3.9
Kenya	76	21	40	7.6
Lesotho	96	73	23	5.3
Liberia	94	62	31	2.5
Madagascar	17	10	7	2.3
Malawi	41	21	7	7.3
Mali	28	13	14	4.2
Mozambique	28	16	5	3.9
Namibia	411	223	6	7.9
Niger	19	10	8	3.0
Nigeria	14	4	10	1.9
Rwanda	35	12	14	5.2
Sao Tome & Principe	45	30	15	3.0
Senegal	61	34	27	4.5
Sierra Leone	17	7	10	3.0
Somalia	11	7	4	2.4
S. Africa	770	364	82	10.3
Sudan	46	10	36	4.4
Swaziland	148	107	41	3.4
Tanzania	21	10	10	5.1
Uganda	42	21	12	3.7
Zambia	45	25	14	6.0
Zimbabwe	242	143	66	9.5

TABLE 3-2 Continued

	Total	Public Sector	Out of Pocket	Total Health Spending % Share of GDP
Memorandum Items				
Australia	1917	1309	309	8.4
France	1994	1550	209	9.4
Germany	2336	1789	361	10.5
Netherlands	1960	1350	142	8.7
United Kingdom	1399	1171	153	6.7
United States	3915	1780	603	13.0

SOURCE: Adapted from (World Health Organization, 2000) and (Commission on Macro-economics and Health Working Group 3, 2002)

yes—although not from personal or corporate income taxes that in Africa have limited tax bases, but from excises, and truly general sales taxes.

Sales taxes (including value-added taxes) can raise substantial sums and increasing their rates, as long as the rise is not draconian, can raise revenues. Excises on gasoline that are relatively easy to levy at point-of-entry or refinery have a significant potential for increasing yields. Much the same is true for taxes on tobacco and alcohol. If governments were committed to increasing the health budget, money could be found; for example, from increased excises or from a rate increase of a truly general sales tax, from improved administration, or from a combination of all three. Using sales taxes to increase revenue will always be criticized on the grounds that it is inequitable. Equity is difficult to achieve using sales taxes, but equity may be better addressed through the spending side of the budget. For example, money raised from a general sales tax and spent on the poor suffering from malaria will almost certainly improve equity.

Traditionally, developing countries have relied on import duties for much of their revenue. The worldwide thrust, through the World Trade Organisation, to lower tariffs means that countries cannot rely on import duties as a way to increase revenue in the future and such taxes are not a desirable base on which to increase social expenditures. Nevertheless, increasing taxes is a sensitive issue in every country.

User Fees

User fees have the potential to provide extra revenue for many government-provided goods and services. The arguments against user fees for health services are well recognized, however, and apply to treating episodes of malaria. Wealth and income are so unequally distributed that charging fees for health care is regressive, and restricts access to medical services, often leading to inappropriate treatment or no treatment at all. This is particularly so in the cases of a catastrophic illness such as malaria. Although a household may have been able to cover the costs of an occasional minor illness, the sudden onset of a life-threatening disease may stretch family finances past the breaking point or, indeed, come at a time when no money is available at all. Charging fees at such a time is unlikely to improve the allocation of resources.

It is true that fees can play a useful role if they derive directly from the locality in which they are collected, and if they are used for locally provided services, for example, the supplementation of nurses' and doctors' wages. Fees have proved successful in some Indian States, but only where procedures exempt the very poorest from having to pay. Fees play a relatively small part in overall contributions to health costs, and the increased costs of new drugs to combat malaria would not seem the desirable peg on which to hang an initiative to expand the use of user fees while at the same time ensuring widespread access to improved treatments.

Other Strategies

Insurance programs, other types of taxes (e.g., carbon taxes, "Tobin taxes" related to currency conversion), and such things as lotteries also are potential sources of revenue for governments, but they are not promising as ways to raise monies that could consistently and reliably fund ACT subsidies.

External Funds Directed toward a Global Subsidy

Most African countries are unlikely to be able to contribute large amounts directly to a global antimalarial subsidy, but they should be able to mobilize external resources to contribute to such a subsidy. This report does not attempt to prescribe how much countries should contribute either directly or through external sources, but it does recognize that such contributions will have to make up some portion of the total.

The Potential for Contributions from
Endemic Countries Outside of Africa

An initial feature of the proposed global antimalarial subsidy is that ACTs be available at subsidized prices to all legitimate consumers. We have discussed the limited resources likely to flow directly from African countries in support of a subsidy. We recognize that Asian countries with endemic malaria will be the other major block of consumers, although the total amount of ACTs needed in Asia is much less than is needed in Africa. Many of the Asian malaria-endemic countries (e.g., Vietnam, Laos, Cambodia, India) are low-income countries, but some (Thailand, China) are among the lower middle-income group. To the extent that the subsidy benefits those in the greatest need, it might be appropriate for governments of the better-off recipient nations to contribute enough to the overall subsidy to offset flows into their countries through both public and private sectors. This arrangement would have the following advantages over not offering subsidized antimalarials to these countries: 1) it would maintain low prices in both the public and private sector for end-users, many of whom are extremely poor, even in somewhat richer countries, and would find unsubsidized prices prohibitive; 2) lower-priced ACTs would undercut monotherapies (which would be cheaper if ACTs were not subsidized); and 3) it would reduce the potential for illegal importation of lower-priced ACTs from other countries.

This report does not prescribe how much countries would be expected to contribute, or the administrative details of how transfers would occur.

The Potential for Greater External Financing to Subsidize ACTs

As a general principle, it seems likely that few, if any, African countries will be able to raise a significant share of the incremental resources required, especially during the first few years of ACT introduction and use. The implication is that endemic countries' development partners are likely to be called upon to play a central role in mobilizing the required resources. These resources represent an important investment in better health in Africa, but also constitute, from the standpoint of those responsible for public budgets, an incremental recurrent expenditure. For this reason alone, a continuing process of national and global costing, and financial planning and monitoring is needed for ACTs, and other new antimalarial therapies.

This is not a revelation, but a fact accepted by the major institutions that are already playing a role, and will play an increasing role, in paying for ACTs—namely, the World Bank, the Global Fund, USAID, and other national aid agencies. Identifying where the funds will be found, and how they will be administered pose major challenges, however; these questions have been the subject of some dissensus within the international community. A related question, also controversial, is whether the funds can be time-limited to just a few years, after which countries would be expected to absorb most of the cost.

The first question is where additional funds totaling US$300-500 million per year (within 2 to 3 years) can be raised. Where the funds come from also dictates, to varying degrees, how they can be used. Potential sources of additional money for antimalarial drugs are the World Bank, and its asso-

---

BOX 3-2
World Bank Instruments and Their Potential for Use in Financing Antimalarial Drugs

Traditionally, the World Bank financed malaria control programs through specific projects, or malaria components of health projects. Today, funds from such projects represent only one-fifth and one-quarter, respectively, of funds estimated currently, and potentially to be available annually from the World Bank for financing of antimalarial drugs. Other World Bank instruments that could be used include:

• *Poverty Reduction Support Loans and Credits (PRSCs).*This instrument provides nonearmarked budget support for countries' poverty reduction strategies. The Uganda PRSC process, to give an example extending over several financial operations, provides a framework for measuring policy and institutional reforms in all service sectors, including health, and a number of cross-cutting areas, such as public procurement. The two PRSCs approved in Uganda each involved commitments of US$150 million (Elmendorf, 2003). A portion of these funds could be available for the purchase of ACTs, which can be promoted by health stakeholders within the domestic PRSC dialogue.

• *Structural Adjustment Loans and Structural Adjustment Credits (SALs and SACs).* SALs and SACs provide quick-disbursing assistance to countries to support structural reforms in one sector or the economy as a whole. They were originally intended to support macroeconomic policy reforms, but have evolved to focus more on structural, financial sector, and social policy reforms, such as establishing social protection funds. Funds are disbursed when the borrower complies with specific release conditions (usually that they not spend money on prohibited items, e.g., military and luxury items) (World Bank, 2001). The fourth structural

---

ciated institutions, the Global Fund, and individual governments. An issue that arises with all of these sources is whether funding can be pooled in some way into the "global subsidy" outlined earlier in this chapter given the usual practice of country-specific funding, discussed below.

Country-Specific versus Global Funding

The World Bank and Affiliated Institutions

Aid and lending institutions have a variety of instruments for transferring funds to recipients (Box 3-2). By and large, funding is specific to countries, most often (but not always) flowing through the governments for use in prescribed ways. African countries are increasingly organizing their externally funded health projects on the basis of a "sector-wide approach" (SWAp) (Cassels, 1997; Peters and Chao, 1998) rather than a series of

adjustment credit (US$50 million) in Guinea, for example, was used to increase accountability and efficiency in public resource use through administrative improvements (World Bank, 2002b). The Bank introduced Higher Impact Adjustment Lending in Africa in 1995, focusing on countries deemed most likely to use it effectively, and reducing conditions by about one-half (World Bank Operations Evaluation Department, 1999).

• *Adaptable Program Loans and Credits (APLs)*. APLs provide phased support, over as long as a decade, to development programs at the sectoral level. They involve a series of loans, contingent on continued progress. The Guinea Population and Reproductive Health Program, e.g., has three phases. The first phase is to set frameworks and processes, and carry out activities including advocacy and health promotion campaigns, and quality assurance. If this is done successfully (based on agreed criteria), the second phase will be triggered, with a goal of reducing high-risk pregnancies by 30 percent, and achieving a national contraceptive prevalence rate of 16 percent. Continued success will trigger the third phase (World Bank, 2002b).

• *Emergency Recovery Loans and Credits*. These are used to support the restoration and reconstruction of economic, social, and physical systems after an extraordinary event such as war, civil disturbance, or natural disaster. The operations may include fast-disbursing components that finance imports needed for effective recovery. The Emergency Multisector Rehabilitation and Reconstruction Project in Democratic Republic of Congo, e.g., committed more than US$450 million from the Bank against total program costs estimated at US$1.7 billion. Health services accounted for an estimated US$154 million, with IDA financing of US$49 million planned. Contracting from UN agencies and prequalified NGOs has been agreed to for medical equipment and supplies for this LICUS country operation (World Bank, 2002a).

specific projects. The SWAp leads countries toward a sector strategy and expenditure program, and away from specific projects for which funds are earmarked. The SWAp is actually a method of organizing relationships between recipients and their donor partners. A memorandum of understanding between the Ministry of Health and its development partners is a common feature, as is a movement toward "basket funding," placing donor funds into a common account to be used by the government to achieve specific goals.[2]

---

[2]The Ghana SWAp is one of the most advanced such arrangements. The World Bank has recently committed US$90 million in IDA Credit and grants in its second support for the SWAp process in Ghana. Under the Tanzania SWAp, a target of reducing the malaria inpatient case fatality rate for children under 5 from 12.8 percent (1997) to 8 percent (2011) has been included among indicators to measure progress. The government of Tanzania allocated US$10 million in IDA SWAp funds for malaria in 2003.

The Global Fund

The Global Fund supports projects within countries through grants for specific activities to control AIDS, tuberculosis, and malaria. Grants may include components for one, two, or all three diseases. One of the key principles of Global Fund grant making is that the funds are not fungible—they may not reduce or replace other sources of funding for the stated diseases or for health in general, but must *add* to the overall amount being spent. In fact, the Global Fund encourages countries to use the grants to leverage still greater funding from other sources. While another principle of Global Fund grants is that the work they support should "evolve from national plans and priorities," and build upon poverty-reduction strategies and SWAps, Global Fund grants lack the fungibility that is a characteristic of those approaches (Global Fund to Fight AIDS, 2003).

The Global Fund has developed a mode of operating that works through "Country Coordinating Mechanisms," which operate at the country level, interacting with the government and other partners in funded projects. Thus far, no grants have been made (or funds otherwise disbursed) for multicountry or global projects, although this would not necessarily be prohibited. It also is the case that money coming into the Global Fund from donors is not conditioned on donor-specified requirements for spending it, e.g., on particular countries (or excluding particular countries), or in specific ways. The allocation among diseases and countries is a matter for the Global Fund, its board, and its advisors to determine. Support of a global subsidy for antimalarial drugs would be consistent with the goals of the Global Fund, even if the type of funding mechanism required does not exist at present.

Bilateral Aid Agencies

The U.S. Agency for International Development (USAID) and its counterparts in other countries also are potential contributors to a global antimalarial drug fund. They currently fund projects and development on a country-specific basis, and contribute to many multilateral programs (e.g., WHO, UNICEF, the Global Fund).

Potential Sources and Amounts of External Funding for an Antimalarial Drug Subsidy

Development cooperation in Africa is characterized by a wide range of financial modalities, terms, and sources (Dollar et al., 2001). Funds can flow from donors through central banks and finance ministries to sectoral departments such as health, which in turn contract with suppliers; or there may be direct financial linkages between donors and suppliers. Large international NGOs often receive funds directly from bilateral donors, especially USAID, and have semiautonomous programs in individual countries, especially those in the LICUS (Low Income Countries Under Stress Initiative) category. Financial terms, too, vary greatly. Bilateral donors and the European Union largely provide grants to African countries. The World Bank and the African Development Bank provide long-term concessional loans through affiliates created for this purpose, the International Development Association (IDA), and the African Development Fund.

Over the past several years, IDA has begun to introduce grants in five categories: 1) HIV/AIDS, 2) natural disaster reconstruction, 3) poorest countries, 4) poorest and debt-vulnerable countries, and 5) post-conflict countries. These grants represent about 20 percent of IDA funds, and more than half of the grants are in the social sectors, including 3-4 percent for HIV/AIDS projects (International Development Association, 2003b).

The introduction of a pilot program of US$450 million per year in FY04-FY05 for regional integration projects to be supported by IDA, and a set-aside of up to 10 percent in the African Development Bank, represents a strong recognition of the positive externalities of regional projects (International Development Association, 2003a). In this connection it should be noted that, to assist countries in nonaccrual status (where the Bank does not extend new financing as a matter of policy), IDA management plans to make IDA grant financing available for regional HIV/AIDS projects through a regional organization, or another country participating in the project (International Development Association, 2003b). These arrangements suggest a certain flexibility that might be exploited for antimalarial drugs.

Beyond the international financial institutions, bilateral donors—including Austria, Belgium, Canada, Denmark, Finland, France, Germany, Ireland, Italy, Japan, the Netherlands, Norway, Sweden, Switzerland, the United Kingdom, and the United States—could conceivably support a global subsidy for antimalarial drugs. Finally, there are the agencies of the United Nations (such as WHO, UNICEF, and the Office of the UN High Commissioner for Refugees), the Global Fund, and the larger foundations, such as the Gates Foundation.

Estimating the amount of funding currently being provided for malaria control (or specifically, antimalarial drugs), much less what *might* be available for subsidies, poses formidable challenges. Systematic tracking of donor expenditures on malaria programs is incomplete. Where data are available, accounting definitions vary, so comparisons are difficult. One recent effort estimated the international aid for malaria control at US$100 million annually, and argued that the sums dedicated to malaria had remained essentially unchanged since the advent of Roll Back Malaria (Narasimhan and Attaran, 2003). The external evaluation of the Roll Back Malaria partnership completed in 2002 estimated external donor disbursements for malaria at US$125 million in 2002 (Feachem, 2002). A separate estimate prepared for the RBM partnership indicates that approximately US$200 million worldwide was earmarked from international and domestic resources for malaria control in 2002 (WHO/UNICEF, 2003).

The IOM Committee commissioned an examination of funds that could potentially be made available for antimalarial drugs from the large international lenders and donors, by Elmendorf and Finn (Elmendorf and Finn, 2003). Where feasible, data collected from external sources were reviewed and corrected with the donor institution. However, it was not possible to obtain information from every donor, particularly European donors. To that extent, the data represent underestimates.

Elmendorf and Finn estimated that approximately US$500 million per year are currently *available*,[3] or somewhat more than US$800 million are *potentially available*[4] to support malaria programs in Africa. Approximately US$160 million per year are estimated to be currently available for financing of antimalarial drugs, and about US$300 million to be potentially available. These funds are judged to be available overall to African countries, but are not equally available to all African countries, nor do they flow from a single source. Similarly, neither the funds defined as "available" or "potentially available" are likely to all end up being spent on malaria control, and of the malaria control expenditures, only a portion will go to drugs.

The estimates of resource availabilities presented above significantly exceed earlier estimates, and the reasons for this merit exploration.

•   First, in most cases the new data do not represent disbursements or even formal financial commitments for malaria programs. As the term implies, the data only represent funds "available" for malaria control *if* recipient countries make the effort needed to access and use them.

---

[3]*Available* is defined as resources that are contractually committed under health sector projects that are expected to be used for malaria programs, plus resources contractually committed for a broader range of purposes that could be applied to malaria programs. This does not mean funds currently disbursed or "used" for malaria and other purposes, nor does this imply in the case of health sector projects that there is a contractual commitment to use the funds for malaria.

[4]*Potentially available* refers to resources that *could* be committed for malaria under health sector projects, and resources that *could* be mobilized for malaria from resources currently committed for a broader range of purposes *if* substantial, additional efforts are made within the recipient country to mobilize and allocate the resources for malaria, and, where necessary, donor institution staff support these efforts. These are resources for which there would be stiff competition among a country's many spending priorities.

- Second, in the case of the World Bank, the data take into account financial resources available to African countries not only under health sector investment projects (the basis of the previous estimates), but also under programmatic lending, structural adjustment and poverty reduction support credits, and emergency loans. For each of these categories, it has not been assumed, of course, that a full financial commitment might accrue to malaria programs. Estimates of the share that might be available for malaria have been made in consultation with the Bank staff concerned. This results in estimated funds currently and potentially available from the World Bank for purchase of antimalarials of US$40 and US$80 million per annum, respectively (see Box 3-2).
- Third, the data take into account funds available to African countries for social programs in connection with the Highly Indebted Poor Countries (HIPC) initiative for debt relief. HIPC funds currently estimated to be available for health programs in Africa on an annual basis exceed US$750 million; for malaria, HIPC resources currently and potentially available annually amount to US$190 and US$250, respectively. HIPC resources available on an annual basis for purchase of antimalarial drugs are estimated currently to be US$96 million, and potentially to be US$125 million. This, however, is the most optimistic estimate. Competition for HIPC funds among the many potential poverty-reduction uses in the social and economic sectors is strong. The likelihood of country authorities allocating this money for a high-level subsidy of the type is probably low.
- Fourth, the funds represent incremental foreign resources to a relatively minor extent. The bulk of the funds reported to be currently or potentially available already are largely under the control of African governments.

It is impossible to estimate how much of the "available" or "potentially available" international funding could be used to support an antimalarial subsidy of the type proposed in this report. Further investigation is needed to determine exactly what next steps are necessary for this to take place. The international finance institutions are, however, a likely source of some significant portion of the requisite funding.

CONCLUSION

Rationale for the Subsidy

The need for the widespread introduction of ACTs is immediate, but there also are immediate obstacles that must be addressed for this to happen. Some are technical—for example, the global capacity to produce artemisinin compounds is currently quite limited, and the processes for making the desired ACTs (i.e., coformulations) are only now being finalized. There are no technical barriers to ramping up production of artemisinins using current technologies (and there is a real possibility of improving yields through better technology (Personal communication, W. Haddad, February 2004). There is every reason to trust that production will increase to meet demand, once the manufacturers know that there is an expanded market for their products and they have mastered the necessary coformulation processes. The demand for the raw material at that point will stimulate agricultural production through standard market forces.

The main piece still missing is getting ACTs from manufacturers to consumers, most of whom will not be able to afford the free-market price (either current or expected, when prices fall). This chapter has laid out the rationale for a "global" subsidy that would be applied very high up in the distribution chain—supranationally—probably through the procurement organization (see chapter 4), or a financial organization affiliated with it. The choice is between using the current pathways for antimalarial distribution—flawed as they are—and accepting some level of misuse, or controlling the introduction of ACTs so that a large proportion of what is provided is used appropriately but, as a result, reaches a minority of the people who need them.

The main reasons for a supranational (as opposed to national) approach are:

• To ensure that ACTs can flow easily into both the public and private sector supply chains with the least disruption of current distribution patterns
• To ensure access in every malaria-endemic country—rather than only those able to act quickly to organize sufficient external funding to pay for them—and internal supply systems to deliver them to the widest possible number of consumers
• To minimize the attractiveness of artemisinin (or other) monotherapies, by having ACTs underprice them

This approach involves tradeoffs: targeted subsidies that allow greater control of the final destination of drugs means that those who do receive and use them correctly would get the greatest possible benefit. Global subsidies, on the other hand, mean that drugs will be wasted and misused. However, a drawback that the targeted subsidy would create (particularly if ACTs reach mainly the public and/or NGO sectors) is that monotherapies (including artemisinins) would undoubtedly dominate the private sector where, unsubsidized, they will be cheaper than ACTs and equally effective, at least initially. From past experience with other drugs, it is likely that monotherapies purchased through the private sector will be taken in partial doses by many people, further compromising the effectiveness of artemisinins.

With a global subsidy of ACTs, monotherapies could be limited in two ways: first, their unsubsidized price would be higher than that of ACTs, so the market itself would work against them. And second, the world's manufacturers of ACTs—who also would be the manufacturers of artemisinin monotherapies—would be dissuaded from producing artemisinin monotherapies in order to benefit from the global ACT subsidy. In this way, the subsidy produces a positive externality: the protection of artemisinins (and other currently effective antimalarials) from the early development of drug-resistant malaria by essentially eliminating the use of artemisinin, and at least some other monotherapies. Countries should, of course, also use their legal authority to control the inappropriate use of monotherapies through complete or partial bans of ACT components, but the degree of control is likely to vary considerably. Regulation alone cannot be expected to succeed in this (recall the availability of many unregistered antimalarials in the examples of drug flows presented in Chapter 1). There also is a need to maintain some monotherapy use in first-line treatment and prevention. There is gathering evidence that artesunate suppositories could save children with severe malaria (which should be treated with an ACT once the child is stable), if readily available for use in the home, as well as in clinics. SP still is needed for intermittent preventive therapy by pregnant women (although in some areas, its effectiveness may be so eroded that it is no longer effective). SP is not, however, recommended as a partner drug in ACTs.

The locus of concern tends toward the high-transmission areas of Africa, where the human toll is so high, but it should be remembered that widespread availability of ACTs in low-transmission areas (in parts of Asia and Latin America, as well as some parts of Africa), together with effective vector control will reduce, and could eliminate malaria, providing sustained economic and humanitarian benefit. More resources could then be concentrated on the more difficult, higher transmission areas.

Changing the status quo toward more rational drug use also is a pressing goal, and one that should be pursued actively through many channels, as recommended in this report. Tying a requirement for dramatic changes in malaria treatment to a subsidy for ACTs does not, however, appear to be a feasible approach in the short term.

Level of Funding Required

We estimate that an annual subsidy of US$300-500 million will be needed to support affordable prices for all ACT consumers. This report does not attempt to apportion the cost of the subsidy among contributors.

It does point out that funds that could be used for ACTs are available from the variety of sources that routinely support health projects. Much of the funding potentially available would be attached to specific countries. Ways to use at least some of that funding as part of a global subsidy would have to be explored.

The issue of sustainability of funding for the subsidy also must be addressed. On the positive side, we can expect the global cost of ACTs to decrease, as economies of scale are reached, and expected technical improvements in the manufacturing process are made. And with very wide access to ACTs, the malaria problem may begin to shrink, further reducing the global price of treating malaria. Those economies notwithstanding, it may be unrealistic to assume that the endemic countries and their populations will, within a few years, be able to afford these drugs any more than they can now. This suggests that the global community should anticipate an ongoing, but declining, need for external funds for this purpose.

Potential Sources of Funding

The prospects are poor for greatly increased funding for antimalarial drugs from existing budgets of endemic countries in sub-Saharan Africa. At the same time, one of the potential objections to a global subsidy is that international development funds will benefit every country with malaria, including some with more robust economies, where the government might be able to afford a larger contribution to a subsidy for its own population. Although there are no high-income countries with substantial malaria problems, some middle-income countries would fall into this group. In general, their burdens (and therefore, demand for antimalarials) are substantially lower than those of sub-Saharan Africa, so their benefit from a subsidy would be proportionately less. Nonetheless, wealthier endemic countries could be approached to contribute directly to the global subsidy fund, amounts bearing some relation to the volume of ACTs likely to be sold in the country at subsidized prices. Data on actual consumption gathered once the subsidy is in place could be used to make adjustments.

There are substantial amounts of money in various streams from the international financing institutions that could be diverted to a global subsidy for antimalarial drugs. It would remain the task of the stewards of the subsidy finances (either the procurement organization or a separate financial entity) to negotiate with the funding institutions and with individual countries to determine the mechanisms through which funds could flow to a central point.

REFERENCES

Cassels A. 1997. *A Guide to Sector-Wide Approaches for Health Development: Concepts, Issues, and Working Arrangements.* Geneva: World Health Organization.

Commission on Macroeconomics and Health Working Group 3. 2002. *Mobilization of Domestic Resources for Health.* Geneva: World Health Organization.

Derriennic Y, Mensah B. 2003. *Financing of Artemisinin-Based Combination Antimalarial Drug Treatment.* Technical Report 023. Bethesda, MD: Abt Associates Inc.

Dollar D, Devarajan S, Holmgren T. 2001. *Aid and Reform in Africa* Washington, DC: World Bank.

Elmendorf AE. 2003. World Bank Policies and Practices and the Financing of Malaria Control Activities and Commodities. Paper commissioned by the Institute of Medicine, Washington, DC.

Elmendorf AE, Finn K. 2003. Estimated external financing of antimalarial drugs in sub-Saharan Africa. Paper commissioned by the Institute of Medicine, Washington, DC.

Feachem R. 2002. *Final Report of the External Evaluation of Roll Back Malaria.* Liverpool: Malaria Consortium.

Global Fund to Fight AIDS, Tuberculosis and Malaria. 2003. *Annual Report 2002/2003.* Geneva: The Global Fund.

Goodman C, Kachur SP, Abdulla S, Bloland P, Mills A. 2004. Investigating competition and regulation in the retail market for malaria treatment in rural Tanzania. Presentation to the Second International Conference on Improving Use of Medicines, Chiang Mai, Thailand, March 30-April 2, 2004.

International Development Association. 2003a. *Allocating IDA Funds Based on Performance.* Washington, DC: International Development Association.

International Development Association. 2003b. *IDA's Commitments, Disbursements and Funding in FY03.* Washington, DC: International Development Association.

Narasimhan V, Attaran A. 2003. Roll Back Malaria? The scarcity of international aid for malaria control. *Malaria Journal* 2(1):8.

Peters D, Chao S. 1998. The sector-wide approach in health: What is it? Where is it leading? *International Journal of Health Planning and Management* 13(2):177-190.

WHO. 2000. *World Health Report 2000.* Geneva: World Health Organization.

WHO/UNICEF. 2003. *The Africa Malaria Report 2003.* Geneva: World Health Organization.

World Bank. 2001. *World Bank Lending Instruments: Resources for Development Impact.* Washington, DC: World Bank.

World Bank. 2002a. *Appendixes to the Technical Annex for a Proposed Credit in the Amount of SDR 358.8 Million to the Democratic Republic of Congo for an Emergency Multisector Rehabilitation and Reconstruction Project. World Bank Report T7551.* Washington, DC: World Bank.

World Bank. 2002b. *Implementation Completion Report on a Credit to the Republic of Guinea for a Fourth Structural Adjustment Credit.* Washington, DC: World Bank.

World Bank Operations Evaluation Department. 1999. *Higher Impact Adjustment Lending (HIAL): Initial Evaluation.* Washington, DC: World Bank.

Worrall E, Wiseman V, Hanson K. 2003. Targeting of subsidies for insecticide treated mosquito nets (ITNs): A conceptual framework, experience from other sectors and lessons for ITNs. HEFP Working Paper 02/03. London School of Hygiene and Tropical Medicine.

4

An International System for Procuring Antimalarial Drugs

INTRODUCTION

No special systems exist internationally to assist either the public or private sectors in procuring antimalarial drugs. Governments generally purchase antimalarials through formal procedures in which companies submit bids according to government specifications. Successful bids are chosen on the basis of various criteria including price, quality, and delivery. Governments also exercise regulatory authority over which drugs are registered for sale in a given country, including aspects of labeling and dispensing (e.g., with or without prescription). The private sector is, of course, required to abide by the laws and regulations, but its operations are independent; private vendors typically import drugs through wholesalers according to perceived demand. How well government dictates are followed in the private sector varies among countries.

In the case of artemisinin combination therapies (ACTs), a more centralized procurement system becomes increasingly attractive—particularly if a large international subsidy is part of the equation. Centralized procurement is not a new idea. UNICEF (United Nations Children's Fund) has been procuring childhood vaccines and other drugs for decades, most recently in collaboration with the Global Alliance for Vaccines and Immunization (GAVI). There is a new "TB Global Drug Facility" with a similar role for procuring drugs that constitute the international standard in tuberculosis treatment. The World Health Organization (WHO) has recently proposed similar entities for malaria and HIV/AIDS. Centralized procurement does not usurp the role of national governments, which retain responsibility over national drug policy and regulatory matters. Centralized procurement will only be effective if countries view it as facilitating their national malaria goals and objectives.

In September 2003, the IOM Committee on the Economics of Antimalarial Drugs cosponsored a meeting with the World Bank and the Roll Back Malaria Partnership to discuss the financing and procurement of ACTs. This chapter is based in large part on discussions that took place at that meeting, and the resulting meeting report (World Bank/Institute of Medicine, 2004).

The chapter discusses the pros and cons of different levels of international procurement of ACTs, and some possible institutional arrangements. For now, the hypothetical organization discussed would only procure ACTs; however, in the future, it also could procure second- and third-generation combination antimalarial treatments. The need for some form of centralized, coordinated procurement is widely acknowledged and relatively uncontroversial. The open questions are these: where should the agency be located? Does it require the creation of a new entity, or can it operate within an existing organization? To what degree should it also manage the international subsidy as opposed to partnering with another group that performs that function? The biggest challenge for an ACT procurement group will be to solidly liaise with the private retail sector in endemic countries. This report strongly endorses the principle of procurement at a high level in the distribution chain (possibly at the level of purchase from manufacturers), but it does not take a position on how it should be organized or administered.

THE BASICS OF DRUG PROCUREMENT

Tasks of Centralized Procurement Organizations

Supranational centralized procurement is attractive because it allows countries to participate in and benefit from a more focused and efficient effort than any single country could individually mount. Even if their drug policies differ, all malarious countries face common challenges. Every country with endemic falciparum malaria will need at least one ACT as first-line treatment for uncomplicated cases. The number of available ACTs in the short-to-medium term will probably number half a dozen, produced by 10-20 manufacturers capable of delivering ACTs of acceptable quality. Therefore, an international procurement organization would likely be charged with the following tasks in greater or lesser degrees of collaboration with governments and WHO, depending on the task:

- Forecasting demand
- Negotiating good prices
- Maintaining healthy competition in the ACT market
- Facilitating wholesale and retail distribution
- Minimizing production of artemisinin (and other) monotherapies
- Assuring quality
- Stimulating the market
- Providing technical assistance
- Conducting monitoring and evaluation
- Handling intellectual property rights issues

Forecasting Demand

There is widespread agreement that accurate forecasts of demand are essential to the success of procurement operations. Agreement is equally widespread that accurately forecasting the demand for antimalarials is nearly impossible. The current figure generally believed to represent worldwide antimalarial demand is 300-500 million adult-equivalent courses of treatment per year. Since funds to subsidize the world's needs are not likely to reach sufficient levels for several years and production scale-up also is just beginning, the best that can be done now is to ratchet up funding and production over several years. Within 5 years, the ability to forecast demand should be greatly improved, however, at which time the procurement organization will have forged relations with major producers, and individual countries will have collected data on the volume of ACTs entering their respective countries and will be in a better position to project demand.

Good Prices and Healthy Competition

There are no firm rules for judging "good" prices, or "healthy" competition, but UNICEF provides some guidance based on their long experience in vaccine procurement (Box 4-1). One key point is the need for multiple suppliers. Furthermore, a single rock-bottom price is not necessarily the best long-term strategy. In the case of ACTs, different prices for different formulations are likely, but there also could be a range of acceptable prices for a given formulation.

One price-lowering option that will not apply to ACTs is tiered pricing because the market for these drugs in high-income countries will be negligible (discussed in Chapter 3).

Facilitating Wholesale and Retail Distribution

The organization should have the capacity to deliver the desired level of subsidy through public, nongovernmental organization (NGO), and private

---

BOX 4-1
UNICEF Principles for Vaccine Procurement

- UNICEF believes that a **healthy industry is vital** to ensure uninterrupted and sustainable supply of vaccines.
- UNICEF believes in **procurement from multiple suppliers** for each vaccine presentation.
- UNICEF believes in procurement from manufacturers in **developing countries**, and **industrialized countries.**
- UNICEF believes in paying a **price that is affordable** to Governments and Donors, and a price that **reasonably covers manufacturers' minimum requirements.**
- UNICEF believes that we should provide manufacturers with **accurate and long-term forecasts**; UNICEF believes that manufactures should provide UNICEF with **accurate and long-term production plans.**
- UNICEF believes that as a public buyer, providing grants to manufacturers is not the most effective method of obtaining capacity increases.
- UNICEF believes that option to quote tiered pricing should be given to manufacturers—in accordance with the World Bank classification of Low, Middle, and High Income countries.

SOURCE: UNICEF, 2003.

---

retail distribution channels. A major challenge will be to assure access and appropriate use of antimalarials purchased through the many facets of the retail private sector. Regardless of how well other systems work, failure of this sector means that the majority of treatment seekers will not obtain effective drugs for themselves and their children.

Minimizing Production of Artemisinin Monotherapy

With its buying power, the procurement organization should be able to prevent producers from manufacturing and selling artemisinin monotherapies, or monotherapies of non-artemisinin partner drugs. In other words, the procurement agency should have the authority to disqualify ACT producers from benefiting from the subsidy if they engage in these activities. The organization also should set guidelines for keeping monotherapies off the market in participating countries. Even without the suasion that buying power brings, if subsidized ACTs become widely available, the economic incentive to produce monotherapies should dry up.

Quality Assurance

Assisting with quality assurance through its prequalification program is one of WHO's strengths. The prequalification requirements for artemisinins and ACTs have been established, but thus far, only one (Coartem) has been prequalified. Several manufacturers of other artemisinin products have applied, but none had passed as of June 2004. WHO is working with these companies (all of them generic manufacturers, mainly in Asia) and there is an expectation that several will become prequalified soon. A persistent problem has been the lack of a standard monograph for the artemisinins, a result of their nonstandard history of development. The product monograph—which usually is assembled by an originator company for a new drug —is important because it specifies quality standards for manufacture, and tests used to verify quality. The companies that have already begun manufacturing and selling artemisinin monotherapies and coformulations in Asia have done so without the benefit of a monograph. WHO has assumed responsibility for developing the monograph, but has not yet completed it (as of June 2004).

Market Stimulation

The establishment of a procurement organization will signal to producers that a market exists, but only if the organization can marshal sufficient funding in the near term. Some participants at the World Bank/RBM/IOM meeting in September 2003 suggested that a minimum of US$10-30 million per year would be needed for the next 3 to 5 years, enough to purchase roughly 10-30 million adult-equivalent courses of treatment. The IOM committee believes this "pump-priming" figure is far below long-run needs, however, which are reflected in the much larger subsidy (US$300-500 million per year) recommended in this report.

In addition to an assured purchase fund, the organization will require funds to organize outreach to current and potential producers of ACTs in order to provide them with information about acceptable products, the WHO prequalification process (including the possibility of technical assistance), the procurement process itself, and the anticipated timetable for purchases.

Technical Assistance

Technical assistance by the procurement organization should cover a wide range of activities to assist both producers and consumers. Assistance may be direct or brokered by the organization (e.g., funding a consultant to visit a plant that needs help with quality control). Countries may require assistance with such tasks as identifying lead ACTs for first-line treatment, product registration and labeling, training regulators and field workers, and setting up monitoring and evaluation systems, to name just a few. Producers also may need help with technical aspects of production, or bidding processes.

Sustainable funding must be identified to provide the technical assistance needed, with or without a cost recovery mechanism.

Monitoring and Evaluation

The organization will need to evaluate its own performance. In addition, it should set standards for countries procuring products through it to determine how well they are meeting the needs of the population, and monitoring antimalarial resistance. The agency should cultivate a strong sense of accountability toward the private sector and its clients.

Intellectual Property Issues

Intellectual property issues for ACTs currently under development should be minor, if they surface at all. The procurement organization must follow the development of new-generation antimalarials, however, which may come with more complex intellectual property backgrounds.

Other Desirable Characteristics of a Procurement Organization for ACTs

ACTs currently have a short shelf-life roughly estimated at 2 years. Therefore, one practical consideration for a procurement agency will be organizing the direct delivery of ACTs from producer to customer with as little delay as possible. This precludes the procurement agency from physically warehousing ACTs and shipping them. Instead, it must devise mechanisms for tracking and accounting for the products as they move without being physically involved in the transfers.

In the beginning, it would be ideal if ACT procurement could be managed by an established organization with sufficient capacity and experience to launch the process whether or not a new institution is later created. UNICEF, for one, could fill the interim role and possibly maintain the program into the future. Another possibility, once functional, is the developing malaria facility being organized under WHO auspices, or yet another new or existing organization. The IOM Committee has taken no position on the specific entity that would be best able to fill this role.

In the early years, a procurement organization also should have guaranteed purchasing power and assume some financial risk for contracts with suppliers. This mirrors UNICEF's role in vaccine procurement. In the case of ACTs, the risk should be small, particularly during early years when demand will greatly outpace supply.

If a global subsidy at the supranational level is implemented, the procurement organization (or a closely allied fiscal entity) should receive funds and be empowered to interact not only with governments but all sectors. We are aware that this approach does not reflect current health development financing, which is largely public-sector oriented (although it sometimes includes NGOs). The procurement organization and its partners (e.g., WHO, The Global Fund) would need to work with major donors to develop ways for donors to contribute to a global subsidy targeted at public and private sectors within the strictures of their organizations.

Degrees of Centralization of Procurement Organizations

The choice between internationally centralized and fully decentralized procurement by individual countries is not a simple dichotomy. A spectrum of possibilities exists, from minimal coordination through full bulk purchasing. Five operating scenarios are described below:

- *Informed buying:* Purchasers share information on prices and suppliers, but purchase individually.
- *Coordinated informed buying:* Purchasers conduct joint market research, share supplier information, and monitor prices but purchase individually.
- *Group contracting:* Purchasers jointly select suppliers and negotiate prices, agreeing to purchase from the selected suppliers. Purchases can be made individually or jointly.
- *Central contracting and purchasing:* Purchasers jointly tender and contract through a global procurement agent.
- *Pooled procurement:* A central organization negotiates and purchases from suppliers, and distributes drugs to next level purchasers.

Participants at the joint meeting in September 2003 (World Bank/Roll Back Malaria/IOM) agreed that efficient procurement of ACTs would require an operation toward the bottom of the list, with far more centralized functions than information sharing.

Examples of Higher Level Procurement Strategies

The GDF

The WHO Global Drug Facility (GDF) for TB drug supply bundles global pooled procurement with pooled financing and includes a network of partners who provide technical assistance to support drug grants. Procurement is one component of four in the GDF framework (Table 4-1). TB drugs are purchased on behalf of countries from a contractual partner of

TABLE 4-1 The Four Functions of the GDF

1. Grant-making to countries and other qualifying recipients.

2. Application review, monitoring, and evaluation, including a monitoring and evaluation process after the grant.

3. Procurement through a contractual partner of the GDF, with shipment to the country's port of entry.

4. Partner mobilization, for technical support in the application process, conducting monitoring and evaluation, and helping with in-country drug management.

SOURCE: World Health Organization (http://www.who.int/gtb/publications/gdf/gdf_factsheets.htm).

the GDF and shipped to countries. At the country level, customs, port clearance, warehousing, and distribution are still handled through the country's own systems. A recent evaluation of the GDF listed three outstanding achievements of the facility (McKinsey and Company, 2003):

1. Expanded access to high-quality TB drugs
2. Facilitation of expanded levels of directly observed treatment (DOTS)
3. System-level benefits resulting in reduced drug prices

The evaluation notes that the combined approach of pooled financing and commodity procurement has been key for the GDF to meet its goals, particularly in providing incentives for countries to adopt the DOTS strategy and to rationalize the choice of drugs used for treatment. The key to stimulating scaled-up drug production was the ability of the GDF to forecast demand.

Coordinated Informed Buying of HIV/AIDS Drugs

A recent example of pooled procurement is found in Management Sciences for Health's (MSH) collaboration with the Rockefeller Foundation and key African institutions on the design of a program for Coordinated Informed Buying of HIV/AIDS-related drugs in programs of regional pooled procurement under the auspices of ACAME (an association of francophone West African countries' central medical stores) and CRHCS (East and Southern Africa Commonwealth Regional Health Community Secretariat). The program will expand beyond HIV/AIDS drugs to a wider selection of drugs on countries' Essential Drugs Lists if the initial experience with HIV/AIDS drugs proves successful. MSH has argued for pooling procurement at the regional level rather than globally, on grounds that this will result in greater ownership by countries and lower levels of requisite political commitment.

Bulk Procurement by UNICEF

UNICEF's Supply Division in Copenhagen has several years of experience in fully centralized purchasing of vaccines under the umbrella of GAVI. UNICEF's program involves both virtual and physical warehousing of commodities, as distinct from pooling of individual orders from countries. UNICEF also is a key partner in the GDF. Like the GDF, UNICEF staff have found demand forecasting the single greatest challenge influencing the success of their efforts in vaccine procurement. Approximately 25 percent of their effort is taken up in forecasting activities.

PROPOSED MALARIA MEDICINES AND SUPPLIES SERVICE

As this study neared completion, in December 2003, the Roll Back Malaria (RBM) partnership issued a "Draft Concept Document" to establish a "Malaria Medicines and Supplies Service" (MMSS) within RBM (WHO, 2003). This, and a companion proposal for HIV/AIDS-related commodities, both modeled on the Global TB Drug Facility, are the initiatives of the new WHO Secretary General, Dr. J.W. Lee.

The RBM draft concept document is not a finished proposal but a starting point for broad consultation to begin honing the plan. This section, therefore, outlines the main characteristics described in the draft with the understanding that it is a living document that may well change before this IOM report is in print.

Characteristics of the Proposed MMSS

The stated purpose of the MMSS is to "facilitate and expand access to high-quality treatment of malaria and preventive measures by improving the supply of medicines and other essential supplies." The products covered will be ACTs and other drugs, diagnostics, and insecticide-treated nets. The functions envisioned fall into three categories:

- Global information products
- Technical tools and assistance to countries and others at all stages of the supply cycle
- Facilitating the procurement of the named products

The procurement function goes as far toward centralization as pooled procurement, but does not mention outright bulk procurement. As described, the MMSS would be responsive to "qualifying national malaria control programs, NGOs, and other private-sector organizations."

The MMSS is proposed as a time-limited endeavor that will phase itself out as capacity is developed in endemic countries to assume the procurement (and other) responsibilities.

Consistency with IOM Recommendations

The MMSS as currently described in the draft document would meet some of the goals of this report's recommendations and could evolve in such a way that it would meet all of them. One obvious difference is that the MMSS is described as a time-limited organization. It is not clear that the need for this function will diminish in the foreseeable future. If working well, it could be a permanent, efficient mechanism for antimalarial procurement.

Another key issue that still must be addressed is the mechanism for injecting a global ACT subsidy into the system in a way that will influence the private retail sector. If this element is not factored into the plan, a number of problems are likely to arise—the biggest one being an inability to discourage the sale and use of monotherapies. The widespread availability of monotherapies would in turn threaten to curtail the useful lifespan of ACTs.

REFERENCES

McKinsey and Company. 2003. *Evaluation of the Global TB Drug Facility*. Geneva: Stop TB Partnership, World Health Organization.

UNICEF. 2003. Overview of UNICEF immunization procurement, 2003. Presentation at World Bank/IOM/RBM meeting, Expert Consultation on the Procurement and Financing of Antimalarial Drugs, September 15-16, 2003.

WHO. 2003. *Proposal for a Malaria Medicines and Supply Service*. Unpublished.

World Bank/Institute of Medicine. 2004. *Expert Consultation on the Procurement and Financing of Antimalarial Drugs, September 15-16, 2003, Washington, DC*. Washington, DC: World Bank.

PART 2

Malaria Basics

5

A Brief History of Malaria

MALARIA'S GLOBAL SAGA

Malaria occupies a unique place in the annals of history. Over millennia, its victims have included Neolithic dwellers, early Chinese and Greeks, princes and paupers. In the 20th century alone, malaria claimed between 150 million and 300 million lives, accounting for 2 to 5 percent of all deaths (Carter and Mendis, 2002). Although its chief sufferers today are the poor of sub-Saharan Africa, Asia, the Amazon basin, and other tropical regions, 40 percent of the world's population still lives in areas where malaria is transmitted.

Ancient writings and artifacts testify to malaria's long reign. Clay tablets with cuneiform script from Mesopotamia mention deadly periodic fevers suggestive of malaria. Malaria antigen was recently detected in Egyptian remains dating from 3200 and 1304 BC (Miller et al., 1994). Indian writings of the Vedic period (1500 to 800 BC) called malaria the "king of diseases." In 270 BC, the Chinese medical canon known as the *Nei Chin* linked tertian (every third day) and quartan (every fourth day) fevers with enlargement of the spleen (a common finding in malaria), and blamed malaria's headaches, chills, and fevers on three demons—one carrying a hammer, another a pail of water, and the third a stove (Bruce-Chwatt, 1988). The Greek poet Homer (circa 750 BC) mentions malaria in *The Iliad*, as does Aristophanes (445-385 BC) in *The Wasps*, and Aristotle (384-322 BC), Plato (428-347 BC), and Sophocles (496-406 BC). Like Homer, Hippocrates (450-370 BC) linked the appearance of Sirius the dog star (in late summer and autumn) with malarial fever and misery (Sherman, 1998).

Malaria's probable arrival in Rome in the first century AD was a turning point in European history. From the African rain forest, the disease most likely traveled down the Nile to the Mediterranean, then spread east to the Fertile Crescent, and north to Greece. Greek traders and colonists brought it to Italy. From there, Roman soldiers and merchants would ultimately carry it as far north as England and Denmark (Karlen, 1995).

For the next 2,000 years, wherever Europe harbored crowded settlements and standing water, malaria flourished, rendering people seasonally ill, and chronically weak and apathetic. Many historians speculate that falciparum malaria (the deadliest form of malaria species in humans) contributed to the fall of Rome. The malaria epidemic of 79 AD devastated the fertile, marshy croplands surrounding the city, causing local farmers to abandon their fields and villages. As late as the 19th century, travelers to these same areas remarked on the feebleness of the population, their squalid life and miserable agriculture (Cartwright, 1991). The Roman Campagna would remain sparsely settled until finally cleared of malaria in the late 1930s.

In India and China, population growth drove people into semitropical southern zones that favored malaria. India's oldest settled region was the relatively dry Indus valley to the north. Migrants to the hot, wet Ganges valley to the south were disproportionately plagued by malaria, and other mosquito- and water-borne diseases. Millions of peasants who left the Yellow River for hot and humid rice paddies bordering the Yangtse encountered similar hazards. Due to the unequal burden of disease, for centuries, the development of China's south lagged behind its north.

Although some scientists speculate that vivax malaria may have accompanied the earliest New World immigrants who arrived via the Bering Strait, there are no records of malaria in the Americas before European explorers, conquistadores, and colonists carried *Plasmodium malariae*, and *P. vivax* as microscopic cargo (Sherman, 1998). Falciparum malaria was subsequently imported to the New World by African slaves initially protected by age-old genetic defenses (sickle cell anemia, and G6PD deficiency) plus partial immunity gained through lifelong exposure. Their descendants, as well as Native Americans and settlers of European ancestry, were more vulnerable, however. Deforestation and "wet" agriculture such as rice farming facilitated breeding of *Anopheles* mosquitoes. By 1750, both vivax and falciparum malaria were common from the tropics of Latin America to the Mississippi valley to New England.

Malaria, both epidemic and endemic, continued to plague the United States until the early 20th century. It struck presidents from Washington to Lincoln, weakened Civil War soldiers by the hundreds of thousands (in 1862, Washington, D.C., and its surroundings were so malarious that General McClellan's Army en route to Yorktown was stopped in its tracks), traveled to California with the Gold Rush, and claimed Native American lives across the continent. Until the Tennessee Valley Authority brought hydroelectric power and modernization to the rural South in the 1930s, malaria drained the physical and economic health of the entire region. Just as the United States was eradicating its last indigenous pockets of infection, malaria reclaimed Americans' attention during World War II. During the early days of the Pacific campaign, more soldiers fell to malaria than to enemy forces. The United States' premier public health agency—the Centers for Disease Control and Prevention—was founded because of malaria. By the time of the Vietnam War, the American military discovered that drug-resistant malaria was already widespread in Southeast Asia, a harbinger of the worldwide hazard it was destined to become.

But nowhere—past or present—has malaria exacted a greater toll than on Africa. A powerful defensive pathogen, it was a leading obstacle to Africa's colonization. Portuguese traders who entered the African coastal plain in the late 1400s and early 1500s were the first foreigners to confront the killing fever. For the next 3 centuries, whenever European powers tried to establish outposts on the continent, they were repelled time and again by malaria, yellow fever, and other tropical scourges. By the 18th century, the dark specter of disease earned West and central Africa the famous epitaph, "the White Man's Grave."

Even stronger testimony to malaria's ancient hold on Africa is the selective survival of hemoglobin S—the cause of the inherited hemoglobin disorder sickle cell anemia. Since individuals who inherit two copies of the hemoglobin S gene (one from each parent) are unlikely to survive and reproduce, the disease should be exceedingly rare. However, in those people who have inherited only one sickle cell gene (such individuals are sickle cell "carriers"—they suffer few if any complications of sickle cell disease), needle-shaped clumps of hemoglobin S within red blood cells confer strong protection against malaria (Bayoumi, 1987). Thus, the sickle cell gene is perpetuated in malarious regions by one set of individuals who reap its benefits while another set pays the price. In some parts of Africa, up to 20 percent of the population carry a single copy of the abnormal gene (Marsh, 2002).

In recent years, by virtue of climate, ecology, and poverty, sub-Saharan Africa has been home to 80 to 90 percent of the world's malaria cases and deaths, although some predict that resurgent malaria in southern Asia is already altering that proportion.

Discovering the Malaria Parasite

Charles Louis Alphonse Laveran (1845-1922) was a French army doctor during the Franco-Prussian War. He later authored a treatise on military medicine. In it he challenged the traditional wisdom regarding malaria's ecology—namely, that the disease was restricted to low-lying humid plains. Laveran noted that malaria also could occur in temperate zones, and that not all tropical areas were plagued by the disease. Although malaria had been linked with swamps ever since the condition known as Roman fever inspired the name *mal'aria* ("bad air"), Laveran knew from contemporary scientific articles that many diseases previously ascribed to miasmas, or evil vapors, were in fact caused by microbes. Thus he predicted: "Swamp fevers are due to a germ" (Jarcho, 1984).

After transferring to a new post on Algeria's North African coast, Laveran investigated his theory. On October 20, 1880, while looking through a crude microscope at the blood of a febrile soldier, he saw crescent-shaped bodies that were nearly transparent except for one small dot of pigment. In preceding decades the brownish-black pigment hemozoin (now known to be the product of hemoglobin digestion by the malaria parasite) had been found in cadaveric spleens and blood of malaria victims by several investigators including Meckel, Virchow, and Frerichs. Laveran subsequently examined blood specimens from 192 malaria patients and saw pigment-containing crescents in 148 sufferers (Laveran, 1978). He ultimately recognized four distinct forms in human blood that would prove to be the malaria parasite in different stages of its life cycle: the female and male gametocyte, schizont and trophozoite stages.

Although his findings were initially viewed with skepticism, 6 years later, Laveran was affirmed. Camillo Golgi (1843-1926) linked the rupture and release of asexual malaria parasites from blood schizonts with the onset of every third- and fourth-day fever due to *P. vivax* and *P. malariae*, respectively. Golgi was awarded the Nobel Prize in 1906 for unrelated studies of the central nervous system. One year later, Laveran received the Nobel Prize for discovering the single-celled protozoan that caused malaria.

Discovering Malaria's Mosquito Stages

August 20, 1897, is the original "Mosquito Day"—so named by Surgeon-Major Ronald Ross (1857-1932) of the British Indian Medical Service. Although Ross had previously spent more than a year fruitlessly studying gray and brindled mosquitoes (probably *Culex fatigans* and *Aedes aegypti*, respectively) incapable of hosting malaria, on that date he discovered a clear, circular body containing malarial pigment in a dapple-winged *Anopheles* mosquito that had previously fed on an infected patient. The next day the doctor-cum-poet/composer/mathematician, who struggled to pass his own medical exams, dissected another *Anopheles* mosquito that had siphoned blood from the same patient on the same day. This time Ross observed even larger pigment-containing bodies. Convinced that malaria parasites were growing in the mosquito, he published his observations ("On some peculiar pigmented cells found in two mosquitoes fed on malarial blood") in the *British Medical Journal* in December 1897.

After transferring to Calcutta, Ross designed experiments involving *Plasmodium relictum*, the malaria parasite of sparrows and crows. Ross identified sporozoites in the salivary glands of mosquitoes that had previously fed on malarious birds. He subsequently infected 21 of 28 fresh sparrows through these mosquitoes (Sherman, 1998). He communicated all of his findings to Patrick Manson who shared them at a meeting of the British Medical Association at the University of Edinburgh in July 1898 (Harrison, 1978). In 1902, Ross received the Nobel Prize for discovering the mosquito stages of malaria.

Ross was not the only investigator who demonstrated the malaria life cycle in the mosquito, however. Credit for confirming that human malaria parasites pass through the same developmental stages in the mosquito as the avian parasites observed by Ross belongs to a group of Italian scientists—in particular, Giovanni Battista Grassi (1854-1925), Amico Bignami, Giovanni Bastianelli, Antonio Dionisi, and Angelo Celli. Following Ross's publication, Grassi (an expert in mosquito taxonomy) not only identified *Anopheles maculipennis* as the vector of human disease in the marshy Roman Campagna, but transmitted the malaria parasite *Plasmodium vivax* to a healthy human volunteer. Because each claimed credit for discovering malaria's life cycle in the mosquito, Grassi and Ross were bitter toward each other for the remainder of their careers.

Parenthetically, Ronald Ross owed much of his success to his teacher and mentor Sir Patrick Manson, considered by many the father of tropical medicine. While working in Amoy and Formosa, Manson was the first researcher to discover that mosquitoes siphon first-stage microfilariae from the bloodstreams of patients with the parasitic disease, filariasis. However, Manson never imagined the final step in the filarial life cycle; namely, that infected mosquitoes might inoculate third-stage filaria larvae back into humans through a subsequent bite. It was left to his protégé Ross to discover that parasites can travel two ways through the proboscis of a mosquito.

Discovering the Parasite in Human Tissue

The third piece of the human malaria puzzle—where sporozoites inoculated by mosquitoes undergo early development in the human host—was solved in 1948. Although previous researchers had found that bird malaria initially reproduced in tissues of the lymph system and the bone marrow, the sanctuary for primate and human malaria outside of red blood cells remained a mystery. Then H. E. Shortt, P. C. C. Garnham, and colleagues

at the Ross Institute of the London School of Hygiene and Tropical Medicine detected malaria parasites in the livers of rhesus monkeys infected with
a primate malaria species. They subsequently found similar stages in liver
biopsy specimens from human volunteers experimentally infected with *P.
vivax*, and confirmed the same early sanctuary for *P. falciparum* (Garnham,
1966).

MILESTONES IN ANTIMALARIAL DRUG
DISCOVERY AND DRUG RESISTANCE

Quinine

*"The Peruvian bark of which the Jesuites powder is made, is
an excellent thing against all sorts of Agues,"*
–William Slamon, Synopsis medicinae (1671)

The pharmaceutical compound known as quinine comes from the bitter bark of a high altitude tree native to South America. As legend has it, the
Spanish Countess of Chinchon was treated with the tree's bark in Peru in
the 1600s. For many years, she was credited with bringing the bark—
variously known as "Jesuit's powder," "Cardinal's powder," or "Peruvian
bark"—back to Spain. However, since she later died in Peru, it is far more
likely that Cardinal Juan de Lugo or another Jesuit priest introduced the
remedy to Europe. In 1742, Linnaeus named the tree *cinchona* after the
Countess, accidentally omitting the first "h" in her name (Meshnick, 1998).

In 1820, the French chemists Joseph Pelletier and Jean Biename
Caventou isolated quinine from cinchona bark. Quinine quickly became a
favored therapy for intermittent fever throughout the world. In the mid-
19th century, British and Dutch botanical explorers combed the Andean
cloud forest for cinchona in order to establish plantations in India, Ceylon,
and the Dutch East Indies. However, many transplants produced only low-
yield quinine crops. Eventually, for a few guilders, the Dutch government
purchased 14 pounds of cinchona seed collected by Charles Ledger, an
Englishman living in Peru. By grafting what was eventually named *C.
ledgeriana* onto the hardier *C. succirubra* (McHale, 1986), the Dutch soon
dominated cinchona cultivation, eventually producing 80 percent of the
world's quinine on the Indonesian island of Java before it was invaded
during World War II.

Quinine remains an important and effective malaria treatment nearly
worldwide to the present day, despite sporadic observations of quinine
resistance. The earliest anecdotal reports of resistance date to 1844 and
1910 (Talisuna et al., 2004). Quinine resistance in *P. falciparum* was first
documented in human volunteers in Brazil and in Southeast Asia in the

1960s (Peters, 1970). Loss of quinine sensitivity and treatment failures became more common in Southeast Asia in the 1980s (Bjorkman and Phillips-Howard, 1990), although, to this day, high-level quinine resistance has not yet been convincingly documented (Personal communication, N. White, Mahidol University, March 2004).

Chloroquine

Because the Allies controlled Java and its valuable quinine stores during World War I, German troops in East Africa suffered heavy casualties from malaria. Determined never to lack for malaria drugs again, the German government commissioned a search for a quinine substitute following Armistice. The center of operations was I.G. Farben, part of the Bayer Dye Works. Farben chemists tested thousands of compounds until they found some that worked. The first promising agent was Plasmochin (pamaquine) in 1926, followed, in 1932, by Atabrine (quinacrine, mepacrine). Plasmochin, an eight-amino quinoline, was quickly abandoned due to toxicity, although its close structural analog primaquine is now used to treat latent liver parasites of *P. vivax* and *P. ovale*. Atabrine was in many ways superior, persisting in the blood for at least a week. However, it too had unacceptable side effects, including yellowing of the skin and, occasionally, psychotic reactions.

The breakthrough came in 1934 with the synthesis of Resochin (chloroquine), followed by Sontochin (3 methyl chloroquine). These compounds belonged to a new class of antimalarials known as four-amino quinolines. Although Farben scientists overestimated the compounds' toxicity and failed to explore them further, ironically, they passed the formula for Resochin to Winthrop Stearns, Farben's U.S. sister company, in the late 1930s. Resochin was then forgotten until the outbreak of World War II, when Allied forces were cut off from quinine—first by the German invasion of Holland, then by the Japanese occupation of Java. After French soldiers raided a supply of German-manufactured Sontochin in Tunis and handed it over to the Americans, Winthrop researchers made slight adjustments to the captured drug to enhance its efficacy. They called their new formulation chloroquine. Only after comparing chloroquine to the older and supposedly toxic Resochin did they realize that the two chemical compounds were identical (Honigsbaum, 2002).

Although the synthesis of chloroquine came too late to help malaria sufferers in the Pacific theater or Sicily (another malaria-ridden front), following World War II, chloroquine and DDT emerged as the two principal weapons in the WHO's ambitious "global eradication" malaria campaign. Subsequently, chloroquine-resistant *P. falciparum* (CRPF) probably arose de novo from four independent geographic locations: the Thai-

Cambodian border around 1957 (Harinasuta et al., 1965); Venezuela and the nearby Magdalena Valley of Colombia around 1960 (Moore and Lanier, 1961); and Port Moresby, Papua New Guinea, in the mid-1970s (Grimmond et al., 1976). In Africa, CRPF was first found in 1978 in nonimmune travelers to Kenya and Tanzania (Lobel et al., 1985), spreading next to inland coastal areas and by 1983, to Sudan, Uganda, Zambia, and Malawi (Talisuna et al., 2004). Current evidence suggests that CRPF strains seen in Africa originated in Asia.

Sulfadoxine-Pyrimethamine

The pyrimidine derivative, proguanil, was another drug that emerged from the antimalarial pipeline during World War II. Proguanil's success in treating humans (Curd et al., 1945) stimulated further study of its pharmaceutical class (agents that block folate synthesis in parasites and bacteria), and the development of pyrimethamine (Falco et al., 1951). However, as both monotherapies came into common use, it became apparent that malaria parasites could quickly alter the target enzyme of the two drugs, leading to resistance. Resistance to proguanil, for example, was observed within a year of introduction in Malaya in 1947 (Peters, 1987).

Sulfones and sulfonamides (drugs which act on another enzyme which helps the malaria parasite synthesize folic acid) were then combined with proguanil or pyrimethamine in the hopes of increasing efficacy, and forestalling or preventing the development of resistance (Cowman, 1998). *P. falciparum* strains resistant to pyrimethamine, and cross-resistant to proguanil and related compounds emerged in 1953 in Muheza, Tanzania; eight years later, these strains constituted 40 percent of *P. falciparum* isolates in a 15-mile radius (Clyde, 1966). Sulfadoxine-pyrimethamine (SP), today the most widely used antifolate antimalarial combination, was introduced in Thailand in 1967. Resistance to SP was first reported in Thailand later that year (Wernsdorfer and Payne, 1991). Although parasite resistance to SP spread quickly throughout Southeast Asia, it remained low in Africa until 5 or 6 years ago. Since then it has rapidly spread throughout Africa as well.

Mefloquine

The development of mefloquine was a collaborative achievement of the U.S. Army Medical Research and Development Command, the World Health Organization (WHO/TDR), and Hoffman-La Roche, Inc. After World War II, about 120 compounds were produced at the Walter Reed Army Institute of Research (WRAIR) in an attempt to find replacements for quinine. Preclinical trials coincided with the appearance of chloroquine-resistant falciparum malaria in areas of American military concern in Southeast Asia, and South America. Ultimately, WRAIR developed WR142490 (mefloquine), a 4-quinoline methanol. Mefloquine's efficacy in preventing falciparum malaria when taken regularly was first reported in 1974 (Rieckmann et al., 1974). Soon after, it also was shown to be a successful treatment agent (Trenholme et al., 1975). Clinical evidence of parasites resistant to mefloquine began to appear in Asia around the time of the drug's general availability in 1985 (Hoffman et al., 1985).

Artemisinin

To reduce fever, "take a handful of sweet wormwood, soak it in a sheng of water, squeeze out the juice and drink it all."
(Ge Hang, AD 340)

Artemisinin is the antimalarial principle isolated by Chinese scientists in 1972 from *Artemisia annua* (sweet wormwood), better known to Chinese herbalists for more than 2000 years as *qing-hao* (Klayman, 1985). Like other members of the family to which it is related (sagebrush, tarragon, absinthe), qing-hao is noted for its aromatic bitterness. The earliest report of its use appears in a Chinese book found in the Mawanhgolui Han dynasty tombs dating to 168 BC, where it was mentioned as a treatment for hemorrhoids. In Zhon Hon Bei ji Jang *(Handbook of Prescriptions for Emergency Treatments)* written by Ge Hang in 340 AD, it was recommended as treatment for chills and fevers (Trigg, 1990). Modern Chinese scientists found that an ethyl ether extract of qing-hao fed to mice infected with the lethal rodent malaria strain, *Plasmodium berghei*, was as effective as chloroquine and quinine at clearing the parasite (Honigsbaum, 2002). Soon after, Mao Tse Tung's scientists began testing qing-hao in humans, publishing their findings in the *Chinese Medical Journal* in 1979.

From a historical perspective, there are several remarkable features to the story of qing-hao's "rediscovery" as a potent antimalarial: 1) the structure of the drug was unlike any other known biological compound at the time; 2) within a few short years Chinese scientists had studied its antimalarial activity from test tube to patient, identified its active structure, then synthesized more active derivatives; and 3) the entire antimalarial drug discovery program resulted from an initial appeal for help from Ho Chi Minh to Zhou En Lai during the Vietnam War.

Today, artemisinin and other artemether-group drugs are the main line of defense against drug-resistant malaria in many areas of southeast Asia. To date, there have been no reported cases of stable, clinically relevant genetic resistance to artemisinin, although tolerance can be produced through repeated in vitro culture of parasites in the presence of the drug (Meshnick, 2002).

REFERENCES

Bayoumi RA. 1987. The sickle-cell trait modifies the intensity and specificity of the immune response against *P. falciparum* malaria and leads to acquired protective immunity. *Medical Hypotheses* 22(3):287-298.

Bjorkman A, Phillips-Howard PA. 1990. The epidemiology of drug-resistant malaria. *Transactions of the Royal Society of Tropical Medicine and Hygiene* 84(2):177-180.

Bruce-Chwatt LJ. 1988. History of malaria from prehistory to eradication. In: Wernsdorfer W, McGregor I, eds. *Malaria: Principles and Practice of Microbiology.* 1st ed. Edinburgh, United Kingdom: Churchill Livingstone.

Carter R, Mendis KN. 2002. Evolutionary and historical aspects of the burden of malaria. *Clinical Microbiology Reviews* 15(4):564-594.

Cartwright F. 1991. *Disease and History.* New York: Dorset Press.

Clyde DF. 1966. Drug resistance of malaria parasites in Tanzania. *East African Medical Journal* 43(10):405-408.

Cowman AF. 1998. The molecular basis of resistance to sulfones, sulfonamides, and dihydrofolate reductase inhibitors. In: Sherman IW, ed. *Malaria: Parasite Biology, Pathogenesis and Protection.* Washington, DC: American Society of Microbiology.

Curd FHS, Davey DG, Rose FL. 1945. Studies on synthetic antimalarial drugs: Some biguanide derivatives as new types of antimalarial substances with both therapeutic and causal prophylactic activity. *Annals of Tropical Medicine and Parasitology* 29:208-216.

Falco EA, Goodwin LG, Hitchings GH, Rollo IM, Russell PB. 1951. 2:4-diaminopyrimidines—a new series of antimalarials. *British Journal of Pharmacology* 6(2):185-200.

Garnham PCC. 1966. *Malaria Parasites and Other Haemosporidia.* Oxford: Blackwell Scientific.

Grimmond TR, Donovan KO, Riley ID. 1976. Chloroquine resistant malaria in Papua New Guinea. *Papua New Guinea Medical Journal* 19(3):184-185.

Harinasuta T, Suntharasamai P, Viravan C. 1965. Chloroquine-resistant falciparum malaria in Thailand. *Lancet* 7414(2):657-660.

Harrison, G. 1978. *Mosquitoes, Malaria and Man: A History of the Hostilities Since 1880.* New York: Dutton.

Hoffman SL, Rustama D, Dimpudus AJ, Punjabi NH, Campbell JR, Oetomo HS, Marwoto HA, Harun S, Sukri N, Heizmann P. 1985. RII and RIII type resistance of *Plasmodium falciparum* to combination of mefloquine and sulfadoxine/pyrimethamine in Indonesia. *Lancet* 2(8463):1039-1040.

Honigsbaum, M. 2002. *The Fever Trail—In Search of the Cure for Malaria.* New York: Farrar Straux and Giroux.

Jarcho S. 1984. Laveran's discovery in the retrospect of a century. *Bulletin of the History of Medicine* 58(2):215-224.

Karlen A. 1995. *Man and Microbes: Disease and Plagues in History and Modern Times.* New York: G.P. Putnam.

Klayman DL. 1985. Qinghaosu (artemisinin): An antimalarial drug from China. *Science* 228(4703):1049-1055.

Laveran CLA. 1978. A newly discovered parasite in the blood of patients suffering from malaria. Parasitic etiology of attacks of malaria. 1880. Translated from the French and reprinted in: Kean BH, Mott KE, Russell AJ, eds. *Tropical Medicine and Parasitology. Classic Investigations.* Vol. 1. 1st ed. Ithaca, New York: Cornell University Press.

Lobel HO, Campbell CC, Schwartz IK, Roberts JM. 1985. Recent trends in the importation of malaria caused by *Plasmodium falciparum* into the United States from Africa. *Journal of Infectious Diseases* 152(3):613-617.

Marsh K. 2002. Immunology of malaria. In: Warrell DA, Gilles HM, eds. *Essential Malariology*. 4th ed. New York: Arnold Press.

McHale D. 1986. The cinchona tree. *Biologist* 33:45-53.

Meshnick S. 1998. From quinine to qinghaosu. In: Sherman IW, ed. *Parasite Biology, Pathogenesis and Protection*. Washington, DC: ASM.

Meshnick SR. 2002. Artemisinin: Mechanisms of action, resistance and toxicity. *International Journal for Parasitology* 32(13):1655-1660.

Miller RL, Ikram S, Armelagos GJ, Walker R, Harer WB, Shiff CJ, Baggett D, Carrigan M, Maret SM. 1994. Diagnosis of *Plasmodium falciparum* infections in mummies using the rapid manual ParaSight-F test. *Transactions of the Royal Society of Tropical Medicine and Hygiene* 88(1):31-32.

Moore DV, Lanier JE. 1961. Observations on two *Plasmodium falciparum* infections with an abnormal response to chloroquine. *American Journal of Tropical Medicine and Hygiene* 10:5-9.

Peters W. 1970. *Chemotherapy and Drug Resistance in Malaria, 1st ed.* London: Academic Press.

Peters W. 1987. *Chemotherapy and Drug Resistance in Malaria, 2nd ed.* London: Academic Press.

Rieckmann KH, Trenholme GM, Williams RL, Carson PE, Frischer H, Desjardins RE. 1974. Prophylactic activity of mefloquine hydrochloride (WR 142490) in drug-resistant malaria. *Bulletin of the World Health Organization* 51(4):375-377.

Sherman IW. 1998. A brief history of malaria and discovery of the parasite's life cycle. In: Sherman IW, ed. *Malaria: Parasite Biology, Pathogenesis and Protection*. Washington, DC: ASM.

Talisuna AO, Bloland P, D'Alessandro U. 2004. History, dynamics, and public health importance of malaria parasite resistance. *Clinical Microbiology Reviews* 17:235-254.

Trenholme CM, Williams RL, Desjardins RE, Frischer H, Carson PE, Rieckmann KH, Canfield CJ. 1975. Mefloquine (WR 142,490) in the treatment of human malaria. *Science* 190(4216):792-794.

Trigg PI. 1990. Quinhaosu (artemisinin) as an antimalarial drug. *Econconomic and Medicinal Plant Research* 3:20-25.

Wernsdorfer WH, Payne D. 1991. The dynamics of drug resistance in *Plasmodium falciparum*. *Pharmacology and Therapeutics* 50(1):95-121.

6

The Parasite, the Mosquito, and the Disease

THE MALARIA PARASITE AND ITS LIFE CYCLE

An Ancient Parasite Shared by Many Vertebrates

Malaria is caused by plasmodia—ancient, single-celled protozoans transmitted to humans by the bites of female *Anopheles* mosquitoes. Plasmodia parasites have complex life cycles involving vertebrate and insect hosts (Figure 6-1). In addition to the four plasmodial species that infect humans, roughly 120 additional species infect various animals from reptiles to birds to higher apes. None of these animal parasites (except, very rarely, certain monkey strains) can be transmitted to humans, however. This degree of host specificity suggests a long association between humans and the four malaria species that infect them.

Four *Plasmodium* Species Cause Human Malaria

The four malaria species that produce human disease are *Plasmodium vivax* (also called tertian malaria), *P. falciparum* (also called malignant tertian malaria), *P. malariae* (also called quartan malaria), and *P. ovale*. *Plasmodium vivax*, which is prevalent in temperate as well as tropical and subtropical zones, has the widest geographical range because it can survive at lower temperatures within a mosquito than the other three parasites that infect humans. *Plasmodium falciparum*, the most lethal strain, is the most prevalent species throughout the tropics and subtropics. *Plasmodium*

136

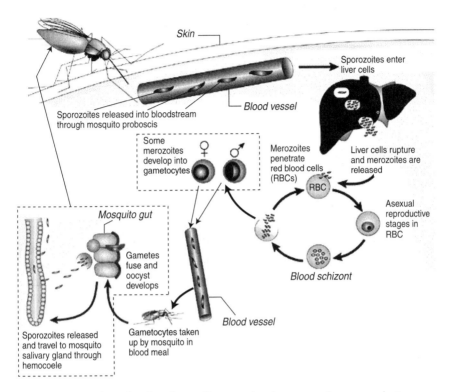

FIGURE 6-1 Life cycle of a *Plasmodium* species that causes human malaria.

malariae is patchily present over the same range as *P. falciparum*. *Plasmodium ovale* is found in tropical Africa, and occasionally in Asia and the western Pacific.

Biologic and Genetic Diversity

One of the remarkable features of human plasmodia is their biology, which allows these small yet genetically complex microbes to survive and exploit several different environments: the liver and blood cells of humans as well as the gut, vascular system, and salivary glands of mosquitoes. With the advent of molecular tools such as polymerase chain reaction (PCR), an understanding of the genetic diversity of plasmodial parasites (in particular *P. falciparum*) has emerged. It is now known that many infected patients from falciparum-endemic areas harbor parasites belonging to more than one genotype. Some carry as many as 10 genotypes detectable by currently available methods (Greenwood, 2002).

The Journey of a Single Malaria Parasite from Mosquito to Human

After mating, female anopheline mosquitoes require blood meals before each egg-laying. Human malaria begins when a female anopheline inoculates malaria acquired from a previous human blood meal. While probing for a capillary with her mouthpiece (basically, a pair of needle-like tubes), the infected female injects thread-like forms called *sporozoites* from her salivary glands. Although sporozoites in the salivary glands of wild-caught mosquitoes usually number around 1,000, only 8 to 10 sporozoites on average are transferred in a single mosquito bite. Nonetheless, even one sporozoite is capable of initiating a malaria infection.

Within 30 to 60 minutes upon entering the human bloodstream, sporozoites migrate through the venous circulation to the liver. Before invading individual liver cells, they attach to cell receptors via a surface molecule known as a circumsporozoite protein. Over the next 5 to 25 days (the length of time depends on the particular malaria species), the sporozoite reproduces by asexual binary fission. Ultimately, each sporozoite generates 10,000 to 30,000 descendants contained within a cyst-like structure called a *liver schizont*. During this developmental period the patient remains symptom-free.

Once the liver schizont ruptures, parasites flood out of the organ and invade circulating red blood cells (RBCs). The process of attachment and entry takes no longer than 30 seconds. Inside RBCs, the parasites derive energy from hemoglobin siphoned from the host cell. Using this metabolic fuel, the invading parasites grow and transform from delicate rings to larger amoeboid forms called trophozoites to a multinucleate *blood schizont* stage containing 8 to 24 daughter parasites.

Mature blood schizonts of *P. falciparum* sequester deep within the venous microvasculature where, unlike ring-stages, they generally are undetectable on routine blood smears. This sequestration of RBCs containing mature stages of *P. falciparum* in the microvasculature of vital organs is the core pathological process in severe falciparum malaria. The organ distribution of sequestration determines the clinical syndrome (Pongponratn et al., 2003). For example, if sufficient numbers of *P. falciparum* schizonts attach to blood vessels in the brain, cerebral malaria can result (Adams et al., 2002), while in the placenta, adherent schizonts may reduce fetal blood supply and thus contribute to impaired fetal growth (Scherf et al., 2001). When the blood schizont finally ruptures, the next generation of parasites is released into the human bloodstream. Each of these parasites then enters a new RBC and continues the cycle of bloodstream infection.

The Release of Bloodstream Parasites Triggers Symptoms and Amplifies Infection

In a nonimmune patient, the release of parasites from blood schizonts triggers recurring attacks of fever, sweats, and chills. The periodicity (every 48 hours in *P. vivax* infection; every 72 hours in *P. malariae* infection) reflects the time needed for a single cycle of intra-erythrocytic growth and development for the respective species. Although *P. falciparum* also has a 48-hour growth cycle, its paroxysms are less predictable because the rupture of blood schizonts occurs in nonsynchronized waves.

With each replicative cycle, the parasite load increases. In the case of *P. falciparum* infection, for example—assuming no host immune factors hold parasite growth in check—the total body parasite load increases roughly 8- to 10-fold every 48 hours. In a child, this rapid replication can yield a lethal parasite burden within a few parasite life cycles.

Sexual-Stage Parasites Perpetuate Malaria in the Mosquito

Certain malaria parasites contained within human RBCs also develop into male and female sexual forms known as *gametocytes*. Although gametocytes do not multiply or cause illness in the human, they perpetuate malaria in mosquitoes. Once siphoned from human blood by a female anopheline, male and female gametocytes produce a mature, fertilized oocyst in the insect midgut over 7 to 10 days. The oocyst then releases sporozoites, which penetrate many body sites, including the mosquito's salivary glands. Assuming she lives long enough to feed again, with her next blood meal, the infected mosquito inoculates salivary sporozoites into a new human host, thus completing the *Plasmodium* life cycle.

Chronically Infected Humans and Malaria Transmission

In order to sustain malaria transmission, new female anophelines must be continuously infected. This requires a human reservoir containing abundant circulating gametocytes. Persons with recently acquired infections have mainly asexual parasites in their blood. However, chronically infected individuals who can tolerate ongoing bloodstream infection with malaria have many gametocytes. The relative contribution of such individuals to overall malaria transmission compared with less immune patients (typically children) in endemic areas has not been determined.

Other Routes of Malaria Infection

Rarely, malaria is acquired through non-mosquito-borne transmission. Infection can follow transfusion of malaria-tainted blood products as well as exposure to RBC-contaminated tissues (such as bone marrow) and transplanted organs. Malaria parasites can also pass through the placental barrier, sometimes leading to congenital infection in newborns.

Recurrent Malaria: Relapse versus Recrudescence

In the absence of reinfection, malaria that recurs following treatment falls into two categories: relapse and recrudescence. Malaria *relapse* is seen exclusively in *P. vivax* and *P. ovale*, and represents a reseeding of the bloodstream by dormant parasites (called *hypnozoites*) contained in the liver. *Plasmodium falciparum* and *P. malariae* do not produce hypnozoites. The recurrence of malaria in these species, conversely, reflects the proliferation of surviving blood-stage parasites from an earlier infection, an event called *recrudescence*.

THE *ANOPHELES* VECTOR

Only female mosquitoes of the genus *Anopheles* transmit human malaria. The genus includes roughly 400 species of *Anopheles* mosquitoes worldwide, of which 60 species are malaria vectors, and some 30 species are of major importance (Bruce-Chwatt, 1985). *Anopheles gambiae*, the principal malaria mosquito in sub-Saharan Africa, is a particularly effective malaria vector because of its strong preference for feeding on humans and its long life compared with some other anopheline species. Up to 10 percent of *A. gambiae* in certain areas of Africa carry *P. falciparum* sporozoites at a given time. A small number of such mosquitoes present a greater hazard to humans than a large number of other anopheline species (such as forest vectors) less likely to bite humans, and in whom sporozoite rates are as low as 0.1 percent.

Worldwide Distribution of Anopheline Mosquitoes and Malaria

Most anopheline mosquitoes live in tropical and subtropical regions, although some species also thrive in temperate climates and even survive the Arctic summer. As a rule, they do not breed at altitudes above 2,000-2,500 meters. Within these geographic bounds, there are many areas free of malaria, however, because transmission is highly dependent on local environmental and epidemiologic conditions.

Table 6-1 lists 12 epidemiological zones of malaria, and their principal and secondary vectors (Bruce Chwatt, 1985).

Anopheline Larval Habitats

The site chosen by mosquitoes for egg-laying and development of larvae is known as the larval habitat. Anophelines prefer relatively clean water as their larval habitat, although species vary in the amount of sun exposure, temperature, salinity, and organic content they prefer in their breeding sites.

Developmental Stages, Mating, Egg-Laying, and Adult Lifespan

The four developmental stages of an anopheline mosquito are egg, larva, pupa, and adult (or imago). Adult males copulate in flight, providing females with sufficient sperm for all subsequent egg-laying. Females need at least two blood meals for their first batch of eggs to develop, and one blood meal for each successive batch. Since egg development takes about 48 hours, blood-seeking is repeated every 2-3 nights.

Under optimal conditions, the average lifespan of an adult female anopheline is 3 weeks or longer (adult males, in contrast, usually live no more than a few days) unless external factors such as temperature, humidity, and natural enemies decrease longevity. When the mean ambient temperature exceeds 35°C, or humidity falls below 50 percent, longevity is significantly reduced, directly influencing the transmission of malaria.

Feeding and Resting Behavior

The male adult anopheline feeds on nectar, while the female adult feeds primarily upon blood. Females of most *Anopheles* species prefer warm-blooded animals, predominantly mammals. Some species prefer humans, and are termed *anthropophagic* or *anthropophilic*. Others prefer animals such as cattle, and are termed *zoophagic* or *zoophilic*. The distance over which a mosquito is attracted to its preferred blood source usually ranges between 7 and 20 meters.

The time of anopheline feeding is, almost without exception, between dusk and dawn. Some species have early peaks of biting (for instance, the Central American vector *A. albimanus*, which feeds between 1900 to 2100 hours). *Anopheles gambiae*, the leading malaria vector in Africa, can feed over a much wider period (2200 to 0600 hours). If biting precedes the local bedtime, insecticide-treated (bed) nets (ITNs) offer little protection against malaria infection.

TABLE 6-1 Twelve Epidemiological Zones of Malaria and Some of the Main and Secondary Vectors

Zone	Extension	Main Malaria Vectors	Local or Secondary Vectors
1 North American	From the Great Lakes to southern Mexico	A.(A.) freeborni A.(A.) quadrimaculatus	A.(N.) albimanus
2 Central American	Southern Mexico, the Caribbean islands, fringe of the South American coast	A.(N.) albimanus A.(N.) aquasalis A.(N.) argyritarsis A.(N.) darlingi	A.(N.) albitarsis A.(N.) allopha A.(A.) aztecus A.(A.) punctimacula
3 South American	Most of the South American continent irregularly beyond the Tropic of Capricorn	A.(N.) albimanus A.(N.) albitarsis A.(N.) aquasalis A.(N.) argyritarsis A.(N.) darlingi A.(A.) pseudopunctipennis A.(A.) punctimacula	A.(K.) bellator A.(N.) braziliensis A.(K.) cruzi A.(N.) nuñez-tovari
4 North Eurasian	Within the Palaearctic region, excluding the Mediterranean coast of Europe	A.(A.) atroparvus	A.(A.) messeae A.(A.) sacharovi A.(A.) sinensis A.(C.) pattoni
5 Mediterranean	Southern coast of Europe, north-western part of Africa, Asia Minor, and east beyond the Arab Sea	A.(A.) atroparvus A.(A.) labranchiae A.(A.) sacharovi	A.(A.) claviger A.(C.) hispaniola A.(A.) messeae A.(C.) pattoni
6 Afro-Arabian	Africa north and south of the Tropic of Cancer including central part of the Arabian peninsula	A.(C.) arabiensis A.(C.) pharoensis A.(C.) sergenti	A.(C.) hispaniola A.(C.) multicolor
7 Afro-Tropical (formerly "Ethiopian")	Southern Arabia, most of the African continent, Madagascar and the islands south and north of it	A.(C.) arabiensis A.(C.) funestus A.(C.) gambiae A.(C.) melas	A.(C.) merus A.(C.) moucheti A.(C.) nili A.(C.) pharoensis
8 Indo-Iranian	Northwest of the Persian Gulf and east of it including the Indian subcontinent	A.(C.) culicifacies A.(C.) fluviatilis A.(C.) stephensi	A.(C.) annularis A.(C.) pulcherrimus A.(A.) sacharovi A.(C.) superpictus

TABLE 6-1 Continued

Zone	Extension	Main Malaria Vectors	Local or Secondary Vectors
			A.(C.) tesselatus
9 Indo-Chinese Hills	A triangular area including the Indo-Chinese peninsula, the north-western fringe beyond the Tropic of Cancer	*A.(C.) dirus* (formerly *A. balabacensis balabacensis*) *A.(C.) fluviatilis* *A.(C.) minimus*	*A.(C.) annularis* *A.(C.) culicifacies* *A.(C.) maculatus* *A.(A.) nigerrimus*
10 Malaysian	Most of Indonesia, Malaysian peninsula Philippines and Timor	*A.(C.) aconitus* *A.(C.) balabacensis* *A.(A.) campestris* *A.(C.) dirus* *A.(A.) donaldi* *A.(C.) leucosphyrus* *A.(A.) letifer* *A.(C.) ludlowae* *A.(C.) maculatus* *A.(C.) minimus* *A.(A.) nigerrimus*	*A.(C.) philippinensis* *A.(C.) subpictus* *A.(C.) sundaicus* *A.(A.) whartoni*
11 Chinese	Largely the coast of mainland China, Korea, Taiwan, Japan	*A.(C.) pattoni* *A.(A.) sinensis*	*A.(A.) lesteri* *A.(A.)nigerrimus*
12 Australasian	Northern Australia, the island of New Guinea and the islands east of it to about 175° east of Greenwich, but excepting the malaria-free zone of the south-central Pacific	*A.(A.) bancrofti* *A.(C.) farauti* *A.(C.) punctulatus*	*A.(C.) hilli* *A.(C.) karwari* *A.(C.) koliensis* *A.(C.) subpictus*

Notes:

1. The malaria-free zone of the south-central Pacific includes New Caledonia, New Zealand, the Caroline Islands, Marianas, up to Hawaiian islands, east to Galapagos and Juan Fernandez, and rejoining the southern tip of New Zealand.

2. This table represents only a crude approximation of distribution of most important vectors of malaria.

3. Subgenera are indicated as follows: *A.* = *Anopheles; C.* = *Cellia; K* = *Kerteszia; N.* = *Nyssorhynchus.*

SOURCE: Adapted from Table 7.2 in Bruce-Chwatt, LJ. 1985. *Essential Malariology.* 2nd ed. New York: John Wiley and Sons.

After blood feeding, some female mosquitoes fly to a nearby wall or ceiling where they rest during daylight, often preferring lower sites within house interiors where the temperatures are cooler, and the humidity is higher. Such species are more suitable targets for indoor residual insecticide spraying (IRS) as a malaria control tool. Other anopheline species that seek secluded outdoor resting places are not suitable targets for IRS.

Entomologic Inoculation Rate (EIR)

A number of investigators, most notably Macdonald (Macdonald, 1952) have developed mathematical models of malaria transmission which attempt to correlate human infection with the prevalence of malaria infection in mosquitoes. The entomologic inoculation rate (EIR), an experimentally determined index, is a key input for such models. Simply put, the EIR equals the number of infectious bites per human per unit time, typically expressed per year.

Across stable endemic areas of malaria transmission in Africa, EIRs vary from one infective bite every 3 years to several infective bites every night (Hay et al., 2000). Even across distances as short as 100 meters, transmission can vary substantially.

PATHOGENICITY, IMMUNITY, AND DISEASE

Species-Specific Risk of Death and Complications

Among the four malaria parasites that infect humans, *P. falciparum* has the greatest risk of complications and death. In brief, the reasons are as follows. The *P. falciparum* merozoite can invade RBCs of all ages, potentially producing bloodstream parasitemias of 250,000/uL or higher. *Plasmodium vivax* and *P. ovale* preferentially infect only young RBCs, yielding parasitemias no higher than 50,000/uL. *Plasmodium malariae* infects only aging RBCs, resulting in parasite loads that generally are below 10,000/uL (Neva, 1977).

All malaria parasites produce anemia due to red cell breakage and other mechanisms. In addition, *P. falciparum*-parasitized RBCs (in particular blood schizonts) are *cytoadherent* to endothelial cells that line small blood vessels throughout the body. In a heavily infected host, the end-organ damage resulting from the intravascular sequestration of parasites can produce a variety of life-threatening complications, most notably involving the brain.

It has been suggested that falciparum parasite "strains" also can differ in virulence, despite the fact that no clear-cut genetic markers for virulence have yet been found in wild malaria parasites (Greenwood, 2002). Parasites causing severe malaria in Thailand, for example, have exhibited higher multiplication capacities as well as nonselective RBC invasion (Simpson et al., 1999; Chotivanich et al., 2000). On the host side of the equation, cytokines, reactive oxygen species, and nitrous oxide generated by the human immune system also contribute to disease severity in malaria (English and Newton, 2002).

The following sections focus primarily on disease due to *P. falciparum.*

Patterns of Immunity to Falciparum Malaria in Children and Adults

Although few if any individuals ever become completely immune to malaria, humans living in *P. falciparum*-endemic areas can and do develop functional immunity (McGregor, 1974). In areas of high transmission, immunity is acquired in two stages: an initial phase of clinical immunity, followed by anti-parasite immunity resulting in limited parasite numbers, replication, and burden within the human host (Schofield, 2002). In other words, functional immunity results in a progressive ability to contain malaria parasitemia.

In general, the acquisition of malaria immunity is slow, requiring numerous infective bites over time. Human and parasite genetic variability, parasite-induced immunosuppression, and other factors contribute to the final degree of protection (Mohan and Stevenson, 1998). Early in life, there is a grace period: in infants born to functionally immune mothers, transplacental antibody (maternal IgG) confers relative resistance to infection and severe clinical episodes of malaria for the first 6 months of life (Edozien et al., 1962). High levels of fetal hemoglobin also provide partial protection (Pasvol et al., 1976). Over the next few years, children exhibit enhanced susceptibility to severe and fatal malaria (Marsh, 1992). After this stage, clinical immunity—manifested as lower rates of disease despite persistent parasitemia—begins to operate, usually continuing into primary school years. This early clinical immunity is sometimes referred to as "clinical tolerance," signifying the ability to remain asymptomatic despite a relatively high number of circulating parasites.

Because individuals in malaria endemic areas rarely go more than a few months without a malaria challenge, immunity, once attained, generally persists as long as an individual remains in an area of stable transmission. This is true even in settings of low annual transmission (Mbogo et al., 1995). There is, however, a shift from severe malarial disease in children younger than 5 years toward severe disease in older age groups when entomological inoculation rates fall below 10 to 20 bites per year (Snow et al., 1997).

Loss of Immunity

The time span over which antimalarial immunity is lost probably varies from host to host. African expatriates (for example, graduate students attending European universities) lose some immunity over 2 to 3 years while remaining protected from severe disease (von Seidlein and Greenwood, 2003). Eventually, however waning immunity increases the risk of life-threatening complications. Rising cases in older-age individuals is generally the first indicator that immunity has been lost in an entire community (Carter and Mendis, 2002).

Ironically, when malaria control in a previously high-transmission area proves successful, whole populations become vulnerable to epidemic malaria. The island of Madagascar, in the Indian Ocean, is a recent example. Malaria transmission was almost completely interrupted in the highlands of Madagascar between 1949 and 1960 by a combination of IRS and mass chloroquine treatment (Hamon et al., 1963). Following reemergence, a severe epidemic of falciparum malaria began in 1986. Over the next 2 years, high death rates occurred in all age groups (Mouchet et al., 1997).

Subclinical Infections in Areas of Stable Transmission

New evidence for chronic, subpatent malaria infection in areas of stable transmission has recently come from studies employing highly sensitive polymerase chain reaction (PCR), a method which amplifies small fragments of parasite DNA present in human blood. Using PCR techniques, two-thirds of blood samples obtained from microscopically negative children from a highly endemic area of Senegal were found to harbor *P. falciparum* parasites (Bottius et al., 1996). Combining PCR and microscopic results, 90 percent of the exposed population proved chronically infected. PCR analysis also has shown that parasites of many different genotypes may circulate simultaneously in individual subjects who are clinically well (Farnert et al., 1997). In areas of seasonal transmission, such as eastern Sudan, low levels of parasitemia detectable only by PCR persisted through the dry season in a surprisingly large proportion of individuals (Roper et al., 1996).

Host Genetics and Malaria

The best known conditions which alter human susceptibility to malaria are red blood cell polymorphisms. In 1948, Haldane hypothesized that the high gene frequencies of hemoglobinopathies in malaria-endemic areas may have resulted from malaria protective effects (Haldane, 1948). This led to an equilibrium, or "balanced polymorphism," in which the homozygote disadvantage was balanced by the heterozygote advantage with respect to malaria. In particular, there is strong epidemiologic evidence that thalassemias (anemias caused by abnormalities in genes encoding hemoglobin), sickle cell hemoglobin, and glucose-6-phosphate dehydrogenase (G6PD) deficiency protect against severe falciparum malaria. Alpha thalassemias (Allen et al., 1997) and G6PD deficiency (Gilles et al., 1967; Ruwende et al., 1995) reduce the risk of death due to *P. falciparum* by about 50 percent, whereas a child with sickle cell trait in West Africa (in other words, a heterozygote) has a 90 percent reduced risk of illness and death from falciparum malaria (Gilles et al., 1967; Hill et al., 1991).

Hemoglobin C, like sickle cell hemoglobin, is another single point mutation found in West Africa. The homozygous state for hemoglobin C also confers a 90 percent protection against falciparum infection (Modiano et al., 2001). Hemoglobin E (which is mainly found in Southeast Asians) lessens the severity of acute falciparum malaria (Hutagalung et al., 1999) and also renders heterozygote RBCs relatively resistant to invasion by *P. falciparum* (Chotivanich et al., 2002).

Individual susceptibility to malaria or cerebral malaria may also be influenced by the genetically governed production of tumor necrosis factor-alpha (McGuire et al., 1994), CD36 (Aitman et al., 2000), nitric oxide synthase-2 (Kun et al., 1998), and the interferon-alpha receptor 1 (Aucan et al., 2003); family-based studies also have linked disease severity to genome regions encoding MHC (major histocompatibility complex), and cytokine genes (Jepson et al., 1997; Rihet et al., 1998). The genetic basis of cell-mediated and antibody-mediated immune responses in malaria is a rapidly evolving area of research.

CLINICAL FEATURES OF FALCIPARUM MALARIA

Falciparum malaria gives rise to a broad spectrum of disease from asymptomatic infection to fatal syndromes such as cerebral malaria, severe anemia, and multi-organ failure. The principal determinant of outcome is the immune status of the infected patient. With respect to its clinical features and consequences, malaria can therefore be broadly considered in three categories: disease in nonimmune individuals (for example, tourists, migrant workers and other non-immune persons in endemic areas); disease in children in endemic areas; and disease in pregnant women. Adults in endemic areas may also suffer periodic attacks, leading to clinical and especially economic consequences.

Malaria in the Nonimmune Host

In a nonimmune host, the traditional symptom complex heralding the onset of infection is the malaria paroxysm, a dramatic constellation of fevers, chills, and sweats that accompanies RBC lysis at the end of a cycle of asexual parasite development. In many medical textbooks, periodic paroxysms (every 48 hours in untreated *P. vivax* and *P. ovale*—"tertian" malaria—and every 72 hours in untreated *P. malariae*—"quartan" malaria) are mentioned as virtually diagnostic of malaria. In fact, in today's era of antimalarial chemotherapy, these periodic syndromes enshrined in the classical terminology of "tertian" and "quartan" malaria are seldom seen. In many patients, the onset of the febrile illness is nonspecific, and therefore indistinguishable from other common causes of fever. *Plasmodium falciparum* in particular causes irregular fevers that may occur daily, or even randomly within a 24-hour period.

In nonimmune subjects with falciparum malaria and overwhelming parasitemias (>10^6 parasitized RBCs per microliter, or more than 20 percent of circulating RBCs), anemia develops within days of the initial paroxysm. Additional clinical features and/or laboratory findings predictive of a "severe" or life-threatening course are prostration, shock, altered consciousness, respiratory distress (from acidotic breathing or pulmonary edema), convulsions, abnormal bleeding, jaundice, excretion of hemoglobin in urine, low blood sugar, elevated blood levels of lactic acid, and worsening kidney function (WHO, 2000).

Table 6-2 compares the frequency and prognostic value of severe manifestations and complications of *P. falciparum* malaria in adults and children.

A Delphi analysis published in 1990 estimated the case fatality risk attributable to highly drug-resistant (R3) *P. falciparum* infection—treated or untreated—at 2 to 5 percent in previously healthy African children aged 6 to 59 months brought to a primary health clinic in an area where malaria was hyperendemic or holoendemic (Sudre et al., 1990). Untreated falciparum malaria in a nonimmune host carries a risk of death of up to 20 to 30 percent (Behrens and Curtis, 1993; Alles et al., 1998; Carter and Mendis, 2002). Untreated *severe* falciparum malaria (as defined by WHO criteria, see Table 6-2) is almost uniformly fatal in all hosts (White and Pongtavornpinyo, 2003).

Malaria in Children

Overview in Endemic Areas

In contrast to the nonimmune adult with falciparum malaria (who will generally suffer one or more malaria paroxysms), the most common clinical manifestation of falciparum malaria in children in endemic settings is an entirely nonspecific febrile illness. In fact, in many parts of Africa, malaria is so ubiquitous—as an asymptomatic blood infection and an illness—that

TABLE 6-2 Severe Manifestations of *P. falciparum* Malaria in Adults and Children[a]

Prognostic Value[b]			Frequency[b]	
Children	Adults		Children	Adults
Clinical manifestations				
+	(?)[c]	Prostration	+++	+++
+++	+	Impaired consciousness	+++	++
+++	+++	Respiratory distress (acidotic breathing)	+++	+
+	++	Multiple convulsions	+++	+
+++	+++	Circulatory collapse	+	+
+++	+++	Pulmonary edema (radiological)	+/-	+
+++	++	Abnormal bleeding	+/-	+
++	+	Jaundice	+	+++
+	+	Hemoglobinuria	+/-	+
Laboratory findings				
+	+	Severe anemia	+++	+
+++	+++	Hypoglycemia	+++	++
+++	+++	Acidosis	+++	++
+++	+++	Hyperlactatemia	+++	++
+/-	++	Hyperparasitemia	++	+
++	++	Renal impairment	+	+++

[a]See the section on severe malaria in children.
[b]On a scale from + to +++; +/- indicates infrequent occurrence.
[c]Data not available.
SOURCE: World Health Organization. 2000. Severe falciparum malaria. *Transactions of the Royal Society of Tropical Medicine and Hygiene.* 94 (suppl 1). Table 1, on p. S1/2 of this supplement, was incomplete. A corrected version was printed and inserted into the supplement.

for practical purposes it cannot be diagnosed solely on clinical features or microscopy.

Why similar infections produce vastly different outcomes in different subjects is one of malaria's central, unsolved mysteries. Even among children with identical parasitemias, one child may be moribund with coma or severe anemia, while another is attending school or playing without apparent illness. One consequence of malaria's often uneventful course in endemic areas is a relative nonchalance on the part of patients, parents, and health care workers toward the disease.

> Some diseases like malaria are so common it's almost like information overload. It's malaria, okay. Malaria again, okay. Malaria again. Once in medical school we had a visiting pathologist—I forgot what country he came from—and he said: I went to the mortuary yesterday and I was doing post mortems, and all the spleens which were being passed off as normal are malaria spleens. [So he asked] why are you passing all of these spleens as normal? And the reply was: well almost everybody here has a spleen like that.
>
> Irene Agyepong, MD, Ghana Health Service (2002)

Viewed objectively, however, malaria exacts a chilling toll of morbidity and mortality on children. Over 90 percent of all cases of life-threatening malaria occur in sub-Saharan African children (Marsh et al., 1995), and malaria causes at least 20 percent of all deaths in children under 5 years of age in Africa (UNICEF, 2002).

Although the original World Health Organization (WHO) proposed definition of "severe malaria" was based on clinical observations in Southeast Asian adults, the multisystem nature of this syndrome also is seen in life-threatening manifestations of falciparum malaria in children in Africa, and other regions (Waller et al., 1995; Marsh et al., 1995; Allen et al., 1996). Common hallmarks of severe malaria in African children are altered consciousness, convulsions, hypoglycemia, acidosis, and anemia. The next sections will review these complications in further detail.

Severe Anemia

Anemia is a consistent marker of severe malaria in children as well as adults. Severe malarial anemia is defined as a hemoglobin concentration less than or equal to 5 g/dL in a patient with *P. falciparum* malaria. Until recently, overt destruction of parasitized RBCs and splenic filtration were thought to be the principal causes of severe malarial anemia. Today, however, an accelerated destruction of *unparasitized* red cells has been identified as a leading contributor to severe malarial anemia as well as anemia in uncomplicated malaria (Price et al., 2001). This destruction reflects reduced red cell deformability and immune-mediated membrane damage (Newton and Krishna, 1998). Malaria also induces bone marrow suppression, leading to decreased production of RBCs (Abdalla et al., 1980). Finally, malaria-specific processes often are compounded by other contributors to tropical childhood anemia such as nutritional iron deficiency and hookworm infection.

There are three principal ways in which malaria can contribute to death in young children. First, an overwhelming acute infection, which frequently presents as seizures or coma (cerebral malaria), may kill a child directly and quickly. Second, repeated malaria infections contribute to the development of severe anaemia, which substantially increases the risk of death. Third, low birth weight—frequently the consequence of malaria infection in pregnant women—is the major risk factor for death in the first month of life.

WHO, Africa Malaria Report, 2003

Children with severe anemia tend to be younger than those with cerebral malaria, but the two conditions often overlap. Overall, case fatality rates for children hospitalized for severe anemia alone range from 5 to 15 percent (Waller et al., 1995). Morbidity and mortality due to malarial anemia have increased with the spread of chloroquine-resistant parasites across Africa (Bloland et al., 1993; Trape et al., 1998).

Respiratory Distress and Metabolic Acidosis

Although respiratory signs and symptoms are common in mild and moderate malaria (O'Dempsey et al., 1993), until recently, metabolic acidosis producing respiratory distress was an underappreciated feature of life-threatening malaria in African children (Taylor et al., 1993; Marsh et al., 1995). Metabolic acidosis carries a 24 percent case fatality rate when it occurs alone, and a 35 percent risk of death when associated with cerebral malaria and/or anemia (Marsh et al., 1995). Many experts now consider respiratory distress to be the single most important prognostic factor and main indication for blood transfusion in children with malaria and severe anemia (Newton et al., 1992).

A second important cause of respiratory distress in children with malaria is lower respiratory tract infection (English et al., 1996). In some cases, this is the principal cause of respiratory symptoms in a patient who also is (coincidentally) parasitemic. Alternatively, there is mounting evidence that many children with severe malaria have dual infections (Berkley et al., 1999).

Cerebral Malaria

"Cerebral malaria" represents an advanced stage in the spectrum of *P. falciparum* asexual parasitemia and altered consciousness. In research settings, the definition is met when a child with bloodstream parasites and no other obvious cause of impaired consciousness (for example, meningitis) is unable to localize a painful stimulus after the correction of hypoglycemia and exclusion of other brain disorders. The Blantyre coma scale (Molyneux et al., 1989) is a clinical research instrument for assessing children not yet able to speak. The Blantyre coma scale produces a total score from 0 (worst) to 5 (best) based on motor response, verbal response, and eye movements. In general, a child with cerebral malaria will register a Blantyre coma score ≤ 2 or occasionally 3 (WHO, 2000).

> I saw this one child—I still remember him—he had cerebral malaria and it was a real struggle for his life but he survived. We were all so excited. Six months later I met this child with his mother. He had developed neurologic sequelae; he was hyperactive, not paying attention in school. I just felt a sense of disappointment. . . . If this child had never had that bad malaria—in spite of having pulled through—maybe he wouldn't be in this state.
>
> Irene Agyepong, Ghana Health Service (2002)

African children with cerebral malaria usually enter a coma following a 1- to 3-day history of fever. The coma may develop quickly, accompanied by one or more convulsions as well as an arched back, posturing, an altered respiratory pattern and/or gaze abnormalities (Molyneux et al., 1989). Other acute neurologic features include a generalized decrease in muscle tone, cranial nerve palsies (Warrell, 1996), and retinal abnormalities including hemorrhage (Lewallen et al., 1999). Convulsions, both generalized and focal, ultimately complicate 50-80 percent of cerebral malaria episodes in children.

In endemic areas, full-blown cerebral malaria typically occurs in children under 5 years of age, and is rarely seen above the age of 10 in children who have been exposed to *P. falciparum* from birth.

Death Due to Cerebral Malaria

The reported hospital case fatality rate of cerebral malaria in children ranges from 10 to 40 percent, but in recent studies it has averaged about 16 percent (White et al., 1987; Molyneux et al., 1989; Waller et al., 1995). Most deaths occur within 24 hours of starting treatment, and are preceded by progressive brainstem dysfunction, respiratory arrest, and/or overwhelming acidosis (Newton and Krishna, 1998). African children with cerebral malaria who survive generally regain consciousness within 48 to 72 hours of appropriate treatment.

Chronic Neurologic Impairment Following Cerebral Malaria

Chronic neurologic sequelae following falciparum malaria are usually seen in patients with protracted seizures, prolonged coma and/or hypoglycemia (Brewster et al., 1990). In Africa, about 13 percent of children who survive cerebral malaria have neurological sequelae, among them ataxia, hemiplegia, speech disorders, and blindness (Taylor and Molyneux, 2002). Late neurologic consequences also include unsteady gait, paralysis, and cognitive and behavioral deficits (Newton and Warrell, 1998). Epilepsy and EEG abnormalities following cerebral malaria have probably been underestimated in past studies; recent data suggest that the relative risk of epileptic discharges following cerebral malaria or malaria plus seizures is increased nearly twofold compared to children who have not suffered severe malaria (Otieno et al., 2002).

> Some students become dull, they don't understand the lessons . . . sometimes they even become like fools, they become abnormal.
>
> Primary school teacher, Muheza, Tanzania (2002)

Some chronic neurologic deficits (for example, gait disturbance, unilateral weakness, and cortical blindness) may resolve after several months. An estimated 2 percent of children who recover from malaria infections affecting the brain suffer from learning impairments and disabilities due to brain damage, including epilepsy, and spasticity (Murphy and Breman, 2001). Furthermore, repeated episodes of fever and illness reduce appetite and restrict play, social interaction, and educational opportunities, thereby contributing to poor development.

People dying of malaria . . . that's over a million deaths a year. But there are ten times, 20 times, 100 times more people that develop severe complications of malaria that are desperately life threatening but do survive. And as part of this survival, there are risks . . . from behavioral disturbances and difficulties in learning through to very severe disabilities such as spasticity, total paralysis down one side of the body . . . to deafness and blindness and epilepsy. Many of those children with epilepsy may die because they fall into fires or down wells."

Bob Snow, Kenya Medical Research Institute (2002)

Hypoglycemia

Prolonged hypoglycemia can produce death and/or chronic neurologic damage. Hypoglycemia associated with falciparum malaria (defined as a blood glucose concentration of less than 2.2 mmol/L or 40 mg/dL) has two discrete etiologies. It may reflect metabolic acidosis (i.e., hyperlactatemia) seen in severe malaria or, in quinine-treated patients, it may reflect quinine-stimulated insulin secretion. Metabolic acidosis is usually present on admission to the hospital and carries a poor prognosis, while hyperinsulinemia tends to appear after the first 12 to 24 hours of treatment (White et al., 1983).

In one study, 13 to 32 percent of children with severe malaria developed hypoglycemia as a complication of their illness (Taylor et al., 1988).

Severe Malaria in Adults versus Children

Most cases of severe malaria in adults occur in regions outside Africa. However, even in malaria-endemic areas of Africa, some adults still suffer and die from severe malaria. The clinical spectrum of illness in these individuals is different from that seen in children. Whereas children are more likely to develop severe anemia, hypoglycemia, or convulsions, adults with severe malaria are more likely to develop jaundice, acute kidney damage, or acute pulmonary edema. Recovery from cerebral malaria in adults is slower than in children although neurologic sequelae are less frequent (occurring in less than 3 percent of adult cases compared with 10 percent of pediatric cases). Kidney failure due to acute tubular necrosis is another important cause of death. Acute pulmonary edema in malaria results from increased capillary permeability, the same pathophysiologic process that leads to acute respiratory distress syndrome. The mortality of severe falciparum malaria in adults who are appropriately treated can reach 15 to 20 percent.

Severe malaria in pregnancy (see below) is associated with additional complications—particularly hypoglycemia, and pulmonary edema—and a higher mortality.

Malaria in Pregnancy

The clinical course of falciparum malaria during pregnancy depends in large part on the immune status of the woman, which, in turn, is influenced by her previous exposure to malaria.

Clinical Consequences in Low-Transmission Areas

In areas of low transmission, falciparum malaria is an important cause of maternal morbidity and mortality in women of all parities. Pregnant women with little or no immunity are two to three times more likely to develop severe disease than non-pregnant adults living under the same conditions (Luxemburger et al., 1997). In addition, if they develop severe disease, they risk a 20 to 30 percent chance of dying (Meek, 1988). Complications to which pregnant malaria-infected women with low immunity are especially susceptible include high fever, low blood sugar, severe hemolytic anemia, cerebral malaria, and pulmonary edema (Looareesuwan et al., 1985).

Malaria in pregnant women with low immunity also affects the developing fetus and the newborn, causing abortion, stillbirth, premature delivery, and low birth weight (Menon, 1972; Nosten et al., 1994). Babies born to nonimmune mothers with malaria at the time of childbirth may develop parasitemia and illness in the first few weeks of life (Quinn et al., 1982). Specific clinical features in infected newborns include fever, lethargy, anemia, and enlargement of liver and spleen.

Clinical Consequences in High-transmission Areas

In sub-Saharan Africa, close to 45 percent of women have malarial infection during pregnancy (Steketee, et al., 1996b), and almost half of women who are pregnant for the first time (primigravidae) will be parasitemic on their first antenatal visit (Menendez, 1995). Pregnant women are more likely to have blood parasites and high parasitemias than non-pregnant women of the same age (Brabin, 1983; Garin et al., 1985; Steketee and Wirima, 1996). For the semi-immune mother, the major risk of malaria during pregnancy is maternal anemia (Shulman et al., 1996), especially during first pregnancies (Greenwood et al., 1994).

In high-transmission areas, placental parasitemia also is common, especially among primigravidae, even when peripheral blood smears are negative (McGregor et al., 1983; Nyirjesy et al., 1993). The most common consequence of placental malaria is intrauterine growth retardation (McGregor et al., 1983; Steketee and Wirima, 1996). In a model based on multiple published studies, Guyatt and Snow (2001) recently found that African babies born to mothers whose placentas were infected at the time of delivery were twice as likely to be underweight at birth, and that their risk of death during the first year of life was three times higher than babies of normal birth weight.

Pathogenesis of Placental Malaria

In placental malaria, the organ is a privileged site of parasite replication. Most (but not all) placental isolates of *P. falciparum* bind to chondroitin sulphate A (CSA) expressed on the surface of maternal placental cells (Duffy and Fried, 2003). Over time, antibodies inhibiting parasite adhesion to CSA develop, reducing the likelihood of heavy placental infection after first or second pregnancies (Fried et al., 1998).

HIV and Malaria

The growing epidemic of HIV/AIDS in malaria-endemic areas of sub-Saharan Africa has prompted many investigators to explore possible interactions between the two infections. Although several early studies—including six hospital-based cross-sectional and longitudinal studies in African children and adults (Nguyen-Dinh et al., 1987; Simooya et al., 1988; Colebunders et al., 1990; Muller and Moser, 1990; Greenberg et al., 1991; Allen et al., 1991; Kalyesubula et al., 1997)—failed to reveal convincing links between malaria and HIV, one study in rural Tanzania found a significantly increased prevalence of asymptomatic malarial parasitemia in HIV-1 positive adults (Atzori et al., 1993), and two studies found higher death rates due to severe malaria in HIV-1 positive adults (Leaver et al., 1990; Niyongabo et al., 1994). In retrospect, small patient numbers, and a failure to take into account the different degrees of immunosuppression found at different stages of HIV-1 infection were weaknesses of many of these early investigations.

More recent case-control (Francesconi et al., 2001) and longitudinal epidemiologic studies (Whitworth et al., 2000; French et al., 2001) have confirmed an association between HIV infection, clinical malaria, and *P. falciparum* parasitemia, particularly among individuals with advanced HIV disease as measured by falling CD4 lymphocyte counts. Symptomatic *P. falciparum* infection also appears to increase HIV-1 viral loads (Hoffman et al., 1999).

HIV, Malaria, and Pregnancy

Currently, the most convincing evidence for a possible interaction between HIV-1 and malaria comes from studies of pregnant women. HIV-1 infected pregnant women in Malawi showed a higher prevalence and density of *P. falciparum* parasitemia than their non-HIV-1 infected counterparts (Steketee et al., 1996). This finding has been confirmed in other studies of pregnant African women (Ladner et al., 2002; van Eijk et al., 2003). Pregnant HIV-infected women also are more likely to be anemic (van den Broek et al., 1998; Meda et al., 1999; van Eijk et al., 2001) and to respond less well to intermittent preventive treatment with sulfadoxine-pyrimethamine than HIV uninfected women (Parise et al., 1998). Postnatal mortality in infants also is increased in mothers co-infected with HIV-1 and malaria than infants of mothers with only one infection (Bloland et al., 1995).

An important question still unanswered is whether or not placental malaria increases mother-to-child HIV transmission. In a recent study of 746 HIV-positive mother-infant pairs in Uganda, the increased risk of mother-to-child transmission associated with placental malaria was 2.89 (Brahmbhatt et al., 2003); however another study completed in Kenya found no association between placental malaria and HIV transmission in utero or peripartum (Inion et al., 2003).

NON-FALCIPARUM MALARIA

Plasmodium vivax

Plasmodium vivax malaria is widely distributed throughout the world—predominantly in Asia, the Western Pacific, and the Americas—and accounts for over half of all malaria infections outside Africa, and roughly 10 percent of infections in Africa (Mendis et al., 2001). It has recently made a comeback in Korea, Peru, Indonesia, and China (Sleigh et al., 1998; Sharma, 1999; Chai, 1999; Roper et al., 2000; Barcus et al., 2002), and currently produces an estimated 75 million acute malarial episodes every year (Sina, 2002).

In humans, the fact that *P. vivax* invades only young RBCs (reticulocytes) limits its total parasite load and disease severity. In addition, *P. vivax* can only attach to human RBCs possessing the Duffy blood group cell surface antigen (Miller et al., 1976). Since most residents of West Africa lack genetic expression of the Duffy blood group antigen, the disease is essentially absent from the region.

The hallmark of vivax malaria is its sudden, dramatic paroxysm, triggered by the cytokines interleukin-6 and tumor necrosis factor alpha (TNF-alpha) (Karunaweera et al., 1992a,b). Paroxysms recur every 48 hours, and may continue for several weeks if patients do not receive appropriate anti-malarial treatment. The most common clinical consequence is anemia, al-though severe and fatal complications associated with lung injury (Torres et al., 1997; Carlini et al., 1999; Tanios et al., 2001), splenic rupture, and associated splenic pathology (Zingman and Viner, 1993) are occasionally reported. Rarely, cerebral complications also have followed pure *P. vivax* infections (Sachdev and Mohan, 1985; Beg et al., 2002). There are rela-tively few reports describing the effect of *P. vivax* malaria on pregnancy, although some investigators have linked it to maternal parasitemia and anemia, as well as low birth weight (Nosten et al., 1999; Singh et al., 1999).

Of the four human malaria species, only *P. vivax* and *P. ovale* undergo true relapse—i.e., reseeding of the bloodstream from dormant parasites (called hypnozoites) in the liver. The likelihood and time interval between primary parasitemia and relapse varies according to environmental vari-ables (Baird and Rieckmann, 2003). In general, strains from temperate regions are less likely to relapse (~30 percent risk), and they exhibit longer latency intervals (>6 months). Tropical strains have an 80 percent risk of relapse, often within several weeks of primary parasitemia (Garnham, 1988; Cogswell, 1992).

Plasmodium malariae

The geographic distribution of *P. malariae*—also called quartan ma-laria—roughly overlaps *P. falciparum*. *Plasmodium malariae* manifests acutely as a febrile illness with anemia. However, the most distinctive fea-ture of *P. malariae* is its decades-long persistence. Chronic, subpatent infec-tions have recrudesced following splenectomy (Tsuchida et al., 1982; Vinetz et al., 1998) or other surgeries unrelated to malaria (Chadee et al., 2000). The parasite also may be transmitted via blood transfusion many years after a blood donor has left an endemic region (Bruce-Chwatt, 1972). In a 20-year review of transfusion-associated malaria in the United States, *P. malariae* accounted for more cases than any other malarial species (Guerrero et al., 1983).

In West Africa and Papua New Guinea, repeated or continuous infec-tion with *P. malariae* infection also is associated with childhood nephro-sis—a syndrome characterized by heavy protein loss in the urine, peripheral edema, and renal impairment (Hendrickse et al., 1972; White, 1996, 1997). The condition is usually steroid-resistant, and may progress to renal failure and death even after successful treatment of infection (Barsoum, 2000). Hyperreactive malarial splenomegaly (HMS, formerly known as tropical splenomegaly syndrome) is another chronic immune-mediated pathology associated with *P. malariae*, as well as *P. falciparum* and *P. vivax* (Hoffman et al., 1984; Piessens et al., 1985). Affected patients experience massive splenomegaly, abdominal pain, episodic prostration, and high mortality due to secondary infections (Crane, 1986).

Plasmodium ovale

Plasmodium ovale is the least studied of the malaria parasites that infect humans. Although transmitted sporadically on all continents, the parasite primarily affects residents of tropical Africa and New Guinea, where its prevalence among children averages between 2 to 10 percent (Faye et al., 2002). Overall, the parasite causes a relatively mild form of malaria that closely resembles *P. vivax* infection and is rarely fatal (Facer and Rouse, 1991).

REFERENCES

Abdalla S, Weatherall DJ, Wickramasinghe SN, Hughes M. 1980. The anaemia of *P. falciparum* malaria. *British Journal of Haematology* 46(2):171-183.

Adams S, Brown H, Turner G. 2002. Breaking down the blood-brain barrier: Signaling a path to cerebral malaria? *Trends in Parasitology* 18(8):360-366.

Aitman TJ, Cooper LD, Norsworthy PJ, Wahid FN, Gray JK, Curtis BR, McKeigue PM, Kwiatkowski D, Greenwood BM, Snow RW, Hill AV, Scott J. 2000. Malaria susceptibility and Cd36 mutation. *Nature* 405(6790):1015-1016.

Allen S, Van de Perre P, Serufilira A, Lepage P, Carael M, DeClercq A, Tice J, Black D, Nsengumuremyi F, Ziegler J. 1991. Human immunodeficiency virus and malaria in a representative sample of childbearing women in Kigali, Rwanda. *Journal of Infectious Diseases* 164(1):67-71.

Allen SJ, O'Donnell A, Alexander ND, Clegg JB. 1996. Severe malaria in children in Papua New Guinea. *Quarterly Journal of Medicine* 89(10):779-788.

Allen SJ, O'Donnell A, Alexander ND, Alpers MP, Peto TE, Clegg JB, Weatherall DJ. 1997. Alpha+-thalassemia protects children against disease caused by other infections as well as malaria. *Proceedings of the National Academy of Sciences of the United States of America* 94(26):14736-14741.

Alles HK, Mendis KN, Carter R. 1998. Malaria mortality rates in south Asia and in Africa: Implications for malaria control. *Parasitology Today* 14(9):369-375.

Atzori C, Bruno A, Chichino G, Cevini C, Bernuzzi AM, Gatti S, Comolli G, Scaglia M. 1993. HIV-1 and parasitic infections in rural Tanzania. *Annals of Tropical Medicine and Parasitology* 87(6):585-593.

Aucan C, Walley AJ, Hennig BJ, Fitness J, Frodsham A, Zhang L, Kwiatkowski D, Hill AV. 2003. Interferon-alpha receptor-1 (IFNAR1) variants are associated with protection against cerebral malaria in The Gambia. *Genes and Immunity* 4:275-282.

Baird JK, Rieckmann KH. 2003. Can primaquine therapy for vivax malaria be improved? *Trends in Parasitology* 19(3):115-120.

Barcus MJ, Laihad F, Sururi M, Sismadi P, Marwoto H, Bangs MJ, Baird JK. 2002. Epidemic malaria in the Menoreh Hills of Central Java. *American Journal of Tropical Medicine and Hygiene* 66(3):287-292.

Barsoum RS. 2000. Malarial acute renal failure. *Journal of the American Society of Nephrology* 11(11):2147-2154.

Beg MA, Khan R, Baig SM, Gulzar Z, Hussain R, Smego RA Jr. 2002. Cerebral involvement in benign tertian malaria. *American Journal of Tropical Medicine and Hygiene* 67(3):230-232.

Behrens RH, Curtis CF. 1993. Malaria in travellers: Epidemiology and prevention. *British Medical Bulletin* 49(2):363-381.

Berkley J, Mwarumba S, Bramham K, Lowe B, Marsh K. 1999. Bacteraemia complicating severe malaria in children. *Transactions of the Royal Society of Tropical Medicine and Hygiene* 93(3):283-286.

Bloland PB, Lackritz EM, Kazembe PN, Were JB, Steketee R, Campbell CC. 1993. Beyond chloroquine: Implications of drug resistance for evaluating malaria therapy efficacy and treatment policy in Africa. *Journal of Infectious Diseases* 167(4):932-937.

Bloland PB, Wirima JJ, Steketee RW, Chilima B, Hightower A, Breman JG. 1995. Maternal HIV infection and infant mortality in Malawi: Evidence for increased mortality due to placental malaria infection. *AIDS* 9(7):721-726.

Bottius E, Guanzirolli A, Trape JF, Rogier C, Konate L, Druilhe P. 1996. Malaria: Even more chronic in nature than previously thought; evidence for subpatent parasitaemia detectable by the polymerase chain reaction. *Transactions of the Royal Society of Tropical Medicine and Hygiene* 90(1):15-19.

Brabin BJ. 1983. An analysis of malaria in pregnancy in Africa. *Bulletin of the World Health Organization* 61(6):1005-1016.

Brahmbhatt H, Kigozi G, Wabwire-Magen F, Serwadda D, Sewankambo N, Lutalo T, Wawer MJ, Abramowsky C, Sullivan D, Gray R. 2003. The effects of placental malaria on mother-to-child HIV transmission in Rakai, Uganda. *AIDS* 17:2539-2541.

Brewster DR, Kwiatkowski D, White NJ. 1990. Neurological sequelae of cerebral malaria in children. *Lancet* 336(8722):1039-1043.

Bruce-Chwatt LJ. 1972. Blood transfusion and tropical disease. *Tropical Diseases Bulletin* 69(9):825-862.

Bruce-Chwatt, LJ. 1985. *Essential Malariology, 2nd ed.* New York: John Wiley and Sons.

Carlini ME, White AC Jr, Atmar RL. 1999. Vivax malaria complicated by adult respiratory distress syndrome. *Clinical Infectious Diseases* 28(5):1182-1183.

Carter R, Mendis KN. 2002. Evolutionary and historical aspects of the burden of malaria. *Clinical Microbiology Reviews* 15(4):564-594.

Chadee DD, Tilluckdharry CC, Maharaj P, Sinanan C. 2000. Reactivation of *Plasmodium malariae* infection in a Trinidadian man after neurosurgery. *New England Journal of Medicine* 342(25):1924.

Chai JY. 1999. Re-emerging *Plasmodium vivax* malaria in the Republic of Korea. *Korean Journal of Parasitology* 37(3):129-143.

Chotivanich K, Udomsangpetch R, Simpson JA, Newton P, Pukrittayakamee S, Looareesuwan S, White NJ. 2000. Parasite multiplication potential and the severity of falciparum malaria. *Journal of Infectious Diseases* 181(3):1206-1209.

Chotivanich K, Udomsangpetch R, Pattanapanyasat K, Chierakul W, Simpson J, Looareesuwan S, White N. 2002. Hemoglobin E: A balanced polymorphism protective against high parasitemias and thus severe *P. falciparum* malaria. *Blood* 100(4):1172-1176.

Cogswell FB. 1992. The hypnozoite and relapse in primate malaria. *Clinical Microbiology Reviews* 5(1):26-35.

Colebunders R, Bahwe Y, Nekwei W, Ryder R, Perriens J, Nsimba K, Turner A, Francis H, Lebughe I, Van der Stuyft P. 1990. Incidence of malaria and efficacy of oral quinine in patients recently infected with human immunodeficiency virus in Kinshasa, Zaire. *Journal of Infection* 21(2):167-173.

Crane CG. 1986. Hyperreactive malarious splenomegaly (tropical splenomegaly syndrome). *Parasitology Today* 2:4-9.

Duffy PE, Fried M. 2003. *Plasmodium falciparum* adhesion in the placenta. *Current Opinion in Microbiology* 6(4):371-376.

Edozien JC, Gilles HM, Udeozo IOK. 1962. Adult and cord-blood gamma globulin and immunity to malaria in Nigerians. *Lancet* 2:951-955.

English M, Newton C. 2002. Malaria: Pathogenicity and disease. *Chemical Immunology* 80:50-69.

English M, Punt J, Mwangi I, McHugh K, Marsh K. 1996. Clinical overlap between malaria and severe pneumonia in Africa children in hospital. *Transactions of the Royal Society of Tropical Medicine and Hygiene* 90(6):658-662.

Facer CA, Rouse D. 1991. Spontaneous splenic rupture due to *Plasmodium ovale* malaria. *Lancet* 338(8771):896.

Farnert A, Snounou G, Rooth I, Bjorkman A. 1997. Daily dynamics of *Plasmodium falciparum* subpopulations in asymptomatic children in a holoendemic area. *American Journal of Tropical Medicine and Hygiene* 56(5):538-547.

Faye FB, Spiegel A, Tall A, Sokhna C, Fontenille D, Rogier C, Trape JF. 2002. Diagnostic criteria and risk factors for *Plasmodium ovale* malaria. *Journal of Infectious Diseases* 186(5):690-695.

Francesconi P, Fabiani M, Dente MG, Lukwiya M, Okwey R, Ouma J, Ochakachon R, Cian F, Declich S. 2001. HIV, malaria parasites, and acute febrile episodes in Ugandan adults: A case-control study. *AIDS* 15(18):2445-2450.

French N, Nakiyingi J, Lugada E, Watera C, Whitworth JA, Gilks CF. 2001. Increasing rates of malarial fever with deteriorating immune status in HIV-1-infected Ugandan adults. *AIDS* 15(7):899-906.

Fried M, Nosten F, Brockman A, Brabin BJ, Duffy PE. 1998. Maternal antibodies block malaria. *Nature* 395(6705):851-852.

Garin YJ, Blot P, Walter P, Pinon JM, Vernes A. 1985. [Malarial infection of the placenta. Parasitologic, clinical and immunologic aspects]. [French]. *Archives Francaises de Pediatrie* 42(Suppl 2):917-920.

Garnham PC. 1988. Swellengrebel Lecture. Hypnozoites and 'relapses' in *Plasmodium vivax* and in vivax-like malaria. *Tropical and Geographical Medicine* 40(3):187-195.

Gilles HM, Fletcher KA, Hendrickse RG, Lindner R, Reddy S, Allan N. 1967. Glucose-6-phosphate-dehydrogenase deficiency, sickling, and malaria in African children in south western Nigeria. *Lancet* 1(7482):138-140.

Greenberg AE, Nsa W, Ryder RW, Medi M, Nzeza M, Kitadi N, Baangi M, Malanda N, Davachi F, Hassig SE. 1991. *Plasmodium falciparum* malaria and perinatally acquired Human Immunodeficiency Virus Type 1 infection in Kinshasa, Zaire. A prospective, longitudinal cohort study of 587 children. *New England Journal of Medicine* 325(2):105-109.

Greenwood AM, Menendez C, Alonso PL, Jaffar S, Langerock P, Lulat S, Todd J, M'Boge B, Francis N, Greenwood BM. 1994. Can malaria chemoprophylaxis be restricted to first pregnancies? *Transactions of the Royal Society of Tropical Medicine and Hygiene* 88(6): 681-682.

Greenwood B. 2002. The molecular epidemiology of malaria. *Tropical Medicine and International Health* 7(12):1012-1021.

Guerrero IC, Weniger BG, Schultz MG. 1983. Transfusion malaria in the United States, 1972-1981. *Annals of Internal Medicine* 99(2):221-226.

Guyatt HL, Snow RW. 2001. Malaria in pregnancy as an indirect cause of infant mortality in sub-Saharan Africa. *Transactions of the Royal Society of Tropical Medicine and Hygiene* 95(6):569-576.

Haldane JBS. 1948. The rate of mutation of human genes. *Hereditas* 35(Suppl):267-273.

Hamon J, Mouchet J, Chauvet G, Lumaret R. 1963. [Review of 14 years of malaria control in the French-speaking countries of tropical Africa and Madagascar. Considerations on the persistence of transmission and future prospects]. *Bulletin de la Societe de Pathologie Exotique Filiales* 56:933-971.

Hay SI, Rogers DJ, Toomer JF, Snow RW. 2000. Annual *Plasmodium falciparum* entomological inoculation rates (EIR) across Africa: Literature survey, internet access and review. *Transactions of the Royal Society of Tropical Medicine and Hygiene* 94(2):113-127.

Hendrickse RG, Adeniyi A, Edington GM, Glasgow EF, White RH, Houba V. 1972. Quartan malarial nephrotic syndrome: Collaborative clinicopathological study in Nigerian children. *Lancet* 1(7761):1143-1149.

Hill AV, Allsopp CE, Kwiatkowski D, Anstey NM, Twumasi P, Rowe PA, Bennett S, Brewster D, McMichael AJ, Greenwood BM. 1991. Common west African HLA antigens are associated with protection from severe malaria. [comment]. *Nature* 352(6336):595-600.

Hoffman IF, Jere CS, Taylor TE, Munthali P, Dyer JR, Wirima JJ, Rogerson SJ, Kumwenda N, Eron JJ, Fiscus SA, Chakraborty H, Taha TE, Cohen MS, Molyneux ME. 1999. The effect of *Plasmodium falciparum* malaria on HIV-1 RNA blood plasma concentration. *AIDS* 13(4):487-494.

Hoffman SL, Piessens WF, Ratiwayanto S, Hussein PR, Kurniawan L, Piessens PW, Campbell JR, Marwoto HA. 1984. Reduction of suppressor T lymphocytes in the tropical splenomegaly syndrome. *New England Journal of Medicine* 310(6):337-341.

Hutagalung R, Wilairatana P, Looareesuwan S, Brittenham GM, Aikawa M, Gordeuk VR. 1999. Influence of hemoglobin E trait on the severity of falciparum malaria. *Journal of Infectious Diseases* 179(1):283-286.

Inion I, Mwanyumba F, Gaillard P, Chohan V, Verhofstede C, Claeys P, Mandaliya K, Van Marck E, Temmerman M. 2003. Placental malaria and perinatal transmission of Human Immunodeficiency Virus Type 1. *Journal of Infectious Diseases* 188(11):1675-1678.

Jepson A, Sisay-Joof F, Banya W, Hassan-King M, Frodsham A, Bennett S, Hill AVS, Whittle H. 1997. Genetic linkage of mild malaria to the major histocompatibility complex in Gambian children: Study of affected sibling pairs. *British Medical Journal* 315(7100):96-97.

Kalyesubula I, Musoke-Mudido P, Marum L, Bagenda D, Aceng E, Ndugwa C, Olness K. 1997. Effects of malaria infection in Human Immunodeficiency Virus Type 1-Infected Ugandan Children. *Pediatric Infectious Disease Journal* 16(9):876-881.

Karunaweera ND, Carter R, Grau GE, Kwiatkowski D, Del Giudice G, Mendis KN. 1992a. Tumour necrosis factor-dependent parasite-killing effects during paroxysms in non-immune *Plasmodium vivax* malaria patients. *Clinical and Experimental Immunology* 88(3):499-505.

Karunaweera ND, Grau GE, Gamage P, Carter R, Mendis KN. 1992b. Dynamics of fever and serum levels of tumor necrosis factor are closely associated during clinical paroxysms in *Plasmodium vivax* malaria. *Proceedings of the National Academy of Sciences of the United States of America* 89(8):3200-3203.

Kun JF, Mordmuller B, Lell B, Lehman LG, Luckner D, Kremsner PG. 1998. Polymorphism in promoter region of inducible nitric oxide synthase gene and protection against malaria. *Lancet* 351(9098):265-266.

Ladner J, Leroy V, Simonon A, Karita E, Bogaerts J, De Clercq A, Van De Perre P, Dabis F, Pregnancy and HIV Study Group (EGE). 2002. HIV infection, malaria, and pregnancy: A prospective cohort study in Kigali, Rwanda. *American Journal of Tropical Medicine and Hygiene* 66(1):56-60.

Leaver RJ, Haile Z, Watters DA. 1990. HIV and cerebral malaria. *Transactions of the Royal Society of Tropical Medicine and Hygiene* 84(2):201.

Lewallen S, Harding SP, Ajewole J, Schulenburg WE, Molyneux ME, Marsh K, Usen S, White NJ, Taylor TE. 1999. A review of the spectrum of clinical ocular fundus findings in *P. falciparum* malaria in African children with a proposed classification and grading system. *Transactions of the Royal Society of Tropical Medicine and Hygiene* 93(6):619-622.

Looareesuwan S, Phillips RE, White NJ, Kietinun S, Karbwang J, Rackow C, Turner RC, Warrell DA. 1985. Quinine and severe falciparum malaria in late pregnancy. *Lancet* 2(8445):4-8.

Luxemburger C, Ricci F, Nosten F, Raimond D, Bathet S, White NJ. 1997. The epidemiology of severe malaria in an area of low transmission in Thailand. *Transactions of the Royal Society of Tropical Medicine and Hygiene* 91(3):256-262.

Macdonald G. 1952. The analysis of the sporozoite rate. *Tropical Diseases Bulletin* 49:569-586.

Marsh K. 1992. Malaria—A neglected disease? *Parasitology* 104(Suppl):S53-S69.

Marsh K, Forster D, Waruiru C, Mwangi I, Winstanley M, Marsh V, Newton C, Winstanley P, Warn P, Peshu N. 1995. Indicators of life-threatening malaria in African children. *New England Journal of Medicine* 332(21):1399-1404.

Mbogo CNM, Snow RW, Khamala CPM, Kabiru EW, Ouma JH, Githure JI, Marsh K, Beier JC. 1995. Relationships between *Plasmodium falciparum* transmission by vector populations and the incidence of severe disease at nine sites on the Kenyan coast. *American Journal of Tropical Medicine and Hygiene* 52(3):201-206.

McGregor IA. 1974. Mechanisms of acquired immunity and epidemiological patterns of antibody responses in malaria in man. *Bulletin of the World Health Organization* 50(3-4):259-266.

McGregor IA, Wilson ME, Billewicz WZ. 1983. Malaria infection of the placenta in the Gambia, West Africa; its incidence and relationship to stillbirth, birthweight and placental weight. *Transactions of the Royal Society of Tropical Medicine and Hygiene* 77(2):232-244.

McGuire W, Hill AV, Allsopp CE, Greenwood BM, Kwiatkowski D. 1994. Variation in the TNF-alpha promoter region associated with susceptibility to cerebral malaria. *Nature* 371(6497):508-510.

Meda N, Mandelbrot L, Cartoux M, Dao B, Ouangre A, Dabis F. 1999. Anaemia during pregnancy in Burkina Faso, West Africa, 1995-96: Prevalence and associated factors. Ditrame Study Group. *Bulletin of the World Health Organization* 77(11):916-922.

Meek SR. 1988. Epidemiology of malaria in displaced Khmers on the Thai-Kampuchean border. *Southeast Asian Journal of Tropical Medicine and Public Health* 19(2):243-252.

Mendis K, Sina BJ, Marchesini P, Carter R. 2001. The neglected burden of *Plasmodium vivax* malaria. *American Journal of Tropical Medicine and Hygiene* 64(1-2 Suppl):97-106.

Menendez C. 1995. Malaria during pregnancy: A priority area of malaria research and control. *Parasitology Today* 11(5):178-183.

Menon R. 1972. Pregnancy and malaria. *Medical Journal of Malaya* 27(2):115-119.

Miller LH, Mason SJ, Clyde DF, McGinniss MH. 1976. The resistance factor to *Plasmodium vivax* in blacks. The Duffy-Blood-Group genotype, Fyfy. *New England Journal of Medicine* 295(6):302-304.

Modiano D, Luoni G, Sirima BS, Simpore J, Verra F, Konate A, Rastrelli E, Olivieri A, Calissano C, Paganotti GM, D'Urbano L, Sanou I, Sawadogo A, Modiano G, Coluzzi M. 2001. Haemoglobin C protects against clinical *Plasmodium falciparum* malaria. *Nature* 414(6861):305-308.

Mohan K, Stevenson MM. 1998. Acquired immunity to asexual blood stages. In: Sherman W, ed. *Parasite Biology, Pathogenesis and Protection.* Washington, DC: ASM Press.

Molyneux ME, Taylor TE, Wirima JJ, Borgstein A. 1989. Clinical features and prognostic indicators in paediatric cerebral malaria: A study of 131 comatose Malawian children. *Quarterly Journal of Medicine* 71(265):441-459.

Mouchet J, Laventure S, Blanchy S, Fioramonti R, Rakotonjanabelo A, Rabarison P, Sircoulon J, Roux J. 1997. [The reconquest of the Madagascar highlands by malaria]. [French]. *Bulletin de la Societe de Pathologie Exotique* 90(3):162-168.

Muller O, Moser R. 1990. The clinical and parasitological presentation of *Plasmodium falciparum* malaria in Uganda is unaffected by HIV-1 infection. *Transactions of the Royal Society of Tropical Medicine and Hygiene* 84(3):336-338.

Murphy SC, Breman JG. 2001. Gaps in the childhood malaria burden in Africa: Cerebral malaria, neurological sequelae, anemia, respiratory distress, hypoglycemia, and complications of pregnancy. *American Journal of Tropical Medicine and Hygiene* 64(1-2 Suppl):57-67.

Neva FA. 1977. Looking back for a view of the future: Observations on immunity to induced malaria. *American Journal of Tropical Medicine and Hygiene* 26(6 Pt 2):211-215.

Newton CR, Krishna S. 1998. Severe falciparum malaria in children: Current understanding of pathophysiology and supportive treatment. *Pharmacology and Therapeutics* 79(1):1-53.

Newton CR, Warrell DA. 1998. Neurological manifestations of falciparum malaria. *Annals of Neurology* 43(6):695-702.

Newton CR, Marsh K, Peshu N, Mwangi I. 1992. Blood transfusions for severe anaemia in African children. *Lancet* 340(8824):917-918.

Nguyen-Dinh P, Greenberg AE, Mann JM, Kabote N, Francis H, Colebunders RL, Huong AY, Quinn TC, Davachi F, Lyamba B. 1987. Absence of association between *Plasmodium falciparum* malaria and Human Immunodeficiency Virus infection in children in Kinshasa, Zaire. *Bulletin of the World Health Organization* 65(5):607-613.

Niyongabo T, Deloron P, Aubry P, Ndarugirire F, Manirakiza F, Muhirwa G, Ndayiragije A, Brelivet JC. 1994. Prognostic indicators in adult cerebral malaria: A study in Burundi, an area of high prevalence of HIV infection. *Acta Tropica* 56(4):299-305.

Nosten F, Ter Kuile F, Maelankiri L, Chongsuphajaisiddhi T, Nopdonrattakoon L, Tangkitchot S, Boudreau E, Bunnag D, White NJ. 1994. Mefloquine prophylaxis prevents malaria during pregnancy: A double-blind, placebo-controlled study. *Journal of Infectious Diseases* 169(3):595-603.

Nosten F, McGready R, Simpson JA, Thwai KL, Balkan S, Cho T, Hkirijaroen L, Looareesuwan S, White NJ. 1999. Effects of *Plasmodium vivax* malaria in pregnancy. *Lancet* 354(9178):546-549.

Nyirjesy P, Kavasya T, Axelrod P, Fischer PR. 1993. Malaria during pregnancy: Neonatal morbidity and mortality and the efficacy of chloroquine chemoprophylaxis. *Clinical Infectious Diseases* 16(1):127-132.

O'Dempsey TJD, McArdle TF, Laurence BE, Lamont AC, Todd JE, Greenwood BM. 1993. Overlap in the clinical features of pneumonia and malaria in African children. *Transactions of the Royal Society of Tropical Medicine and Hygiene* 87(6):662-665.

Otieno GO, Carter J, Mturi N, White S, Newton CJRC. 2002. Electroencephalographic findings post-severe childhood malaria. *The Third MIM Pan-African Malaria Conference—Arusha, Tanzania. Global Advances in Malaria Research: Evidence-Based Decision Making for Malaria Control and Policy* 117, Abstract 168.

Parise ME, Ayisi JG, Nahlen BL, Schultz LJ, Roberts JM, Misore A, Muga R, Oloo AJ, Steketee RW. 1998. Efficacy of sulfadoxine-pyrimethamine for prevention of placental malaria in an area of Kenya with a high prevalence of malaria and Human Immunodeficiency Virus infection. *American Journal of Tropical Medicine and Hygiene* 59(5):813-822.

Pasvol G, Weatherall DJ, Wilson RJ, Smith DH, Gilles HM. 1976. Fetal haemoglobin and malaria. *Lancet* 1(7972):1269-1272.

Piessens WF, Hoffman SL, Wadee AA, Piessens PW, Ratiwayanto S, Kurniawan L, Campbell JR, Marwoto HA, Laughlin LL. 1985. Antibody-mediated killing of suppressor T lymphocytes as a possible cause of macroglobulinemia in the tropical splenomegaly syndrome. *Journal of Clinical Investigation* 75(6):1821-1827.

Pongponratn E, Turner GD, Day NP, Phu NH, Simpson JA, Stepniewska K, Mai NT, Viriyavejakul P, Looareesuwan S, Hien TT, Ferguson DJ, White NJ. 2003. An ultrastructural study of the brain in fatal *Plasmodium falciparum* malaria. *American Journal of Tropical Medicine and Hygiene* 69(4):345-359.

Price RN, Simpson JA, Nosten F, Luxemburger C, Hkirjaroen L, ter Kuile F, Chongsuphajaisiddhi T, White NJ. 2001. Factors contributing to anemia after uncomplicated falciparum malaria. *American Journal of Tropical Medicine and Hygiene* 65(5): 614-622.

Quinn TC, Jacobs RF, Mertz GJ, Hook EW III, Locklsey RM. 1982. Congenital malaria: A report of four cases and a review. *Journal of Pediatrics* 101(2):229-232.

Rihet P, Traore Y, Abel L, Aucan C, Traore-Leroux T, Fumoux F. 1998. Malaria in humans: *Plasmodium falciparum* blood infection levels are linked to chromosome 5q31-Q33. *American Journal of Human Genetics* 63(2):498-505.

Roper C, Elhassan IM, Hviid L, Giha H, Richardson W, Babiker H, Satti GM, Theander TG, Arnot DE. 1996. Detection of very low level *Plasmodium falciparum* infections using the nested polymerase chain reaction and a reassessment of the epidemiology of unstable malaria in Sudan. *American Journal of Tropical Medicine and Hygiene*. 54(4):325-331.

Roper MH, Torres RS, Goicochea CG, Andersen EM, Guarda JS, Calampa C, Hightower AW, Magill AJ. 2000. The epidemiology of malaria in an epidemic area of the Peruvian Amazon. *American Journal of Tropical Medicine and Hygiene* 62(2):247-256.

Ruwende C, Khoo SC, Snow RW, Yates SN, Kwiatkowski D, Gupta S, Warn P, Allsopp CE, Gilbert SC, Peschu N. 1995. Natural selection of hemi- and heterozygotes for G6PD deficiency in Africa by resistance to severe malaria. *Nature* 376(6537):246-249.

Sachdev HS, Mohan M. 1985. Vivax cerebral malaria. *Journal of Tropical Pediatrics* 31(4):213-215.

Scherf A, Pouvelle B, Buffet PA, Gysin J. 2001. Molecular mechanisms of *Plasmodium falciparum* placental adhesion. *Cellular Microbiology* 3(3):125-131.

Schofield L. 2002. Antidisease vaccines. *Chemical Immunology* 80:322-342.

Sharma VP. 1999. Current scenario of malaria in India. *Parassitologia* 41(1-3):349-353.

Shulman CE, Graham WJ, Jilo H, Lowe BS, New L, Obiero J, Snow RW, Marsh K. 1996. Malaria is an important cause of anaemia in primigravidae: Evidence from a district hospital in coastal Kenya. *Transactions of the Royal Society of Tropical Medicine and Hygiene* 90(5):535-539.

Simooya OO, Mwendapole RM, Siziya S, Fleming AF. 1988. Relation between falciparum malaria and HIV seropositivity in Ndola, Zambia. *British Medical Journal* 297(6640):30-31.

Simpson JA, Silamut K, Chotivanich K, Pukrittayakamee S, White NJ. 1999. Red cell selectivity in malaria: A study of multiple-infected erythrocytes. *Transactions of the Royal Society of Tropical Medicine and Hygiene* 93(2):165-168.

Sina B. 2002. Focus on Plasmodium vivax. *Trends in Parasitology* 18(7):287-289.

Singh N, Shukla MM, Sharma VP. 1999. Epidemiology of malaria in pregnancy in central India. *Bulletin of the World Health Organization* 77(7):567-572.

Sleigh AC, Liu XL, Jackson S, Li P, Shang LY. 1998. Resurgence of vivax malaria in Henan Province, China. *Bulletin of the World Health Organization* 76(3):265-270.

Snow RW, Omumbo JA, Lowe B, Molyneux CS, Obiero JO, Palmer A, Weber MW, Pinder M, Nahlen B, Obonyo C, Newbold C, Gupta S, Marsh K. 1997. Relation between severe malaria morbidity in children and level of *Plasmodium falciparum* transmission in Africa. *Lancet* 349(9066):1650-1654.

Steketee RW, Wirima JJ, Bloland PB, Chilima B, Mermin JH, Chitsulo L, Breman JG. 1996a. Impairment of a pregnant woman's acquired ability to limit *Plasmodium falciparum* by infection with Human Immunodeficiency Virus type-1. *American Journal of Tropical Medicine and Hygiene* 55(1 Suppl):42-49.

Steketee RW, Wirima JJ, Slutsker L, Khoromana CO, Breman JG, Heymann DL. 1996b. Objectives and methodology in a study of malaria treatment and prevention in pregnancy in rural Malawi: The Mangochi Malaria Research Project. *American Journal of Tropical Medicine and Hygiene* 55(1 Suppl):8-16.

Sudre P, Breman JG, Koplan JP. 1990. Delphi survey of malaria mortality and drug resistance in Africa. *Lancet* 335(8691):722.

Tanios MA, Kogelman L, McGovern B, Hassoun PM. 2001. Acute respiratory distress syndrome complicating *Plasmodium vivax* malaria. *Critical Care Medicine* 29(3):665-667.

Taylor TE, Molyneux ME. 2002. Clinical features of malaria in children. In: Warrell DA, Gilles HM, eds. *Essential Malariology*. London: Arnold Publishers.

Taylor TE, Molyneux ME, Wirima JJ, Fletcher KA, Morris K. 1988. Blood glucose levels in Malawian children before and during the administration of intravenous quinine for severe falciparum malaria. *New England Journal of Medicine* 319(16):1040-1047.

Taylor TE, Borgstein A, Molyneux ME. 1993. Acid-base status in paediatric *Plasmodium falciparum* malaria. *Quarterly Journal of Medicine* 86(2):99-109.

Torres JR, Perez H, Postigo MM, Silva JR. 1997. Acute non-cardiogenic lung injury in benign tertian malaria. *Lancet* 350(9070):31-32.

Trape JF, Rogier C. 1996. Combatting malaria morbidity and mortality by reducing transmission. *Parasitology Today* 12(6):236-240.

Trape JF, Pison G, Preziosi MP, Enel C, Desgrees du Lou A, Delaunay V, Samb B, Lagarde E, Molez JF, Simondon F. 1998. Impact of chloroquine resistance on malaria mortality. *Comptes Rendus de L'Academie des Sciences—Serie III, Sciences de la Vie* 321(8):689-697.

Tsuchida H, Yamaguchi K, Yamamoto S, Ebisawa I. 1982. Quartan malaria following splenectomy 36 years after infection. *American Journal of Tropical Medicine and Hygiene* 31(1):163-165.

UNICEF. 2002. *State of the World's Children 2003*. New York: UNICEF.

van den Broek NR, White SA, Neilson JP. 1998. The relationship between asymptomatic Human Immunodeficiency Virus infection and the prevalence and severity of anemia in pregnant Malawian women. *American Journal of Tropical Medicine and Hygiene* 59(6):1004-1007.

van Eijk AM, Ayisi JG, ter Kuile FO, Misore A, Otieno JA, Kolczak MS, Kager PA, Steketee RW, Nahlen BL. 2001. Human Immunodeficiency Virus seropositivity and malaria as risk factors for third-trimester anemia in asymptomatic pregnant women in western Kenya. *American Journal of Tropical Medicine and Hygiene* 65(5):623-630.

van Eijk AM, Ayisi JG, ter Kuile FO, Misore AO, Otieno JA, Rosen DH, Kager PA, Steketee RW, Nahlen BL. 2003. HIV increases the risk of malaria in women of all gravidities in Kisumu, Kenya. *AIDS* 17(4):595-603.

Vinetz JM, Li J, McCutchan TF, Kaslow DC. 1998. *Plasmodium malariae* infection in an asymptomatic 74-year-old Greek woman with splenomegaly. *New England Journal of Medicine* 338(6):367-371.

von Seidlein L, Greenwood BM. 2003. Mass administrations of antimalarial drugs. *Trends in Parasitology* 19(10):452-460.

Waller D, Krishna S, Crawley J, Miller K, Nosten F, Chapman D, ter Kuile FO, Craddock C, Berry C, Holloway PA. 1995. Clinical features and outcome of severe malaria in Gambian children. *Clinical Infectious Diseases* 21(3):577-587.

Warrell DA. 1996. Cerebral malaria. In: Shakir RA, Newman PK, Poser CM, eds. *Tropical Neurology.* London: W.B. Saunders.

White NJ. 1996. Malaria. In: Cook GC, ed. *Manson's Tropical Diseases.* 20th ed. London: W.B. Saunders.

White NJ. 1997. Assessment of the pharmacodynamic properties of antimalarial drugs in vivo. *Antimicrobial Agents and Chemotherapy* 41(7):1413-1422.

White NJ, Pongtavornpinyo W. 2003. The de novo selection of drug-resistant malaria parasites. *Proceedings of the Royal Society of London—Series B: Biological Sciences* 270(1514):545-554.

White NJ, Warrell DA, Chanthavanich P, Looareesuwan S, Warrell MJ, Krishna S, Williamson DH, Turner RC. 1983. Severe hypoglycemia and hyperinsulinemia in falciparum malaria. *New England Journal of Medicine* 309(2):61-66.

White NJ, Miller KD, Marsh K, Berry CD, Turner RC, Williamson DH, Brown J. 1987. Hypoglycaemia in African children with severe malaria. *Lancet* 1(8535):708-711.

Whitworth J, Morgan D, Quigley M, Smith A, Mayanja B, Eotu H, Omoding N, Okongo M, Malamba S, Ojwiya A. 2000. Effect of HIV-1 and increasing immunosuppression on malaria parasitaemia and clinical episodes in adults in rural Uganda: A cohort study. *Lancet* 356(9235):1051-1056.

WHO. 2000. Severe falciparum malaria. *Transactions of the Royal Society of Tropical Medicine and Hygiene* 94(Suppl 1):S1-S90.

Zingman BS, Viner BL. 1993. Splenic complications in malaria: Case report and review. *Clinical Infectious Diseases* 16(2):223-232.

7

The Human and Economic
Burden of Malaria

INTRODUCTION

The cost of malaria can be measured in lives lost, in time spent ill with fever, and in economic terms. Money spent on preventing and treating malaria, the indirect costs of lost wages, time home from school, and time spent caring for sick children, adds up at the personal level. In the public sector, large fractions of health sector budgets are spent on malaria control and treatment. And at the macroeconomic level, a heavy national burden of malaria dampens economic development, sometimes subtly, but pervasively. All of these effects are recognized and accepted widely, but their magnitude has been poorly documented.

Studies of the effects of malaria have most often been motivated by a desire to understand the costs of the disease to individuals and society, and frequently to justify public expenditures to diminish the burden. This type of work has only grown in importance, as competition for resources is ever more explicit, both within the spectrum of malaria activities (research vs. control, prevention vs. treatment) and between malaria and other diseases.

THE HEALTH BURDEN OF MALARIA IN AFRICA

In Africa, most people are born, live, and die without leaving a trace in the official record.

Don de Savigny, Tanzania Essential Health Interventions Project

Estimates of Deaths from Malaria

Deaths are not well counted in much of the world, and the situation is worst where people are poorest—which is where malaria takes its greatest toll. This has begun to change—Snow and colleagues (2003) date recognition of the importance of reliable estimates to the World Health Organization's (WHO's) Global Burden of Disease program of the early 1990s—but the figures available are still approximate.

Some 50 years ago, Leonard Bruce-Chwatt estimated the annual African death toll from malaria at one million. The figure was an extrapolation to the continent based on the civil registration of deaths in Lagos in 1950 (Bruce-Chwatt, 1952). Other numbers have been produced since then—between 0.5 million and 2 million deaths per year—using a variety of more and less evidence-based methods (Sturchler, 1989; Greenwood, 1990; WHO, 1996; Schwartlander, 1997). The most plausible current estimates come from Snow and colleagues, and their work on the Burden of Malaria in Africa (BOMA) project (Snow et al., 2003), which builds on the MARA (Mapping Malaria Risk in Africa) risk mapping, as well as mining of a wide range of other data sources. Their best estimate is 1,144,572 deaths attributable directly to malaria in Africa in the year 2000 (Table 7-1).

WHO's most recent estimate of malaria deaths is similar—a worldwide total of 1,124,000 deaths due directly to malaria in 2001, of which about 970,000 would have been in Africa (WHO, 2002). The estimate also includes about 90,000 malaria deaths in Southeast Asia, 56,000 in the Eastern Mediterranean region, 11,000 in the Western Pacific, and about 1,000 in the Americas. While in the same overall range, the estimates do differ in their distribution among age groups: Snow and colleagues figures suggest that about 65 percent of deaths among children under 5, and the corresponding figure from WHO is much higher at 86 percent.

Estimates of Malaria Cases

There are no direct counts of the number of cases of malaria that occur each year. A very wide range of estimates has been made, using a variety of definitions. The lack of precision is problematic for this report, because an estimate of how many courses of malaria treatment are used is needed to estimate how much a global ACT subsidy will cost. The number of cases and the number of treatments are not the same but are related.

Malaria cases may be overestimated because few cases are definitively diagnosed before treatment (whether prescribed or self-selected), so quite a large number of fevers that are not malaria may be counted as such. The number also may be underestimated because people may get no treatment, either through choice or economic default, and in any case, episodes of malaria are not kept track of formally anywhere.

TABLE 7-1 Estimated Malaria-Specific Mortality during 2000, best estimate and IQR range

	0-4 years	5-14 years	15+ years	Total
Southern Africa malaria risk (Class 4)	266 [164–430]	482 [297–779]	1,129 [695–1,824]	1,877 [1,156–3,033]
Rest of Africa— low stable/ epidemic risk (Classes 2+3)	57,688	32,588	49,079	139,355
Rest of Africa— stable endemic risk (Class 4)	684,364 [541,330– 1,068,723]	182,113 [76,072– 319,274]	136,863 [84,399– 214,419]	1,003,340 [701,801– 1,1602,415]
Total	742,318 [541,494– 1,069,153]	214,701 [76,369– 320,053]	187,071 [85,094– 216,253]	1,144,572 [702,957– 1,605,448]

IQR = Interquartile range, which represents the range of values from the 25th percentile to the 75th percentile, essentially the range of the middle 50% of the data. Because it uses the middle 50%, the IQR is not affected by extreme values.

Classification of areas:

   Class 1: no human settlement, or unsuitable climate for malaria transmission.

   Class 2: populations exposed to marginal risks of malaria transmission, uncommon in an average year.

   Class 3: populations exposed to acute seasonal transmission with a tendency toward epidemics.

   Class 4: populations exposed to stable, endemic malaria transmission. In southern Africa (Namibia, Swaziland, South Africa, Botswana, Zimbabwe) Class 4 areas, malaria still poses a risk but its extent and transmission potential are determined by aggressive vector control.

SOURCE: Snow et al. (2003).

Snow and colleagues, using the general pattern of risk and population as they used to estimate deaths for the Disease Control Priorities Project, also estimated the number of malaria episodes likely to occur in Africa in a year (the year 2000). In this case, they used the BOMA database to search for prospective studies of the incidence of fever (i.e., axillary or rectal body temperature $\geq 37.5°$) since the 1980s.[1] Studies were included if they met the following criteria:

---

[1]Prospective studies have been carried out as part of controlled trials or for descriptive purposes. In such studies, a defined population is monitored continuously or periodically.

•　They were cross-sectional studies with at least two rounds of observations on a single cohort to reflect seasonal differences in risk.

•　Subjects were recruited randomly from the community, and not from a clinic population.

•　For cohorts involved in randomized trials, only the control arm participants (i.e., those not receiving a study intervention) were included.

•　Clinical episodes were defined by quantified parasite levels (although levels differed among studies, ranging from 1,000 to 10,000 parasites/μl blood).

Definitions and methods of detection differed among the studies, and it was not possible to standardize them; some lack of comparability and imprecision had to be accepted.

The results are summarized in Table 7-2, ending with a median estimate of 213,549,000 episodes per year in Africa (with the estimate ranging from 134,322,000 to 324,617,000). Among young children in stable endemic areas, data from 28 studies led to a median estimate of 1,424 episodes per 1,000 children each year (i.e., nearly 1.5 episodes per child). The

TABLE 7-2 Estimated Number [IQR] of Clinical Attacks (thousands) of Malaria during 2000

	0-4 years	5-14 years	15+ years	Total
Southern Africa malaria risk (Class 4)	60 [20– 265]	109 [36– 479]	255 [84– 1,122]	424 [140– 1,866]
Rest of Africa— low stable/ epidemic risk (Classes 2+3)	4,007 [2,752– 4,756]	6,310 [4,333– 7,488]	6,291 [4,320– 7,466]	16,608 [11,405– 19,710]
Rest of Africa— stable endemic risk (Class 4)	104,452 [61,468– 158,952]	67,658 [44,145– 112,610]	24,407 [16,880– 31,479]	196,517 [122,493– 303,041]
Totals	108,519 [64,240– 163,982]	74,077 [48,514– 120,577]	30,953 [21,284– 40,067]	213,549 [134,322– 324,617]

SOURCE: Snow et al. (2003).

19 studies that included older children led to an estimate of 587 per 1,000 (on average, about one episode every other year). The median estimate for non-pregnant adults (based on only seven studies) was 107 per 1,000 people each year. Rates in low-transmission and fringe areas were correspondingly lower.

The Effect of Antimalarial Drug Resistance on the Burden of Malaria

Given the fragmentary statistics on malaria morbidity and mortality, it may seem presumptuous to attempt an assessment of how the spread of resistance to chloroquine and sulfadoxine-pyrimethamine (SP) has affected these measures over the past decades. There is, in fact, little direct information on how the number of cases of malaria has changed in the most endemic areas. What has been documented, however, are stark bellwethers of worsening conditions: a well-documented instance is the malaria epidemic of 1999-2000 in KwaZulu Natal, South Africa, which was a direct result of failing antimalarial drugs—SP had a failure rate of 88 percent. Other factors—increased vector resistance to the pyrethroid insecticides that were introduced in 1996, and the reinvasion of the highly anthropophilic *Anopholes funestus* vector—further exacerbated this epidemic (Muheki et al., 2003). The introduction of ACTs (and other control measures) brought the epidemic under control. And the question of changes in mortality has been addressed by thorough reviews of the data that do exist, in two major efforts. The first, the long view across the 20th century, used a variety of historical records from the BOMA project (Snow et al., 2001). The other case is an examination of trends in the 1980s and 1990s on a finer scale, contrasting East and West Africa (Korenromp et al., 2003), using the relatively uniform data reported in African Demographic Surveillance Systems (DSS).

Trends Through the 20th Century

The BOMA project provides the best opportunity to chart malaria's past in Africa, and how drug resistance has affected its course over the final decades of the 20th century. The BOMA project began in 1998 with the aim of assembling in a single database all available evidence on morbidity, disability, and mortality associated with falciparum malaria in Africa, starting as far back as possible. The data come not only from the usual electronic databases, but from hand searches of early, unindexed papers in English and French tropical medicine journals, and a mass of unpublished material from local and regional conference proceedings, libraries, and Ministries of Health records (Snow et al., 2001).

In 2001, Snow and colleagues selected as much information as possible from the BOMA database to inform an analysis of malaria mortality in Africa from 1900 through the 1990s (Snow et al., 2001). They took mortality reports from areas with documented, stable endemic transmission, where the prevalence of parasitemia in children was at least 30 percent, and which had recorded both all-cause mortality and malaria-specific mortality. Thirty-nine studies in 13 countries of sub-Saharan Africa [2] met the criteria, spanning the period from 1912 to 1995. A year-by-year analysis was not possible with these scattered, sparse data. Instead, the time span was divided into three periods, corresponding approximately to changes of probable significance to malaria control. The period before 1960 represents a time of limited access to primary health care and hence, to effective antimalarial drugs. From 1960 until 1990, after the beginning of independence for most countries, health care expanded across Africa and chloroquine became widely available, both from health services and as self-medication. The 1990s saw the widespread emergence of chloroquine resistance in many parts of Africa.

The picture painted by these data suggests a continuing downward trend in *total* child mortality over the three periods, but a downward and then ascending course for *malaria-specific* mortality, with the lowest rates in the middle period, and similar rates pre-1960 and post-1990 (Figure 7-1). With a 34 percent decline in overall mortality from before 1960 into the 1990s, and the fall and rise of malaria death rates into the 1990s, the *proportion* of all deaths due to malaria first fell from 18 percent pre-1960 to 12 percent in 1960-1990 but rose to 30 percent during the 1990s. Snow and colleagues (2001) cite data from Tanzania, Senegal, and Kenya comprising more detailed time series, which are consistent with the findings overall.

The data used to describe these trends, are by their nature, limited and not entirely comparable. The pre-1960 data are mainly from colonial Anglophone Africa, where malaria deaths were tracked through civil notification systems operating in defined populations. The pre-1960 systems probably missed a greater proportion of deaths than the later prospective surveillance studies, which have high rates of ascertainment of the fact of death. However, identification of deaths from "malaria" may actually have been more accurate in the earlier period because deaths often were followed up by a medical officer to determine their cause. The later surveillance systems rely on assigning cause of death retrospectively, mainly through verbal autopsies.

The declines in childhood mortality during the second half of the 20th

---

[2]Senegal, The Gambia, Guinea Bissau, Sierra Leone, Ghana, Nigeria, Benin, Democratic Republic of Congo, Burundi, Uganda, Kenya, Tanzania, and Malawi.

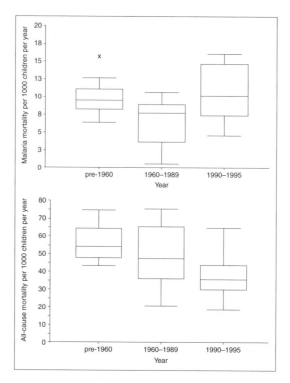

FIGURE 7-1 Malaria mortality and all cause mortality per 1000 children under 5 years in three time periods: pre-1960, 1960–1989, and 1990–1995. Central thick lines represent median estimates, box height represents 25%–75% quartile range, and extensions represent upper and lower confidence intervals.
SOURCES: Trape and Marsh, 2001; Snow, Trape, and Marsh, 2001.

century are well documented and accepted. The biggest declines have been in deaths from diarrheal disease, widely attributed to the development and dissemination of oral rehydration therapy, largely through WHO-sponsored programs. Declines also occurred in deaths from pneumonia and other infectious diseases. The declines are not uniform, and there are even places where trends are reversing in overall child mortality, but by and large, the trends have been positive. Malaria appears to be an exception.

   How can the observed trends in malaria mortality among African children be explained? The positive effects on total mortality are a plausible result of expanded basic health services, including vaccinations, the widespread adoption of oral rehydration therapy, expanded access to antibiotics, and at least in places, improved sanitation and general living conditions. In the mid-20th century, chloroquine would have counted among new beneficial drugs, even in the absence of a major campaign against malaria. The rise in malaria-specific mortality coincides with the spread of chloroquine-resistant strains of falciparum malaria. Although it is virtually impossible to demonstrate a causal link, in the absence of any other compelling reason, chloroquine resistance is the most plausible explanation for the increase.

Trends in the 1980s and 1990s

Resistance to chloroquine first became apparent in Africa in the late 1970s, more than a decade after its appearance in Asia. By 1990, resistant strains had been reported from all the endemic countries in Africa (Trape, 2001). The spread of drug resistance was implicated in the previous section as responsible for reversing the improvement in childhood mortality from malaria. The inference was made because mortality patterns in large population groups coincided with the general patterns of drug resistance, but the measurements of drug resistance were not available to make the link definitive.

There are data—albeit limited—that address the question more directly, although again, not definitively. Trape (2001) identified population- and hospital-based studies that recorded annual malaria mortality in Africa, based on continuous monitoring. He chose for analysis all those that spanned a period during which chloroquine resistance was known to be emerging in that area. Some of the hospital-based studies also had information on the prevalence of severe malaria over time. The remainder of this section is based on Trape's report.

Population-Based Studies

Three studies tracked childhood malaria mortality in populations over the period in which chloroquine resistance emerged, from the mid-1980s to the mid-1990s. All were in Senegal, in different climatic areas: Mlomp area (rain forest), Niakhar area (Sahel), and Bandafassi area (savanna). In all three areas, the malaria mortality rates increased from the early to the later periods (Table 7-3). They more than doubled in all three sites and in Mlomp, increased 10-fold. Over the same period, standardized clinical protocols for assessing drug failures were carried out at least twice. In all cases, the degree of resistance intensified.

In one other place, Bagamoyo, on the Tanzania coast, deaths were investigated in 1984-1985, and again in 1992-1994 (i.e., not continuous, as in Senegal), bounding a period of increasing chloroquine resistance. Overall child mortality remained the same, but the proportion attributed to malaria was twofold higher in the later period.

TABLE 7-3 Childhood Malaria Mortality in Three Sites in Senegal

		Year first CQ therapy failures reported		
Mlomp (hypoendemic)	1985-1989	1990-1992	1993-1995	1990
<5 malaria death rate (per 1,000)	0.5	3.4	5.5	
Resistance from standardized surveys		RII/RIII: 36% (1991)	RII/RIII: 46% (1995)	
Niakhar (mesoendemic)	1984-1991	1992-1995		1992
<10 malaria death rate (per 1,000)	4.0	8.2		
Resistance from standardized surveys		RII/RIII: 10% (1993)	RII/RIII: 29% (1996)	
Bandafassi (holoendemic)	1984-1992	1993-1995		1993
<5 malaria death rate (per 1,000)	4.2	11.4		
Resistance from standardized surveys		RII/RIII: 6% (1994); RII/RIII: 16% (1995)		

SOURCE: Trape, 2001.

Hospital-Based Evidence

Data from hospitals in several countries offer another glimpse at trends in malaria incidence and death, with definite limitations. A hospital population consists only of those who decide—often through a complex decision-making process—to seek care there. Trends in the proportion of people with malaria who go to a hospital may relate to changes in incentives for hospital-based versus other sites of care (e.g., the population may know that hospitals are out of drugs at a particular time, a competing provider may be more attractive, or money for the hospital is unavailable in a given season or year) and changes in the incidence of other diseases, as well as to changes in the epidemiology of malaria. Hospitals also have advantages because of their range of expertise and technologies, and their record keeping.

Malawi. Malawi has national records for hospital admissions and deaths. From 1978 through 1983, the incidence of admissions for malaria for children under 5 years of age more than doubled. Throughout the period, about 5 percent of those children died (Khoromana et al., 1986). The spread of chloroquine resistance in Malawi during this time was well documented.

Tanzania. The mission hospitals in Tanzania recorded steep increases in the proportion of admissions for malaria from 1968 through 1985. In the 1970s, about 10 percent of admissions were for malaria, and by the mid-1980s, had risen to 23 percent (Kilama and Kihamia, 1991). This also coincides with the rapid increase in chloroquine-resistant malaria in Tanzania.

Congo. In the hospital that was the main referral center in Kinshasa, the proportion of overall pediatric admissions for malaria increased each year, from 29.5 percent in 1982, to 56.4 percent in 1986, and the proportion of deaths increased from 4.8 to 15.3 percent over the same period (Greenberg et al., 1989). Again, this was the period during which chloroquine resistance emerged and spread quickly in Kinshasa.

Malaria admissions and deaths at the four hospitals in Brazzaville were studied for the years 1983-1989, during which (in 1985) chloroquine resistance was first detected there. From 1983 through 1986, pediatric admissions for malaria increased from 22 to 54 percent of all pediatric admissions, and then remained stable. Deaths from cerebral malaria more than doubled from the first to the second half of the study period (Carme et al., 1992).

Nigeria. A similar pattern was seen in the pediatric emergency room of Calabar Hospital in Nigeria, where the number of cases of malaria-related convulsions doubled during the years 1986 through 1988. In 81 percent of these cases, chloroquine was ineffective (Asindi et al., 1993).

Other Types of Evidence from Hospital-Based Studies

Various other studies, including one of trends in severe anemia in Kenya, and another of changes in hospital case fatality rates for malaria after a switch from chloroquine to SP, provide corroborating evidence that chloroquine resistance has led to increases in severe malaria and malaria deaths (Trape, 2001).

THE ECONOMIC BURDEN OF MALARIA

It has long been recognized that a malarious community is an impoverished community.

T. H. Weller, Nobel Laureate in Medicine, 1958

> We remain woefully ignorant of the social and economic effect of malaria in those countries of the world where it is prevalent.
>
> Andreano and Helminiak, 1988
>
> . . . from the preventive point of view this [the cost of malaria] is perhaps the most important question before us; because, obviously, it governs the question of the expenditure which may be demanded for the anti-malarial campaign.
>
> Ronald Ross, 1911

The human costs of malaria are high, in lives that are lost and many more that are diminished. The immediate monetary costs of treating and trying to prevent disease are obvious and large, for governments and families. Those costs are far from the whole economic story, though. Malaria's presence has—subtly, and overtly—influenced the nature of economic activities that define levels of development, and ultimately health and wellbeing in the broadest sense. For centuries, malaria's pervasive effects have been recognized, and people have tried to estimate the costs in economic terms (Box 7-1).

Ideally, to understand the influence of malaria, one would start with a top-down approach, deriving dollar figures that represent the aggregate economic effects of malaria in a nation or region—the macroeconomic approach—and then working from the ground up, uncovering the detailed chains of causation leading to various streams of cost—the microeconomic approach. Such a coherent economic picture of the whole and its parts is not what exists today, however. The information is richer in quantity and quality than it was in 1991, when the Institute of Medicine last reported on this topic (IOM, 1991), but the knowledge base remains small compared with the size of the problem.

In fact, it is not only results that are lacking but the methods for generating them. In a recent review of approaches to evaluating the economic burden of malaria, Malaney (2003) observes:

> . . . the state of the art for costing a disease like malaria has not progressed to the point where a dominant paradigm can be said to exist. Rather there are competing schools of thought, each of which directly addresses some piece of the puzzle at the expense of leaving some other aspect of the problem for a competing methodology.

BOX 7-1
Historical Estimates of the Costs of Malaria

In 1911, Sir Ronald Ross proposed to calculate the economic loss to the community based on malaria mortality and morbidity and "the local values of human life and labour at various ages and in various social classes." But even then, Ross wrote that "many such estimates" had already been attempted (Najera and Hempel, 1996). He cited as previous work the calculations of Dr. Bolton, who estimated that hospital, and other direct expenses for malaria were about 2.6 rupees[a] per capita in the island-nation of Mauritius, a total of about one million rupees for the entire population of about 383,000. This figure excluded the indirect costs of illness (Najera and Hempel, 1996). Ross also quoted an estimate from Howard that malaria cost "surely not less than $100,000,000 per year" for the United States in 1909 (Najera and Hempel, 1996).

Sinton examined the costs of malaria "nationally, socially and economically" in India in the 1930s, based on a national malaria survey. He found malaria responsible for at least one million deaths directly, and at least two million if indirect effects were included, based on between 100 million and 200 million cases, with a case fatality rate of 1 percent (Najera and Hempel, 1996). He also was among the earliest to explicitly document areas where malaria prevented expansion of agriculture, with concomitant forgone income (IOM, 1991).

Najera and Hempel (1996) observed:

> The development of health statistics during the 19th century, the economic motivations of the European colonial enterprise, the obvious recognition of malaria as a serious obstacle and the need of important investments for its control, lead to early efforts to define the malaria problem as a burden on society, measurable first in economic terms, such as lost productivity, and later including more general social values, such as learning ability and impact on education.

Perhaps even more obvious than the continual, insidious costs of endemic malaria, the high human and financial costs associated with malaria epidemics have been recognized since antiquity. Organized malaria control was one of the earliest activities of emerging public health services in endemic countries as it became clear that certain human activities, such as rice cultivation, triggered malaria epidemics (Najera and Hempel, 1996).

---

[a]One rupee was worth about 1/15th of a British pound.

Understanding the economic effects of malaria has practical significance for prioritizing overall health spending, and at the program level, for identifying the mix of interventions most likely to benefit people, both in human and economic terms. Not knowing the current costs of malaria—what they represent, and how they are distributed—makes these decisions less certain. And having no baseline hampers an assessment of economic benefits derived from new programs.

Recent Estimates of the Costs of Malaria

The remainder of this chapter describes recent work on defining the economic costs of malaria. The macroeconomic effects—more elusive but unquestionably greater than the aggregate of currently measured microeconomic effects—include economic losses to nations from lack of foreign investment, drains of human capital, and other large-scale effects that hamper overall economic development. The microeconomic costs most often measured include the direct expense, to both government and individuals, of preventing and treating the disease, and the indirect costs of being sick with malaria.

The Effects of Malaria at the Macroeconomic Level

Malaria and poverty occupy common ground. Where the burden of malaria is highest, economic prosperity is lowest. Both are concentrated today in tropical and subtropical zones. Quantifying the relationship between malaria and country-level economics has posed an analytical challenge, first addressed just a few years ago. Analyses approached with several different datasets representing malaria and economic indices confirmed a strong relationship, although the magnitude of effect has varied. A recent review by one of the leaders in the field, Jeffrey Sachs, estimates that the average per-capita gross domestic product (GDP) of malaria-endemic countries in 1995, at about $US1,500 (adjusted for purchasing power parity[3]), was roughly one-fifth the average across the nonmalarious world (Sachs and Malaney, 2002). Annual economic growth in malarious countries between 1965 and 1990 averaged 0.4% of per-capita GDP, compared with 2.3% in the rest of the world, after controlling for the other standard growth determinants used in macroeconomic models. Over the long run, this decrement suggests that malaria could reduce GDP by nearly one-half in highly endemic countries.

These analyses do not constitute proof that malaria is a *cause* of low incomes and poor economic growth, but that the disease must be considered at least a legitimate contributor, and possibly the major contributor. It is true at the microeconomic level that poverty can lead to a heavier burden of malaria, and that malaria can deepen poverty, if a lack of money equals an inability to protect oneself against malaria or to properly treat it. Relationships at the macroeconomic level are real, but—possibly because the

---

[3]Purchasing power parities are derived by pricing a "market basket" of goods in different countries, to adjust for the differences in price. They are used to more accurately compare standards of living across countries, although they also can introduce some distortions in their comparisons.

chains of causation are obscured—easier to dismiss (Sachs and Malaney, 2002). Some of the ways in which malaria may hinder economic development are discussed in the sections that follow. An empirical study of the effect of reducing the numbers of malaria cases and related deaths in Vietnam (Box 7-2) found a generalized positive effect on household living standards (as measured by expenditures), which was greatest for areas with the greatest malaria reductions, and less so for areas with lesser malaria improvement (Laxminarayan, 2003).

Some Pathways Through Which Malaria May Hinder Economic Development

Demographic Effects

The deaths of one million children each year in sub-Saharan Africa affects demographic patterns, directly and indirectly. The direct effects are obvious. Indirectly, they lead to high fertility and large family sizes. Whether to ensure surviving heirs or caretakers for old age, the relationship between high infant and child mortality, and high fertility, is strong. Many children per family means fewer resources—including education, and health care—for each one. Girls often are given lowest priority for education, which adds fuel to the high fertility cycle. Employment choices are limited for women with many children; poorer health resulting from multiple pregnancies also detracts from women's capacity to work. Over the long term, these conditions lead to high costs at the national and family level.

Effects on Human Capital

Infants and children carry the greatest burden of malaria morbidity and mortality. Those who survive may have lasting effects on their physical and mental—hence, economic—potential. The physical and cognitive effects are recognized, though poorly quantified. Even without direct effects of the disease, however, children with malaria lose out by missing school. In the few studies that have examined the relationship, upward of 10 percent (up to 50 percent) of school days lost to illness in sub-Saharan Africa are due to malaria (Sachs and Malaney, 2002). Across a population, this means higher failure rates, higher dropout rates, and poorer achievement. The total decrement in human capital development due to malaria is, however, unknown.

Trade and Foreign Direct Investment

The failure of malarious countries to attract foreign investment has undoubtedly had a major influence on economic development. As with

---

BOX 7-2
Does Reducing Malaria Improve Household Living Standards?

During the 1990s the government of Vietnam invested in malaria control mainly through insecticide, re-treatment of bednets, and by providing effective treatment for clinical episodes. The result was a dramatic overall decline in cases of malaria, but varying in magnitude among areas. Laxminarayan (2003) recognized this as a "natural experiment," to see whether the malaria declines in each province could be related to subsequent improvements in living standards for the province as a whole (not only among the households that had experienced malaria recently). Specifically, he related changes in malaria incidence at the provincial level to changes in household living standards in that province over a 6-year period (controlling for other household characteristics). The "panel approach" design was meant to minimize the effect of unobserved variables on the results.

Household living standards were based on a measure of household consumption, extracted from the Vietnam Living Standards Surveys (VLSS) for 1992-93 and 1997-98. The 1992-93 survey included 4,800 households and 23,839 individuals, and the later survey 6,000 households and 28,518 individuals, sampled from across the country. The study was based on the roughly 4,300 households and 18,000 individuals surveyed in both periods. Province-level data were used for the numbers of malaria cases, malaria deaths, and population size.

Between the two periods, malaria incidence declined by 68 percent averaged over the country, and malaria mortality declined, on average, by 91 percent across the country, varying by province. Incidence in the earlier period ranged from roughly 1 percent to 16 percent among geographic regions. In the later period, malaria had been virtually eliminated in some areas, and was down to about 5 percent in the Central Highlands, the area with the highest incidence earlier. This trend reinforces that the study was not simply capturing the benefits of saving money not spent directly on malaria, since most households were unlikely to experience even a single episode in a given year.

Results

For all households in the sample, a 10 percent decrease in malaria cases at the provincial level resulted in a 0.3 percent increase in consumption ($p<0.001$).[a] Poorer households were likely to benefit more, so a convergence in the consump-

---

other macroeconomic effects, it is impossible to estimate the size of the effect, but examples of the problems malaria brings to projects are well known. At an aluminum smelter built recently in Mozambique by a British corporation (Billiton) which invested US$1.4 billion, the first 2 years of operation saw 13 malaria-related deaths among expatriate employees and 7,000 cases of malaria (Sachs and Malaney, 2002). The tourist trade also can be a casualty of endemic malaria. In general, malaria confines both the domestic and foreign workforce, which constrains development.

tion data was noted. In terms of household health expenditures, a 10 percent decrease in malaria cases translated to a 0.63 percent decrease (average US$0.16 per household). Poorer households did not see significant savings, consistent with their lower use of health services to begin with. Wealthier households had the greatest declines in health expenditures.

Discussion

The 1990s were a period of increasing prosperity in Vietnam, but by and large, the rapid gains against malaria can be attributed to government programs. Between 1991 and 1998, the number of people sleeping under insecticide-treated bednets increased from 300,000 to about 10.8 million. In the clinics, artemisinin-based antimalarials replaced failing chloroquine and SP. These measures cost the central and local governments a total of US$28 million between 1991 and 1997. Were these investments worthwhile?

There were about 850,000 fewer cases of malaria annually in 1997-98 than in 1992-93. At a cost to the government of about US$11 for a clinic visit plus drugs (1998 costs) to treat an episode, the direct costs saved were about US$9.5 million, which is about twice the amount spent on malaria control each year. To this is added about US$14 million in reduced out-of-pocket health care costs to households.

The study was designed to look beyond these direct expenditures, however, at the generalized effect of freeing people from malaria. Accordingly, the 60 percent decline in malaria cases was associated with a 1.8 percent increase in annual household consumption. Applied nationwide, this amounts to a US$12.60 benefit to each household, for an aggregate benefit of US$183 million each year. The study demonstrates that households in areas with the greatest declines in malaria benefited to a greater extent than households where the decline was smaller.

Looking only at the direct costs of preventing and treating malaria appears to grossly underestimate the overall effect of the disease, and the extent to which controlling it benefits people. Even if some of the benefit observed in this study resulted from other factors that were not measured, a large share is almost certainly due to the generalized effects of malaria control.

---

*a*See original paper for details of the analyses.

Microeconomic Studies of the Effect of Malaria[4]

Most microeconomic studies of malaria use the "human capital" approach, which involves tallying the apparent costs of malaria borne privately by individuals and their families, by various levels of government,

---

[4]Much of this section is based on a paper by Chima and colleagues (Chima et al., 2003), which reviews recent studies. The authors converted all costs to 1999 values for purposes of comparability, and these also are reported here.

and by other providers of services (e.g., nongovernmental organizations of various kinds, organizations financing malaria programs). Other methods to get at the costs of malaria are possible, including the "willingness-to-pay" approach, an example of which is described later in this section.

In the human capital approach, the immediate costs of treating or preventing an episode of illness consist of the "direct" costs—money spent for malaria prevention and treatment, including, for example, the cost of bednets and mosquito repellents in the first instance, and of consulting a health provider, buying drugs, and paying for transportation, in the second. Indirect costs represent loss of income (or productive labor, even if the benefits are not monetized, e.g., lost agricultural production because of an inability to plant or harvest crops) due to illness. Indirect costs also include periods of being too sick to work, time spent caring for others who are sick, and time spent seeking care. Some drawbacks of the method, as used, are discussed after a review of the findings of recent studies.

Direct Costs

Household Expenditures on Prevention   Households and health services are the usual focus in studies of spending on the prevention and treatment of malaria. Households purchase prevention items such as mosquito coils, sprays and repellents, and bednets (with or without insecticide treatment), although these items also are desired for nuisance insect control and not just malaria prevention. Expenditures for these items have been studied in a few places, and range, per month, from US$0.05 per person in rural Malawi (Ettling et al., 1994) to US$2.10 per person in urban Cameroon (equivalent to a range of US$0.24 to US$15 per household) (Desfontaine et al., 1989). These average values mask tremendous variation across time and populations. Not surprisingly, studies have shown that expenditures are strongly correlated with income, and that the lowest income households spend the least. In one study in Malawi, 4 percent of very low-income households spent any money at all on malaria prevention, compared with 16 percent of other households (Ettling et al., 1994).

Household Expenditures on Treatment   Malaria treatment can incur expenditures for consultation fees, drugs, transportation to health facilities, and, in some cases, the cost of staying at the facility, for patient and family member. A few studies document the monthly expenditures for treatment, ranging from US$0.41 (all of Malawi) (Ettling et al., 1994) to US$3.88 per person (urban Cameroon) (equivalent to a range of US$1.88 to US$26 per household) (Desfontaine et al., 1989). What evidence exists suggests that expenditures consume a much larger proportion of income in poorer households. In Malawi in the early 1990s, the direct costs of malaria treatment amounted to 28 percent of household income for very low-income house-holds, and 2 percent for the rest (Ettling et al., 1994).

Government Expenditures on Prevention and Treatment   Little informa-tion exists on levels of public spending for malaria prevention and treat-ment. Health care budgets, of course, are not developed for specific dis-eases, and no specific studies of overall public spending for malaria appear to have been done. There are, however, indicators of how much malaria costs, at least in relative terms. About 20-40 percent of all outpatient visits in sub-Saharan Africa are for "fever," a substantial (but varying) fraction of which is malaria. And 0.5 to 50 percent of all inpatients in different settings have been found to have malaria. The total resources consumed are sub-stantial, even if they are not easily quantified.

Indirect Costs

When people are too sick to work, or their work capacity is reduced by illness, there are economic consequences: wage earners are paid less; agri-culturists may produce less (particularly if illness coincides with the har-vest); sick children themselves cannot work (even some very young children work) and may cause parents to lose work time. Deaths from malaria also have clear economic consequences. The death of an adult has obvious economic consequences, leaving families without needed resources. The death of a child involves a different set of economic losses. Illness and death from malaria diminish the stock of "human capital" in many ways. Conly (1975) conducted what is considered a classic study of the effect of malaria on agricultural settlers in Paraguay, finding major effects on the productiv-ity of families (Box 7-3).

Studies of the indirect costs of illness vary in their methods, and in what is included as time lost. Although some include only time spent seeking treatment, most include some period of morbidity; some also include the costs of mortality (lifetime lost income) (Table 7-4). The value placed on lost time also varies among studies (as it does in life), but in all cases, simplifying assumptions are made to try to capture average experience, generally by age group. In the relatively few studies that attempted to calculate indirect costs of malaria, the cost for each episode ranges from US$0.68 for children under 10 years of age in Malawi (Ettling et al., 1994) to US$23 for an adult in Ethiopia (Cropper et al., 1999).

Total Direct and Indirect Costs

A few researchers have estimated "total" costs of malaria. One of the earliest studies, published in 1966, estimated the total cost of malaria in

BOX 7-3
Conly's Classic Microeconomic Study in Paraguay[a]

In the early 1970s, Conly spent 22 months in the field observing and recording data on malaria (and health more generally), work of all kinds, and finances among farmers in Paraguay in newly-settled areas (Conly, 1975). She divided the families into three groups: "little malaria," "moderate-incidence," and "much malaria." The divisions, to a great extent, reflected immune status, with the "much malaria" families being the most recently arrived from nonmalarious areas, and thus most vulnerable immunologically in all age groups.

Conly found immediate effects of malaria on the work a family was able to do, as well as more far-reaching effects. During the period of illness, agricultural labor input declined, crops were neglected, and work done was less efficient than when people were well. In many cases, families were able to make up the lost work, and harvests did not suffer. But she also demonstrated that the threat of malaria caused families to shift from more labor-intensive (and valuable) crops to less labor-intensive ones, to minimize the risk of loss in case malaria kept family members from working at key times, particularly during the harvest.

Conly describes the effects on "much malaria" families during their first year of farming:

> These farmers, even after making use of all available hands, skilled or not, were unable to do enough even to protect their immediate returns. It was not merely a matter of letting the condition of the farm deteriorate in a way that would mean much catching up later on: it was a question of losing crops that had been planted, of not being able to stop the weeds from stunting and choking the growing crops, of being unable to strip off the tobacco leaves at the right moment or get the burst of pods of cotton in before the rain. . . . In the intervals between bouts of illness these farmers—and their wives, children, parents and other relatives as well—worked long hours, but their yields at harvest time . . . were 36 percent lower than they should have been.

By the second year, they began to adapt their farming in various ways and no doubt, also acquired some immunity to malaria, which would have protected at least some individuals from the debilitating episodes of the first year.

This study has the strength of collecting data continuously over nearly two years. Most subsequent work has been based on shorter periods, and on individuals' recall of illness episodes and their consequences.

---

[a] This description of Conly's work is taken from Gomes (1993).

Pakistan (Khan, 1966), based on approximately 4.2 million people experiencing malaria per year, of whom 2.5 million were assumed to be workers. The costs included direct costs of treatment for everyone plus lost workdays (valued at an average daily wage rate) for the workers. This totaled to 81 million rupees, which was about 0.75 percent of GNP.

Two studies have estimated total household direct and indirect costs. In Malawi, the total annual household cost was estimated at about US$40, which was 7 percent of household income (Ettling et al., 1994). Total household costs were estimated at 9-18 percent of annual income for small farmers in Kenya, and 7-13 percent in Nigeria (Leighton and Foster, 1993).

One multicountry study has attempted an Africa-wide estimate of direct plus indirect costs of malaria based on extrapolations from four case studies of areas in Burkina Faso, Chad, Congo, and Rwanda. The totals reported were US$1,064 million overall, which translates to US$3.15 per capita and 0.6 percent of total sub-Saharan Africa GDP (in 1987, inflated to 1999 U.S. dollars) (Shepard et al., 1991). Two of the country case studies estimated household plus government costs (including the direct costs of treatment, but not prevention; and including indirect mortality costs). The national cost per capita was estimated at US$1.55 in Burkina Faso (Sauerborn et al., 1991), and US$3.87 in Rwanda (Ettling and Shepard, 1991), figures that were roughly equivalent to 3.5 days of individual production.

Drawbacks of the Human Capital Method for Estimating Costs of Malaria

The studies reported here vary widely in the details of the methodology, their sources of data, and in their perspectives. Comprehensive studies of this type are difficult to conceive and to carry out, given inherent limits on data available in the places most affected, general difficulties in carrying out research in such places, and a lack of funding for such studies. Even when done well, however, the methods often require assumptions about such things as employment levels (which affect whether wages are actually lost), the value of leisure time, and substitutability of work by other families. Some of the aspects not generally captured by the human capital method relate to coping strategies adopted by families, which affect their economic well-being in ways not usually measured through direct and indirect costs usually measured.

Coping Strategies with Effects Not Captured by the Human Capital Method

In addition to paying for malaria prevention and treatment with cash-on-hand, and losing wages and other productive labor, families cope with malaria in ways that diminish their overall economic wellbeing. They respond not only to actual episodes of illness, but to the risk of illness with "anticipatory" coping strategies. These are often ignored in quantitative analyses because they may be hidden, and are at best, difficult to quantify.

Families faced with paying extraordinary costs for malaria treatment may:

TABLE 7-4 Calculations of Productivity Costs of Morbidity from a
Malaria Episode Using the Wage Rate Method

Authors	Country	Method of Valuing Time
Atkins (1995)	The Gambia	Marginal value of work time on crops cultivated by women
Asenso-Okeyre et al (1997)	Ghana	Average agricultural wage differential by age and gender
Bruce-Chwatt (1963)	Nigeria (psychiatric patients, Lagos)	–
Cropper et al. (1999)	Ethiopia	50% or 100% of the average daily wage
Ettling et al. (1991)	Rwanda	85% of average rural wage
Ettling et al. (1994)	Malawi	Mean per capita income from household survey
Gazin et al. (1988)	Burkina Faso (factory)	–
Guiguemde et al. (1997)	Burkina Faso	Mean annual income per worker by occupational group and age
Leighton and Foster (1993)	Kenya	Weighted average wage rate in agricultural, service and industrial sectors
Leighton and Foster (1993)	Nigeria	Weighted average wage rate in agricultural, service and industrial sectors
Miller (1958)	West African men	–
Nur and Mahran (1988)	Gezira, Sudan	–
Sauerborn et al. (1991)	Burkina Faso	Market value of average output per person for main produce in each of three seasons

SOURCE: Chima et al., 2003.

Time Lost per Episode by Sick Adult	Time Lost per Episode by Carrier or Sick Child	Average Indirect Cost per Episode (1999 US$)
–	2.16 h per day per child for 4 days plus time lost seeking treatment	–
5 days	5 days	57.63
2.6 days (untreated)	–	–
18 days (total of 21 days lost, taking account of labor substitution)	2 days (total of 12 days lost, taking account of labor substitution)	$6–23 for adults & teenagers; $3–12 for children (including net effects of labor substitution)
1 day for each hospitalized day plus 3 additional days	1 day for each hospitalized day plus 1 additional day	–
2.7 days	1.2 days	$1.54 for patients over 10 years of age; $0.68 for patients age 10 and under
3.5 days	–	–
4 days (all ages; 73% were <5)	1.2 days	$4.21
2–4 days (plus allowance for lower productivity for 2 days)	2–4 days	–
1–3 days (plus allowance for lower productivity for 2 days)	2–4 days	–
4.2 days per episode	–	–
6 days of disability, plus 5 at 50% productivity		–
Mild illness 1 day; severe 5 days	1/3 of adult illness time	$0.73

- deplete savings;
- sell assets important to the household asset base, e.g., livestock;
- receive cash gifts from family and friends; or
- take out loans, which can lead to serious debt.

When a family member is sick with malaria, other family or community members may compensate for the loss of work time. Where unemployment or underemployment is common, the loss may be fully compensated without difficulty, so the economic loss might be less than otherwise estimated. This is particularly true in agricultural and other nonwage communal settings, but can even be the case for wage laborers whose family members substitute for them. On the other hand, the family of a small-scale farmer who falls ill may not be able to complete the work he would have done. In any case where children are substituting for adult laborers, they also may lose time from school, which is rarely quantified.

The anticipatory coping strategies are more subtle, but can have major economic consequences. In a labor market where illness is common, these may include limiting staff specialization or maintaining labor reserves to ensure a sufficient workforce, both of which reduce overall average productivity.

Families may limit their investments to maintain cash for malaria emergencies, or invest in assets that can be easily turned into cash. Families also may modify their farming practices, to avoid crops that require intensive work during the high-transmission seasons. Another family coping strategy is having larger numbers of children to ensure that a reasonable number will survive, with all of the obvious and subtle economic consequences entailed.

Malaney (Malaney, 2003) observes that the human capital approach "strains under the weight of a disease that affects entire societies on an effectively permanent basis," a context for which these methods were not originally designed. But she also proposes ways of beginning to broaden the human capital approach to integrate these effects.

The Willingness-to-Pay Approach to Disease Valuation

Individuals and families regularly make decisions with economic consequences, like deciding to seek treatment for disease as opposed to watching and waiting, deciding whether or not to buy a bednet to prevent malaria, and deciding to plant one crop versus another with different labor requirements and different economic yield when harvested. Clearly, economic realities constrain these decisions, although some are forced upon families, such as a child in convulsions, who must be given attention.

The willingness-to-pay approach attempts to estimate the costs of disease by determining the value people would place on avoiding it. The assumption is that this approach would incorporate the burden of treatment and prevention, of lost productivity, lost leisure time, and the value of not having to cope with malaria in other ways. But the way in which this valuation happens is subject to individual interpretation, and assumes that people's economic choices are rational and related to costs and other consequences. Nonetheless, the amount people are willing to pay to avoid disease—if captured in a reliable way—is a useful measure of how important the disease is, and can help make it a priority for public policy.

Studies of this type are very difficult to carry out reliably. The study described here is one of the few examples in malaria.

The Tigray Study

Malaria is endemic to the Tigray region of northern Ethiopia, with seasonal transmission throughout the rainy season (June through September), peaking toward the end of it (October and November). Malaria is a visible health problem to those who live there. The government encourages community control measures (mainly limiting mosquito breeding sites). It also carries out spraying, and trains community health workers to recognize and treat malaria.

Cropper and her colleagues studied the monetary value that households in Tigray place on preventing malaria through a "willingness-to-pay" scenario. They also made conventional "cost of illness" estimates for malaria (direct and indirect costs), in order to compare those figures with how much people were willing to pay to prevent malaria. If accurate, the amount that people are willing to pay to prevent malaria would capture the value placed on the economic losses as well as the pain and suffering caused by malaria, within the financial means of real families.

Study Design

The survey took place in January 1997 in the Tembien sector of Tigray region, where most people live by subsistence agriculture, plus some income from livestock. One person in each participating household (selection of survey households is described below) was interviewed with a three-part questionnaire. The first and third parts were the same everywhere: first, a "cost-of-illness" section with questions about the household's current health status, knowledge of malaria, and expenditures on malaria prevention and treatment, mainly in the previous 2 years. The other constant section asked about socioeconomic characteristics of the household and its members, including education, income, assets, occupation, and housing construction. The middle section measured willingness to pay, with questions that varied in order to build a coherent story. To do this, respondents were introduced to one of two scenarios: one regarding a hypothetical malaria vaccine that would prevent the disease entirely for one year, and the other, about bednets. For each scenario, a respondent was asked whether they would buy the intervention (the vaccine or the bednet) at a given price, and how many they would buy, recognizing that a dose of vaccine would protect one person, and a single bednet could be used for one or more people. The price each respondent was given for the intervention was one of five, assigned randomly, so that estimates could be made about the effect of price on willingness to pay.

Eighteen study villages were chosen (to represent a range of malaria incidence), and randomly assigned either the vaccine (12 villages) or the bednet (six villages) scenario. The target was to interview one respondent in 50 households chosen in each village (although it was not possible to select random samples of households because of a lack of records, the sampling method appears to have been unbiased). Of the intended 900 interviews, 889 were completed but 41 were dropped from the sample because the respondent was not familiar with malaria. This left 569 in the vaccine sample (about 114 for each of the five price levels) and 279 in the bednet sample (about 56 for each price level).

Results

Malaria and the Cost of Illness   Malaria was common. More than half of the respondents (58 percent) reported having malaria in the previous 2 years; in half of the households, another adult (besides the respondent) had had malaria, and in half, a child or teenager had had malaria. Using the detailed information collected on these episodes, the costs of malaria per episode and per household were calculated (Table 7-5). Direct costs to the household included out-of-pocket expenditures to see a health practitioner, buy medicines, and pay for transportation, amounting to about US$1.60 for an adult episode, and about half that for a child. Indirect costs of illness are based on productive time lost by patients themselves, other family members caring for patients, and family members substituting for patients at their work. The average adult loss per episode was 21 days. Dollar values were assigned to the days lost, for adults, equivalent to the average daily wage for a healthy, unskilled worker. Under the "high productivity" assumption this amounted to US$24 for an adult, and under the "low productivity" assumption, half that amount. The rates for teenagers were half the adult rates, and for children, one quarter.

Willingness to Pay to Prevent Malaria   As would be expected, for both the hypothetical vaccine and bednets, the lower the price offered to respon-

TABLE 7-5 Cost of Malaria to Households in Tigray, Ethiopia

| Age Group | Direct Costs (1997 US$) | | | Indirect Costs | | Average Cost (1997 US$)[d] | Total Annual Costs (1997 US$) | |
	Consult[a]	Medicine[b]	Transport	Total Direct	Workdays Lost[c]		High Prod	Low Prod
Adults	1.30	.20	.10	1.60	21	7-24		
Teenagers	.80	.20	.04	1.10	26	7-23		
Children	.60	.20	.02	.82	12	4-12		
Household							31	9

[a]Out-of-pocket costs to see a practitioner.
[b]Out-of pocket costs of medicines.
[c]Average number of days of productivity loss per episode.
[d]Average cost of illness per episode, using high- and low-productivity assumptions.
SOURCE: Cropper et al. (1999).

dents, the more said they would buy, and the number they would buy was greater the lower the price (keeping in mind that each respondent was offered the intervention at one specific price). For vaccines, at the lowest price offered (US$0.80), three-quarters of households would buy at least one dose, but at the highest price (US$32), only 10 would buy at least one. For bednets, at the lowest price (US$1.30), about 80 percent of households would acquire at least one, and at the highest price (US$16), about 40 percent.

These results were compared with the cost-of-illness figures using three different models (see original paper for details), with similar results: people appear to be willing to pay about three times the annual cost of illness for total malaria prevention (the vaccine). For partial prevention (bednets), willingness to pay was less, about 72 percent of the value for vaccines.

Comments

People living in malarious areas are willing to spend dearly—according to this study, about 15 percent of their annual household income—to prevent malaria. This is two to three times the expected annual economic losses per household from malaria (and this does not count the amount spent by government). The amount itself does not necessarily have an economic basis, but it makes clear that people view malaria as much more than simply the sum of its obvious economic consequences, which themselves are substantial.

Summing Up

The "true" economic costs of malaria are undeniably large, but just how large is not known. Admittedly, the information base is small, which accounts for part of the problem, but the methods themselves are not as well developed as needed. Adding up all of the effects from the best microeconomic studies using the human capital method, the totals do not begin to approach the magnitude of effect seen with top-down macroeconomic approaches. The human capital method, as practiced, underestimates costs in ways that are identifiable, as well as some that have yet to be defined. With macroeconomic methods, it is impossible to know whether other factors, inadequately controlled for, are inflating the numbers.

Understanding both the magnitude of malaria's economic effects as well as its operative pathways will accomplish two goals. It will better place malaria in its appropriate economic context and it will improve strategies by which to combat it.

REFERENCES

Asenso-Okyere WK, and Dzator JA. 1997. Household cost of seeking malaria care. A retrospective study of two districts in Ghana. *Social Science and Medicine* 45(5):659-667.

Asindi AA, Ekanem EE, Ibia EO, Nwangwa MA. 1993. Upsurge of malaria-related convulsions in a paediatric emergency room in Nigeria. Consequence of emergence of chloroquine-resistant *Plasmodium falciparum. Tropical and Geographical Medicine* 45(3):110-113.

Bruce-Chwatt LJ. 1952. Malaria in African infants and children in southern Nigeria. *Annals of Tropical Medicine and Parasitology* 46:173-200.

Bruce-Chwatt LJ. 1963. A longitudinal survey of natural malaria infection in a group of West African adults, Parts I & II. *West African Medical Journal* 12:141-173, 199-217.

Carme B, Yombi B, Bouquety JC, Plassard H, Nzingoula S, Senga J, Akani I. 1992. Child morbidity and mortality due to cerebral malaria in Brazzaville, Congo. A retrospective and prospective hospital-based study, 1983-1989. *Tropical Medicine and Parasitology* 43(3):173-176.

Chima RI, Goodman CA, Mills A. 2003. The economic impact of malaria in Africa: A critical review of the evidence. *Health Policy* 63(1):17-36.

Conly, G. 1975. *The Impact of Malaria on Economic Development: A Case Study.* Washington, DC: Pan American Health Organization.

Cropper ML, Haile MLJA, Poulos C, Whittington D. 1999. *The Value of Preventing Malaria in Tembien, Ethiopia, Working Paper.* Washington, DC: The World Bank.

Desfontaine M, Gelas H, Goghomu A, Kouka-Bemba D, Carnevale P. 1989. Evaluation of practices and costs of vector control at the family level in central Africa, I. Yaounde City (March 1988). [French]. *Bulletin de la Societe de Pathologie Exotique et de Ses Filiales* 82(4):558-565.

Ettling M, McFarland DA, Schultz LJ, Chitsulo L. 1994. Economic impact of malaria in Malawian households. *Tropical Medicine and Parasitology* 45(1):74-79.

Ettling MB, Shepard DS. 1991. Economic cost of malaria in Rwanda. *Tropical Medicine and Parasitology* 42(3):214-218.

Gallup JL, Sachs JD. 2001. The economic burden of malaria. *American Journal of Tropical Medicine and Hygiene* 64(1-2 Suppl):85-96.

Gazin P, Freier C, Turk P, Gineste B, Carnevale P. 1988. [Malaria in employees of an African industrial enterprise (Bobo Dioulasso, Burkina Faso)]. [French]. *Annales de la Societe Belge de Medecine Tropicale* 68(4):285-292.

Gomes M. 1993. Economic and demographic research on malaria: A review of the evidence. *Social Science and Medicine* 37(9):1093-1108.

Greenberg AE, Ntumbanzondo M, Ntula N, Mawa L, Howell J, Davachi F. 1989. Hospital-based surveillance of malaria-related paediatric morbidity and mortality in Kinshasa, Zaire. *Bulletin of the World Health Organization* 67(2):189-196.

Greenwood BM. 1990. Populations at risk. *Parasitology Today* 6(6):188.

Guiguemde TR, Coulibaly N, Coulibaly SO, Quedraogo JB, Gbary AR. 1997. A precise method to estimate the cost of malaria: The application to a rural area in Burkina Faso (West Africa). [French]. *Tropical Medicine and International Health* 2(7):646-653.

IOM (Institute of Medicine). 1991. *Malaria: Obstacles and Opportunities.* Oakes SC, Mitchell VS, Pearson GW, Carpenter CCJ, eds. Washington, DC: National Academy Press.

Khan MJ. 1966. Estimate of economic loss due to malaria in West Pakistan. *Pakistan Journal of Health* 16:187-193.

Khoromana CH, Campbell CC, Wirima JJ, Heymann DL. 1986. In vivo efficacy of chloroquine treatment for *Plasmodium falciparum* in Malawian children under five years of age. *American Journal of Tropical Medicine and Hygiene* 35(3):465-471.

Kilama WL, Kihamia CM. 1991. Malaria. In: Mwaluko GMP, Kilama WL, Mandara MP, Muru M, Macpherson CNL, eds. *Health and Diseases in Tanzania*. London: Harper Collins Academic.

Korenromp EL, Williams BG, Gouws E, Dye C, Snow RW. 2003. Measurement of trends in childhood malaria mortality in Africa: An assessment of progress toward targets based on verbal autopsy. *The Lancet Infectious Diseases* 3(6):349-358.

Laxminarayan R. 2004. Does reducing malaria improve household living standards? *Tropical Medicine and International Health* 9(2):267-272.

Leighton C, Foster R. 1993. *Economic Impacts of Malaria in Kenya and Nigeria*. Bethesda, MD: Abt Associates.

Malaney P. 2003. *Micro-Economic Approaches to Evaluating the Burden of Malaria*. CID Working Paper No. 99 ed. Boston: Center for International Development at Harvard University.

Miller MJ. 1958. Observations of the natural history of malaria in the semi-resistant West African. *Transactions of the Royal Society of Tropical Medicine and Hygiene* 52(2):152-168.

Muheki C, Barnes K, McIntyre D. 2003. *Economic Evaluation of Recent Malaria Control Interventions in KwaZulu Natal, South Africa: SEACAT Evaluation*. Cape Town: SEACAT.

Najera JA, Hempel J. 1996. *The Burden of Malaria*. CTD/MAL/96.10th ed. Geneva: World Health Organization.

Sachs J, Malaney P. 2002. The economic and social burden of malaria. *Nature* 415(6872):680-685.

Sauerborn R, Shepard DS, Ettling MB, Brinkmann U, Nougtara A, Diesfeld HJ. 1991. Estimating the direct and indirect economic costs of malaria in a rural district of Burkina Faso. *Tropical Medicine and Parasitology* 42(3):219-223.

Schwartlander B. 1997. Global burden of disease [letter]. *Lancet* 350(9071):141-142.

Shepard DS, Ettling MB, Brinkmann U, Sauerborn R. 1991. The economic cost of malaria in Africa. *Tropical Medicine and Parasitology* 42(3):199-203.

Snow RW, Trape JF, Marsh K. 2001. The past, present and future of childhood malaria mortality in Africa. *Trends in Parasitology* 17(12):593-597.

Snow RW, Craig MH, Newton CRJC, Steketee RW. 2003. *The Public Health Burden of Plasmodium Falciparum Malaria in Africa: Deriving the Numbers*. Bethesda, MD: Disease Control Priorities Project.

Sturchler D. 1989. Estimates of malaria incidence: Reply. *Parasitology Today* 5(12):384.

Trape JF. 2001. The public health impact of chloroquine resistance in Africa. *American Journal of Tropical Medicine and Hygiene* 64(1-2 Suppl):12-17.

WHO (World Health Organization). 1996. *Investing in Health Research and Development: Report of the Ad Hoc Committee on Health Research Relating to Future Intervention Options. TDR/Gen/96.1*. Geneva: World Health Organization.

WHO. 2002. *World Health Report 2002*. Geneva: World Health Organization.

8

Malaria Control

INTRODUCTION

This chapter reviews malaria control over the last century, tracking malaria's retreat from much of the world to its current lines of demarcation. It also describes individual control methods targeting both the mosquito vector and the human reservoir of infection and the current status of diagnosis and vaccine development. The chapter concludes with a discussion of malaria control *strategies*, including national and regional policies and programs operating today.

HISTORICAL OVERVIEW

Historically, malaria's reach extended far beyond the tropics. Until the 19th century, transmission occurred in much of the temperate world, including parts of England, Holland, Germany, central and southeastern Europe, Asia, India, China, and the Americas (Shiff, 2002). In North America, the disease reached as far north as New York, and even Montreal (Barber, 1929). In the early 20th century, the Tennessee Valley Authority brought hydroelectric power to the southeastern United States, modernizing the region. As housing and lifestyles improved, and the human reservoir of infection decreased, malaria retreated (Desowitz, 1999). Malaria also disappeared during the first half of the 20th century from most of Europe following changes in land use, agricultural practices, house construction, and targeted vector control (Greenwood and Mutabingwa, 2002).

Then came the golden days of DDT, a highly effective insecticide first used as a delousing agent at the end of World War II. During the 1950s and 1960s, indoor residual spraying with DDT was the centerpiece of global malaria eradication efforts. DDT's months-long ability to kill or deter adult female mosquitoes resting on treated walls after feeding led to further declines in malaria in India, Sri Lanka, the former Soviet Union, and other countries. By 1966, campaigns using DDT spraying, elimination of mosquito breeding sites, and mass treatment had freed more than 500 million people (roughly one-third of the population previously living in malarious areas) from the threat of disease (Shiff, 2002). Unfortunately, eradication was not sustained due to high program costs, community resistance to repeated house spraying, and the emergence of resistance to DDT. By the late 1960s, the hope of eradicating malaria through vector control was finally abandoned (Guerin et al., 2002). In many countries, the pendulum then swung to overreliance on chloroquine, a widely available antimalarial drug.

Sub-Saharan Africa was always a special case. With the exception of a few pilot programs, no sustained malaria control efforts were ever mounted there (Greenwood and Mutabingwa, 2002). The biggest obstacle was the widespread distribution of *Anopheles gambiae*, a long-lived and aggressive malaria vector. The entomological inoculation rate (EIR) (which measures the frequency with which a human is bitten by an infectious mosquito) rarely exceeds five per year in Asia or South America. In contrast, EIRs of over 1,000 have been recorded in several parts of sub-Saharan Africa (Greenwood and Mutabingwa, 2002).

Today, the global burden of malaria is concentrated in sub-Saharan Africa where stable, endemic disease is linked to poverty and highly efficient vectors. The insecticide-treated bednet (ITN)—first shown in The Gambia to reduce overall childhood mortality by 60 percent when combined with malaria chemoprophylaxis (Alonso et al., 1991)—is the vector control tool with the greatest promise for Africa. At the Africa Summit on Roll Back Malaria in Abuja, Nigeria in 2000, leaders from 44 African countries set a target of 60 percent ITN coverage of pregnant women and infants in Africa by 2005, an ambitious goal requiring roughly 160 million ITNs at an estimated cost of US$1.12 billion (Nahlen et al., 2003). Sadly, the goal is still far from being met. At the same time, insecticide resistance (involving pyrethroids and DDT) is a growing problem in Africa, along with environmental change brought by agriculture and other types of development that foster mosquito breeding. International sponsors also have withdrawn support for DDT due to environmental concerns.

With respect to malaria's human reservoir, the overriding challenge facing Africa is the development of drug resistance by *Plasmodium falciparum* to cheap and effective treatments (chloroquine and sulfadoxine-pyrimethamine [SP]), compounded by large and, in some cases, mobile infected populations.

BASIC PRINCIPLES OF MALARIA CONTROL

Successful malaria control programs traditionally use multiple interventions. In 1952, Paul Russell (a noted Rockefeller Foundation malariologist, and former head of the Allied antimalaria campaign in Italy) listed five approaches to malaria eradication (Russell, 1952):

1. Measures to prevent mosquitoes from feeding on humans (human-vector contact)
2. Measures to prevent or reduce the breeding of mosquitoes
3. Measures to destroy mosquito larvae
4. Measures to kill or reduce the lifespan of adult mosquitoes
5. Measures to eliminate malaria parasites from humans

Since Russell's era, an increasing emphasis on the control of human disease has produced three additional strategies (Beales and Gilles, 2002):

6. Measures to prevent and reduce malaria mortality (especially in high-risk groups)
7. Measures to reduce malaria morbidity
8. Measures to reduce malaria transmission

Today's control efforts mainly rely upon the interruption of human-vector contact and treatment of infected persons. Personal protection via ITNs or curtains is generally preferred in settings where vectors feed indoors during nighttime sleeping hours. ITNs also kill malaria vectors and reduce the local intensity of transmission (the "mass effect"). Indoor residual spraying (IRS) with DDT or a pyrethroid insecticide is another way to reduce bites by vectors whose feeding and resting habits render them susceptible, as long as the majority of houses in a targeted community are sprayed. IRS also is the preferred vector control method during malaria epidemics and in refugee camps since trained spray teams can rapidly cover likely areas of transmission.

Case management—which encompasses prompt access to health care, an accurate diagnosis, and effective treatment—is the other cornerstone of malaria control. The current failure to control malaria with drugs often starts with a failure to deliver appropriate case management to many malaria sufferers, particularly at the periphery of health systems.

Other control strategies outlined by the World Health Organization (WHO) in 1993 include early forecasting of malaria epidemics and the development of epidemiological information systems; capacity-building in basic and applied research; and ongoing assessment of ecological, social, and economic determinants of disease within affected countries and regions (WHO, 1993). Effective field operations also require expertise and teamwork. Qualified personnel with the scientific knowledge, skills, and authority are perhaps the single most important resource needed for effective vector control (Roberts et al., 2000). The same need for knowledge applies to those rendering clinical care to malaria patients: from parents, village health care workers, drug sellers, and traditional healers to laboratory workers, nurses, doctors, and other health care professionals.

INSECTICIDES AND INSECTICIDE RESISTANCE

Insecticides in Public Health

Immediately after World War II, DDT and other chlorinated hydrocarbon insecticides formed the mainstay of malaria control. DDT was initially developed as a public health insecticide prior to its widespread agricultural use and recognition as an environmental pollutant (Curtis and Lines, 2000). Of note, when used indoors in limited quantities, DDT's entry into the global food chain is minimal (Attaran et al., 2000). (For a full summary of DDT's role in public health, readers are referred to a recent review [Taverne, 1999]).

Today, despite concerns over their environmental effects and possible inactivation by mosquito vectors, chemical insecticides remain key elements in malaria control.

A WHO-coordinated research program is now in place to develop new candidate insecticides and test their activity and safety(WHO, 1996a). The specifications for pesticides used in public health are part of the WHO Pesticide Evaluation Scheme (WHOPES).

Classified by chemical characteristics, the most common insecticides currently used in public health practice are:

- Petroleum oils and their derivatives
- Active constituents of flowers of pyrethrum (pyrethrins) or newer synthetic compounds of this group (pyrethroids)
- Chlorinated hydrocarbons (e.g., dichloro-diphenyl-trichloroethane (DDT), hexachlorocyclohexane (HCH), and dieldrin)
- Organophosphorous insecticides (e.g., malathion, and temephos)
- Carbamates (e.g., propoxur, and carbaryl)
- Insect growth regulators (e.g., diflubenzuron, methoprene, and pyriproxyfen)

Pyrethrum, an extract of dried chrysanthemum flowers, is the oldest effective insecticide known. Both pyrethrum and its natural and synthetic relatives (pyrethrins and pyrethroids) are nerve poisons that rapidly permeate and kill adult insects with high margins of mammalian safety. They also demonstrate rapid knock down (i.e., immobilizing) and repellant effects. The chief drawback of the class is its relatively short-lived action, although newer synthetic compounds such as permethrin and deltamethrin are more stable than naturally occurring products. The residues of DDT, in contrast, remain active for up to a year following application to impervious surfaces such as plastered walls (on mud brick, DDT loses its insecticidal effect faster). DDT's long-term repellant, and contact irritant effects probably contribute as much or more than its direct insecticidal action in controlling malaria transmission (Roberts et al., 2000).

On a molecular level, all major classes of chemical insecticide exert their principal effects within the nerve tissue of targeted insects. DDT and pyrethroids cause persistent activation of sodium channels (Soderlund and Bloomquist, 1989), while pyrethroids also act on receptors that normally govern inhibitory neurotransmission, and organophosphates and carbamates target acetylcholinesterase.

Insecticide Resistance

Levels of resistance in insect populations reflect the amount and frequency of insecticide contact as well as inherent characteristics of the target species. Thus far, DDT resistance has not developed in long-lived disease vectors such as tsetse flies or triatomid bugs (definitive hosts of African sleeping sickness and Chagas' disease, respectively). Mosquitoes, in contrast, have several characteristics suited to rapid development of resistance, including a short life cycle and abundant progeny.

In 1946, only two species of malaria vector were resistant to DDT. However, by 1966 the emergence of resistance was clear: 15 species were resistant to DDT, and 36 species were resistant to dieldrin (WHO Expert Committee on Insecticides, 1970). By 1991, 55 anopheline vectors demonstrated resistance to one or more insecticides. Of these, 53 were resistant to DDT, 27 to organophosphates, 17 to carbamates, and 10 to pyrethroids (WHO, 1992a,b). A decade later, some form of pyrethroid resistance (either decreased mortality, or decreased excito-repellancy of mosquitoes by pyrethroid-impregnated ITNs) had been reported from countries in Asia, Africa, and South America (Takken, 2002).

Three major groups of inactivating enzymes (glutathione S-transferases, esterases, and monooxygenases) are responsible for metabolic resistance to DDT, pyrethroids, organophosphates, and carbamates in *Anopheles* mosquitoes. Knock-down resistance (kdr) is a separate resistance phenotype linked to a point mutation in sodium channels targeted by both pyrethroids and DDT. Although prevalent in *A. gambiae* in West Africa, kdr has not impaired ITN efficacy in the region (Sina and Aultman, 2001; Hemingway and Bates, 2003). In southern Africa, in contrast, the local vector *A. funestus* has acquired metabolic resistance to pyrethroids, rendering ITNs ineffective (Chandre et al., 1999; Brooke et al., 2001). A looming concern for the future is that *A. gambiae* in equatorial Africa will acquire the same metabolic resistance to pyrethroids seen in *A. funestus* in southern Africa. Currently, metabolic resistance to pyrethroids in *A. gambiae* is limited to focal areas of West Africa and Kenya (Ranson et al., 2002).

In coming years, strategies to decrease insecticide resistance may include rotations, mosaics, and mixtures of agricultural and environmental insecticides guided by mathematical models (Tabashnik, 1989). Until now, little field-testing of models has been conducted; however, with new biochemical and molecular field tools, large-scale trials of resistance management are feasible. Treating ITNs with two insecticides with differing mechanisms of action is another approach that may be implemented in the near future. In West Africa, bi-treated nets pairing pyrethroids with carbosulfan (a carbamate insecticide), or chlorpyrifos-methyl (an organophosphate insecticide) are currently under evaluation (Muller et al., 2002).

INSECTICIDE-TREATED BEDNETS AND INDOOR RESIDUAL SPRAYING

History of ITNs

More than two thousand years before Ronald Ross and Giovanni Battista Grassi showed that mosquitoes transmit malaria, human beings used nets to fend off night-biting insects. Mosquito nets appear in historical records from the Middle East to West Africa to Papua New Guinea (Lindsay and Gibson, 1988). The Greek writer Herodotus (484 - ?425 BC) described how Egyptians living in marshy lowlands protected themselves with fishing nets.

Every man there has a net which he uses in the daytime for fishing, but at night he finds another use for it: he drapes it over the bed . . . and then crawls in under and goes to sleep. Mosquitoes can bite through any cover or linen blanket . . . but they do not even try to bite through the net.

Herodotus, *The Histories*

By the early 19th century, British colonists in India—most likely inspired by the example of Punjabi fishermen—also were sleeping under nets. However, it was not until World War II that textiles and insecticides were combined. In central Asia, the Soviet army applied juniper oil to bednets to repel mosquitoes, and sand flies bearing malaria and leishmaniasis (Blagoveschensky et al., 1945), while the American military in the Pacific theater impregnated bednets and jungle hammocks with 5 percent DDT to ward off malaria and filariasis (Harper et al., 1947).

Interest in insecticide-impregnated nets as a malaria control tool resurfaced in the late 1970s and early 1980s. By then, synthetic pyrethroids were the logical insecticide choice because of their low mammalian toxicity and known efficacy in killing and repelling a variety of nuisance and disease-bearing insects. Several governments including the Philippines, Solomon Islands, and Vanuatu began to include ITN promotion as one of their malaria control objectives (Chavasse et al., 1999). However the most successful government-financed ITN programs today are found in China and Vietnam, where the public sector's chief contribution is to offer regular net re-treatment services. When re-treatment is provided free of charge (e.g., China and Vietnam), coverage is generally high (Curtis et al., 1992). Conversely, in Africa, where many nets and insecticides have been provided free or at subsidized prices through local projects and NGOs, less than 5 to 20 percent of nets are re-treated (Snow et al., 1999; Rowley et al., 1999; Guillet et al., 2001).

Individual and Community Effects of ITNs

Child Mortality

After a number of small-scale studies in the 1980s showed favorable effects, the first large-scale study of ITNs plus chemoprophylaxis reported a 60 percent reduction of all-cause child mortality (Alonso et al., 1991). These results prompted the UNDP/World Bank/WHO Special Programme for Research and Training in Tropical Diseases (TDR) to sponsor four randomized controlled trials in Africa to assess the effect of ITNs on all-cause mortality in African children in different epidemiologic settings. A cluster randomization design was used in all four trials. In The Gambia (D'Alessandro et al., 1995), a 25 percent reduction in all-cause mortality was seen in children less than 9 years old. In Kenya (Nevill et al., 1996) and Ghana (Binka et al., 1996), the introduction of ITNs was associated with 33 and 17 percent reductions in all-cause child mortality, respectively, in children under 5 years of age. Study populations in all three sites ranged from 60,000 to 120,000 (Table 8-1).

The fourth randomized controlled trial in Burkina Faso (Habluetzel et

TABLE 8-1 Protective Efficacy of ITNs: Reductions in Child Mortality in Five Randomized Controlled Trials

Country in Which Study Was Performed	Percent Reduction in Child Mortality	EIR
The Gambia (D'Alessandro et al., 1995)[a]	25%	1-10
Kenya (Nevill et al., 1996)	33%	10-30
Ghana (Binka et al., 1996)	17%	100-300
Burkina Faso (Habluetzel et al., 1997)	15%	300-500
Kenya (Phillips-Howard et al., 2003)	16%	200-300

[a]This study was considered an effectiveness, as opposed to an efficacy, study.

al., 1997) examined insecticide-treated curtains (ITCs) rather than bednets in roughly 100,000 residents of a region with alternating high and low malaria seasons. Baseline mortality, approaching 45 per thousand, was the highest to date among the four African ITN trials (Diallo et al., 1999). After 2 years of tracking, the use of ITCs was associated with a 15 percent decrease in all-cause mortality in Burkina Faso, concentrated in the first year of use.

Viewed as a group, the four TDR-sponsored randomized controlled trials demonstrate decreasing ITN efficacy with increasing transmission pressure, since sites experiencing higher EIRs (100-500 infective bites per person per year, i.e., Ghana, and Burkina Faso) witnessed lower ITN benefits.

The most recent group-randomized controlled trial of permethrin-treated bednets conducted in western Kenya (Hawley et al., 2003a) was designed to assess ITN efficacy at an upper range of year-round transmission. This study yielded an overall protective efficacy of 16 percent in all-cause child mortality; thus, ITN benefits were validated in an area of very high transmission. Maximum effect was dependent on regular re-treatment of ITNs, however. For example, the protective efficacy of ITNs in children aged 1-11 months fell from 26 to 17 percent when re-treatment was delayed beyond 6 months. The Kenyan trials also demonstrated roughly 90 percent transmission reduction from a baseline EIR of 60-300 (Gimnig et al., 2003b). When ITNs are combined with highly effective therapy such as artemisinin combination therapies (ACTs)—even in highly endemic areas—it is possible that the EIR could decline even further, approaching 0 (Personal communication, N. White, Mahidol University, February, 2004).

Child and Maternal Morbidity

Acute and chronic consequences of childhood malaria include uncomplicated febrile episodes with parasitemia, and anemia. Data from a large meta-analysis suggest that ITN use under stable transmission conditions roughly halves mild malaria episodes in children under five (Lengeler, 2001). In a nonrandomized trial of ITNs in southwestern Tanzania, treated nets conferred protective efficacy of 62 and 63 percent, respectively, on parasitemia and anemia in children under 5 (Abdulla et al., 2001). In an area of high perennial transmission in western Kenya, ITNs delayed the time to first infection in infants from 4.5 to 10.7 months (ter Kuile et al., 2003a).

Repeated malaria infection also causes anemia and morbidity in pregnant women and newborns. Four randomized controlled trials of ITNs in pregnancy have shown variable benefits in different transmission settings. In Thailand and The Gambia (areas with lower, seasonal transmission), ITNs significantly reduced malaria parasitemia and maternal anemia (Dolan et al., 1993; D'Alessandro et al., 1996); in The Gambia, they also increased birth weight (D'Alessandro et al., 1996). However, similar benefits were not seen in areas with more intense transmission (coastal Kenya and Ghana) (Shulman et al., 1998; Browne et al., 2001), raising concern that ITNs might not protect pregnant women in areas with a very high EIR. This concern was allayed by the most recent findings.

In the western Kenya trial, complete data were available in nearly 3,000 pregnancies (ter Kuile et al., 2003b). Before the study began, up to one-third of all infants were born preterm, small for gestational age, or with low birth weight. ITN-using pregnant women (gravidae 1-4) experienced a 38 percent reduction in maternal parasitemia, a 47 percent reduction in malarial anemia, and a 35 percent reduction in placental malaria at the time of delivery, while their newborns demonstrated a 28 percent reduction in low birth weight.

Community and Population Effects

In addition to conferring benefits upon individual users, ITNs can protect nonusers within ITN households as well as nonusers in nearby houses. Such effects were first noted in early village-scale ITN trials in Burkina Faso (Robert and Carnevale, 1991), Tanzania (Magesa et al., 1991), Kenya (Beach et al., 1993), and Zaire (Karch et al., 1993). More recent ITN studies have confirmed community-wide reductions in vector populations (Hii et al., 1997; Binka et al., 1998; Hii et al., 2000; Howard et al., 2000; Maxwell et al., 2002). Some ITN trial data have even demonstrated spatial effects on health. In Ghana, child mortality increased by 6.7 percent for every 100 m away from an intervention compound (Binka et al., 1998), while in western Kenya, mortality, parasitemia, and anemia decreased in unprotected children living within 300 m of households from ITN villages (Gimnig et al., 2003a). The minimum ITN coverage needed to achieve community benefits is 50 to 60 percent of households within a neighborhood with suitable indoor, night-biting vectors (Hawley et al., 2003b). In Asia, in contrast, ITNs have had mixed results because vectors often bite outdoors in the late evening (or sometimes in the early morning), and both children and adults are susceptible.

Long-Lasting Insecticidal Nets

At present a single insecticide treatment of a conventional cotton or nylon mosquito net lasts for 6 to 12 months. "Long-lasting insecticidal nets" (with insecticide incorporated directly in net fibers) would eliminate the need for regular re-treatment. Two prototypes (Olyset and Permanet) are now on the market while others are being developed (Moerman et al., 2003). One early problem with the Vestergaard-manufactured Permanet was inconsistency among batches; in a study of randomly-sampled new unwashed, traditionally washed, and up to 18 months field-used products, insecticide concentration was much reduced after two washes, and mosquito mortality reached unacceptably low levels after only 12 months (Muller et al., 2002). These problems have presumably been rectified since Permanets produced by Vestergaard are now approved by WHO and production is slated to increase to one million nets per month (Personal communication, B. Greenwood, London School of Hygiene and Tropical Medicine, March 2004).

Indoor Residual Insecticide Spraying

Sprayed insecticides to kill adult mosquitoes were introduced on a large scale in the mid-1930s. Pyrethrum was first used for indoor residual spraying (IRS) in southern Africa and India and later replaced by DDT after World War II. IRS is most effective in reducing mosquitoes that rest indoors following a blood meal. To be effective, IRS does not have to kill all *Anopheles* at once but simply prevent a large proportion from surviving 12 to 14 days (the time it takes for a malaria parasite to develop to the infective stage within the mosquito). Even with the hardiest vectors, this can be achieved with a daily mortality of 40 to 50 percent. In places with lower malaria endemicity, daily mosquito mortality of 20 to 25 percent generally is adequate (Beales and Gilles, 2002).

Just as ITNs extend benefits to nonusers in the community, IRS is especially effective when applied on a large scale, since this maximizes the reduction in mosquito lifespan, and overall transmission. This so-called mass effect has been well documented in a number of IRS trials. Specific examples include three demonstration projects in Africa: an observational study in the Pare-Taveta Malaria Scheme in Tanzania where dieldrin reduced malaria transmission from an annual EIR of 10-50 to <1 (Pringle, 1969; Bradley, 1991); a trial in Kisumu, Kenya, where IRS with fenitrothion reduced malaria transmission by 96 percent compared to baseline over 2 years (Payne et al., 1976); and the Garki project in northern Nigeria where IRS with propoxur also substantially decreased transmission and improved infant and child mortality (Molineaux, 1985) (Box 8-1).

Over the last 30 years, DDT-based IRS has declined, in part, because of DDT resistance among malaria vectors. A lack of sustained government support and financing as well as general disapproval of DDT by the international community also have contributed to IRS's restricted use in sub-Saharan Africa. In parts of Asia, Latin America, and southern and northeastern Africa where IRS is still used, it is typically organized and paid for by governments (for example, government-funded DDT house spraying was recently reinstated in KwaZulu Natal, South Africa, and the Madagascar highlands because of rising prevalence of pyrethroid-resistant *A. funestus* vectors and human malaria cases [Hargreaves et al., 2000]). IRS also is used in urban epidemics and refugee camps worldwide, and sometimes provided by foreign and multinational companies for the protection of employees and local communities in malaria-endemic areas (Sharp et al., 2002a).

The implementation of IRS is not trivial, and, if incorrectly performed, may be quite ineffective (Shiff, 2002). Houses and animal shelters within a target area should receive IRS before the start of the transmission season and at regular intervals thereafter. Before application of insecticide, all furniture, hanging clothing, cooking utensils, food and other items should be removed from human habitations, and left covered outside. Emulsions or solutions of insecticide are often preferred over suspensions of water-dispersible powders, which leave whitish deposits. Mud and porous plaster walls retain less IRS insecticide than wood or non-absorptive surfaces.

Barriers to ITN and IRS Use

ITNs and IRS both require user cooperation, albeit in different ways. Current-generation ITNs must be properly installed, faithfully used, and retreated with insecticide every 6 to 12 months in order to maintain extended efficacy. IRS, in comparison, is passive but intrusive. Some residents of endemic areas forfeit IRS benefits by painting or replastering sprayed walls, while other families evade IRS altogether by locking their houses during the spraying round (Mnzava et al., 2001; Goodman et al., 2001). In addition, some housing or shelter materials such as plastic sheeting are not amenable to residual spraying.

BOX 8-1
The Garki Project

In the early 1970s, an ambitious malaria control experiment was undertaken to determine whether malaria transmission could be interrupted in a highly endemic area of Africa. The experiment was conducted in a group of villages near the town of Garki in northern Nigeria. Villages were allocated to three intervention groups.

- Villages in group A1 received household spraying with propoxur plus mass drug administration (MDA) with sulfalene-pyrimethamine every 2 weeks plus limited larval control with temephos (Abate).
- Villages in group A2 received household spraying with propoxur plus MDA with sulfalene-pyrimethamine every ten weeks.
- Villages in group B received only household spraying with propoxur.
- Villages in group C served as controls.

The main findings of the Garki project were as follows:

1. Household spraying with propoxur was relatively inefficient in reducing local populations of *Anopheles gambiae*, possibly due to outdoor resting behavior, and/or as a result of high sporozoite rate.
2. In villages where residual spraying was combined with MDA—especially in group A1 where MDA was given every two weeks throughout the transmission season—there was a marked fall in *Plasmodium falciparum* parasitemia below 1 percent.
3. Deaths were reduced in both control and intervention areas although some evidence suggested a more marked effect in intervention villages.
4. After the interventions stopped, parasitemia increased in intervention compared with control villages. However, the increase was not marked, and limited post-intervention surveillance did not reveal a rebound in clinical cases or deaths.

The Garki project was planned at a time when eradication of malaria was still viewed as a serious option for highly endemic areas such as Nigeria. The experiment showed that interrupting transmission was not possible even when a full armamentarium of malaria control tools was applied. Its findings helped to redirect attention from eradication to controlling the clinical effect of malaria in Africa. Although the study did not focus on malaria-related morbidity and mortality to the same degree as would be likely today, its parasitemia data suggest that mortality and morbidity from malaria would have fallen dramatically in study villages during the 2-year period of integrated malaria control.

Brian Greenwood, London School of Hygiene and Tropical Medicine

Despite its proven benefits, current ITN use in sub-Saharan Africa also is low. Most households in malaria endemic areas do not possess any net, insecticide-treated or not. In nine African countries surveyed between 1997 and 2001, a median 13 percent of households had one or more nets of any kind; a median 1.3 percent of households in three countries owned at least one ITN; and across 28 countries, only 15 percent of children under age 5 were sleeping under any net (WHO/UNICEF, 2003). Not surprisingly, net ownership and use are lowest in poor households.

In addition to purchase cost and re-treatment, one additional barrier to ITN use is the common misconception that ITNs are meant to control mosquitoes as opposed to malaria. In urban areas with untreated wastewater and high year-round populations of "nuisance" culicine mosquitoes, this misconception favors ITN use. In rural areas, however, mosquito densities and mosquito nuisance are generally lower despite year-round biting by clandestine female anophelines. As a result, ITN use is rarely sustained night after night, especially during the dry season (Gyapong et al., 1996; Binka et al., 1996; Binka and Adongo, 1997).

In western Kenya, the use of ITNs was observed directly in nearly 800 households (Alaii et al., 2003a). About 30 percent of ITNs in homes were unused. Children less than 5 years of age were less likely to use ITNs than older individuals, and ITNs were more likely to be used in cooler weather. Neither mosquito numbers, relative wealth, number of house occupants, nor educational level of the head of the household influenced adherence. Excessive heat was often cited as a reason for not using a child's ITN. Researchers also commented on the effort required of caregivers to store and rehang the ITN on a daily basis (Alaii et al., 2003a).

Finally, misunderstandings about malaria also lower incentives to use ITNs and/or IRS. In southern Ghana, the Adangbe people believe that *asra*, a local disease that resembles malaria, is the result of prolonged exposure to heat (Agyepong, 1992). In Bagamoyo District, Tanzania, *degedege*—a local term for fever and convulsions—is often blamed on a bird-spirit instead of cerebral malaria (Makemba et al., 1996). In western Kenya, many ITN trial participants believed that malaria was a multicausal disease and that ITNs were therefore only partly effective (Alaii et al., 2003b).

OTHER VECTOR CONTROL MEASURES

Household and Community Measures

In areas of high malaria transmission, prevalence of infection may vary significantly over relatively short distances. This has been observed not only in Africa (Greenwood, 1999) but in other countries, such as Papua New

Guinea (Graves et al., 1988), and Pakistan (Strickland et al., 1987). Local factors (in addition to IRS and insecticide-impregnated materials) that affect the microepidemiology of malaria are house siting, screening and construction, proximity of animals to human dwellings, and use of mosquito deterrents such as repellants, aerosols, and fumigants.

House Siting and Construction

Despite the fact that anopheline mosquitoes can fly substantial distances, the proximity of houses or villages to a breeding site strongly influences malaria risk, especially where breeding sites are restricted. In a suburb of Dakar, Senegal, malaria prevalence rose steeply from the center to the edge of town adjacent to marshy breeding sites of *Anopheles arabiensis* (Trape et al., 1992). In Sri Lanka, the risk of malaria was much higher among those who lived in poor quality houses within 2.5 km of a river where *A. culicifacies* bred (Gunawardena et al., 1998).

House design and construction also influence the risk of malaria (Schofield and White, 1984). Eaves—which allow interior ventilation, and the escape of smoke from cooking fires—are a common feature that facilitate mosquito access to sleeping areas in houses in the tropics. Using mud or plaster to fill in eaves (Lindsay and Snow, 1988), or hanging eaves curtains (Curtis et al., 1992) reduce human-vector contact. In Sri Lanka, Gunawardena et al. (1998) estimated that the cost of upgrading all low-quality housing (whose residents suffered a fourfold risk of malaria compared to families living in well-constructed houses in the same locale) would be balanced by savings in malaria treatment costs over a period of 7 years.

Animals

In some communities, animals live in or near houses. *Zooprophylaxis* is a term that suggests the possible diversion of mosquito bites from humans to nearby animals. However, this diversion depends entirely on the biting habits of the local vector and varies from species to species. In some cases, livestock may actually attract certain mosquitoes that would otherwise avoid human habitats, resulting in increased malaria exposure to household members (Hewitt et al., 1994; Bouma and Rowland, 1995; Mouchet, 1998). In Pakistani and Afghan refugee camps, malaria cases were concentrated in communities that kept cattle, presumably because the local vectors *A. culicifacies* and *A. stephensi* were preferentially attracted to these households (Bouma and Rowland, 1995).

Repellants, Aerosols, and Fumigants

Many communities use aromatic smokes to deter mosquitoes. In The Gambia, tree bark combined with synthetic perfumes (locally known as *churai*) reduced the number of mosquitoes entering a room but not the incidence of malaria (Snow et al., 1987). In contrast, traditional fumigants in Sri Lanka decreased malaria (van der Hoek et al., 1998). In Thailand, a mixture of DEET (N,N-diethyl-m toluamide) and a paste made from a local tree (wood apple) was an effective repellant when applied to the skin (Lindsay et al., 1998).

Commercially manufactured coils containing pyrethroids or DDT also repel mosquitoes (Charlwood and Jolley, 1984; Bockarie et al., 1994). Although coils are cheap, households may spend substantial sums of money on items of this kind. In Dar es Salaam, Tanzania, average household expenditure on antimosquito measures was in the region of US$2-3 per month (Chavasse et al., 1999).

Environmental and Biologic Management

Since *A. gambiae* can breed in virtually any puddle, larval control in sub-Saharan Africa has always been challenging. Where vector breeding sites are few in number and easily identified, however, environmental or biologic control of larval breeding sites is often feasible. Petroleum oil larvicides have played an important part in mosquito control since the beginning of the 20th century. Breeding sites also may be eliminated by draining or filling in pools, modifying the boundaries of rivers or their run-off systems, and creating impoundments (reservoirs behind dams). Intermittent drying of rice fields, stream sluicing or flushing, salination of coastal marshes or lagoons (for example, using tidegates), shading of stream banks, and clearing of vegetation are naturalistic manipulations that proved beneficial in controlling certain vectors, primarily in India and southeast Asia. Although eclipsed by residual insecticides for several decades, many of these environmental methods of vector control are now back in vogue with strong WHO endorsement.

Biological control strategies, including use of bacteria such as *Bacillus thuringiensis subsp. israelensis* (Bti), or larvivorous fish, also have been combined with other control measures with variable success (Romi et al., 1993; Karch et al., 1993; WHO, 1999; Kaneko et al., 2000). Bti spores produce a toxin that is poisonous to mosquitoes and other aquatic insects but harmless to plants, animals, and humans. *Bacillus sphaericus* (Bsph) multiplies in polluted waters, and produces a longer-acting toxin than Bti; however, resistance to Bsph toxin is present in some mosquito populations in India, Brazil, and France (WHO, 1999).

Genetic Control

Genetic control refers to any method that reduces an insect's reproductive or disease-transmitting potential through alteration of its hereditary material. The oldest form of genetic control is sterile insect technology (SIT), a proven strategy in past campaigns against screw worm, tsetse flies, and Mediterranean fruitflies. Unfortunately, when mass hybrid sterility was tried against *A. gambiae* in Burkina Faso, West Africa, few matings actually took place between the sterile males and wild female anophelines. Producing large numbers of sterile yet competitive male mosquitoes, and successfully releasing them in the wild remain major operational hurdles.

First predicted decades ago by Curtis (Curtis, 1968), genetically modified mosquitoes are now another potential means of vector control. The reasoning is as follows. Since only some anopheline mosquitoes transmit malaria, genes encoding the nontransmitting phenotype, or genes that prevent malaria parasites from developing within mosquitoes altogether, could be inserted into vector genomes (Collins, 1994; James et al., 1999). The feasibility of this approach was recently shown when a synthetic gene inserted into *A. stephensi* almost fully prevented its ability to transmit a strain of rodent malaria (Ito et al., 2002). However, the same practical obstacle facing SIT—namely, the rapid replacement of native mosquito populations—affects genetically modified mosquitoes. Concerns also have been raised about the fitness of genetically modified mosquitoes, the negative consequences of unstable genetic modifications, and public reservations regarding deployment of genetically altered organisms (Clarke, 2002).

TREATMENT AND CHEMOPREVENTION

The primary aim of malaria treatment is saving lives. Prompt, effective treatment in the early stages of falciparum malaria reduces the risk of death as much as 50-fold, whereas effective treatment after progression to severe illness produces only a five-fold reduction in the risk of dying (White, 1999). However, malaria treatment also can reduce malaria transmission in endemic areas. This section reviews the role of treatment as a control measure capable of reducing malaria transmission, as well as past and present chemoprevention strategies in residents of malaria-endemic areas. (See Chapter 9 for more detailed information regarding antimalarial drugs, drug resistance, and treatment protocols.)

Antimalarials and Reduction of Malaria Transmission

A key objective of many early studies of widespread antimalarial distribution was interrupting malaria transmission (Greenwood, 2004). Two approaches were tried: treatment of symptomatic cases; and mass drug administration, which included mass chemoprophylaxis, and the Pinotti method—the systematic addition of antimalarial drugs to salt.

Treatment of Symptomatic Cases

The notion that treating symptomatic individuals might indirectly protect an entire malaria-exposed population dates back to Robert Koch and the early years of the 20th century (Harrison, 1978). At that time, with this goal partly in mind, quinine was used extensively in Italy and elsewhere. Since quinine has little effect on gametocytes, however, it had little effect on transmission overall.

Today, in contrast, artemisinin-based drugs (which do kill early-stage gametocytes as well as asexual parasites) have helped to decrease transmission in selected areas of Asia and Africa. On the Thai-Burmese border, where field studies using ACTs were first undertaken in 1991, replacing mefloquine with mefloquine-artesunate as first-line treatment for symptomatic malaria substantially reduced the incidence of local *P. falciparum* infection (Nosten et al., 2000). Widespread use of artemisinins and ACTs—along with ITNs or IRS—also contributed to a marked decline in the overall incidence of falciparum malaria in Vietnam (Hung et al., 2002) and South Africa (Barnes et al., 2003) (Box 8-2)—both areas with relatively low EIRs. Whether widespread use of ACTs will bring about a similar outcome in areas of higher malaria transmission (EIR > 100) is still unknown.

Mass Drug Administration

Unlike Southeast Asia and South Africa, many malaria infections in sub-Saharan Africa—especially in older children and adults—are asymptomatic and untreated but have parasite densities sufficient for transmission (von Seidlein et al., 2002). Under these conditions, reducing malaria transmission by use of a gametocytocidal drug requires that asymptomatic as well as symptomatic carriers be treated. This led to the concept of mass drug administration (MDA). During MDA, the entire population of a community known to contain many asymptomatic infected subjects receives treatment without first determining who is actually parasitemic.

MDA as a method of reducing malaria transmission gained momentum after the 8-aminoquinolones (of which primaquine is the leading prototype) were discovered. This class of drugs is highly effective at killing gametocytes of *P. falciparum*. One of the first trials to investigate 8-aminoquinolones as MDA agents took place in a Liberian rubber plantation in 1930. Mass treatment with plasmoquine led to a marked decrease in parasite prevalence and a reduction in infected mosquitoes in two treated camps (Barber et al., 1932). During the 1960s and 1970s, several more

BOX 8-2
Malaria Morbidity and Mortality in KwaZulu Natal

Ingwavuma district in northern KwaZulu Natal carried the highest malaria burden in South Africa until 2000. This changed after improvements in vector control in KwaZulu Natal and neighboring southern Mozambique during 2000, and the implementation of an artemisinin combination therapy (ACT), artemether-lumefantrine (AL), in January 2001. These interventions were followed by a 78 percent decrease in malaria case notifications in the province within 1 year. There was a further 75 percent decrease in notifications in 2002, and this decrease was sustained throughout 2003 (Figure 8.2-1).

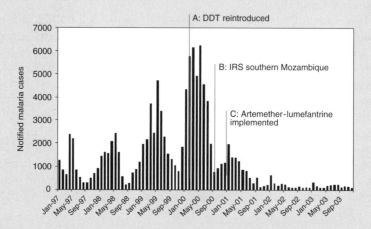

FIGURE 8.2-1 *The synergistic effect of improved vector control and artemisinin combination therapy, artemether-lumefantrine, on malaria transmission in KwaZulu Natal, South Africa.*

A. Reintroduction of DDT for indoor residual spraying (IRS) of traditional structures in KZN in March 2000.
B. Introduction of IRS in southern Mozambique in October 2000.
C. Implementation of artemether-lumefantrine (AL) for the treatment of uncomplicated falciparum malaria in KZN in January 2001.

SOURCE: Muheki C, Barnes K, McIntyre D. 2003. *Economic Evaluation of Recent Malaria Control Interventions in KwaZulu, South Africa: SEACAT Evaluation.* SEACAT.

The success of this dual intervention is further reflected by the 89 percent decrease in both malaria-related hospital admissions (range 81-92 percent), and deaths (range 78-93 percent) across the three rural district hospitals that serve the Ingwavuma community. Despite KwaZulu Natal also carrying South Africa's highest burden of the HIV/AIDS epidemic, the total number of "all cause" hospital admissions also was reduced following improved malaria control. Dr Hervey Vaughan Williams, medical superintendent of Mosvold hospital, a rural district hospital in Ingwavuma, reports that "during the peak of the 2000 malaria epidemic, hospital admissions were averaging three patients per bed." Following the reduction in the overall number of hospital admissions, it is expected that the standard of care for all patients could be improved.

These improvements in malaria control also have been welcomed by the local communities. During focus group discussions on malaria, there was general enthusiasm for the change in malaria treatment. One female household head reported "Every year I used to have malaria. This year I heard that new pills were coming. I was very sick with malaria. They gave me the new pills . . . the (next) morning I was very fine. . . . I have cultivated and harvested and I've never had malaria again this year." These comments are in contrast with the opinion of female household heads on SP, e.g., "Those tablets that were used before the present ones . . . most of us didn't like taking them . . . because after taking them you would feel as if the malaria has become more severe than before." The community perceptions that those with malaria should seek health care urgently at public-sector facilities, is likely to have contributed to the marked public health effect observed following the implementation of AL. These perceptions were described during focus group discussions: "There is no way to treat malaria besides taking him to the clinic"; "Once you waste time at the *sangoma* [traditional healer], you die."

The sustained benefits to public health following the implementation of artemether-lumefantrine in KwaZulu Natal are most encouraging. These reflect the benefits of ACT in significantly decreasing treatment failure and gametocyte carriage rates, within a context of effective vector control, and a relatively well developed rural primary health care infrastructure.

Karen Barnes, University of Cape Town (2003)

MDA trials took place in Africa and Asia with the primary aim of interrupting transmission (von Seidlein and Greenwood, 2003). By today's standards, the studies were poorly designed and their results difficult to assess; however, in nearly all cases, MDA failed to interrupt transmission, although it did markedly reduce parasite prevalence (Greenwood, 2004) (Box 8-1, The Garki Project). In 1981, the largest-ever MDA program produced essentially the same outcome. After a single round of chloroquine plus primaquine was given to roughly eight million people in Nicaragua, there was an immediate, marked decrease in clinical *P. vivax* malaria, but transmission continued and the incidence of malaria soon returned to its previous level (Garfield and Vermund, 1983).

In most MDAs, tablets have been given, sometimes under supervision. Although this ensures effective dosing, it is onerous. As an alternative to tablets, Pinotti devised the concept of drug delivery using medicated salt (Pinotti, 1954). During the 1950s, a number of trials of medicated salt were conducted in malaria-endemic areas (Payne, 1988); they generally led to a reduced incidence of clinical episodes of malaria at the cost of rapid emergence of antimalarial resistance (Meuwissen, 1964; Giglioli et al., 1967). It is now known that exposing malaria parasites to suboptimal doses of antimalarial drugs over time is an ideal way to induce resistance. Thus, medicated salt has no place in malaria control today.

One MDA program that incorporated other control interventions was recently reported from the island of Aneityum, Vanuatu. In this case, the effort was successful. Eight rounds of MDA with chloroquine-SP-primaquine combined with ITNs and environmental control measures eliminated falciparum infection from the island (Kaneko et al., 2000).

Chemoprophylaxis

Antimalarial chemoprophylaxis is often used by short-term, nonimmune visitors to high-risk areas. Its direct benefits to individuals are obvious, while its indirect benefits include expanded international tourism, business travel, and economic development of malarious regions. However, the use of antimalarial drugs to protect the resident population of malaria-endemic areas has always been more controversial (Greenwood, 2004). The following two sections summarize past data and current trends regarding the use of drugs to protect high-risk individuals within *P. falciparum* endemic areas from acute infection.

Chemoprophylaxis in Children

In 1956, McGregor and others reported the results of a trial in The Gambia in which children received chloroquine weekly from birth until age 2. Children who received chemoprophylaxis had fewer episodes of malaria, grew better, and had higher mean hemoglobin values than children in the control group (McGregor et al., 1956). These findings were later reproduced in studies in several other African countries (Prinsen Geerligs et al., 2003).

In the 1980s, a 5-year trial using weekly Maloprim (pyrimethamine plus dapsone) during the rainy season in children under 5 was conducted in The Gambia (Greenwood et al., 1988). Overall mortality was approximately 35 percent lower in children on prophylaxis. Protected children also had fewer clinical attacks of malaria, and a higher mean packed cell volume than control children. These results were sustained over several years (Allen et al., 1990), and are at least as impressive as results obtained with ITNs. A more recent study in Tanzanian infants using Maloprim also showed a marked reduction in clinical attacks of malaria, and the incidence of severe anemia (Menendez et al., 1997).

Chemoprophylaxis in Pregnant Women

Antimalarial chemoprophylaxis in pregnant women was first studied in a Nigerian mission hospital in 1964 (Morley et al., 1964). Chemoprophylaxis with pyrimethamine substantially increased birth weight overall, but particularly in infants born to primigravidae (women pregnant for the first time). Later studies in other African countries confirmed chemoprophylaxis's positive effects on birth weight (Garner and Gulmezoglu, 2000), and maternal hemoglobin levels (Greenwood et al., 1989), particularly during first and second pregnancies (Greenwood, 2004). Drugs used for chemoprophylaxis in pregnancy include chloroquine, pyrimethamine, proguanil, Maloprim, and mefloquine. Although rarely implemented on any scale until recently, WHO recommended that all pregnant women in areas of moderate or high malaria transmission receive weekly chemoprophylaxis with chloroquine during their second and third trimesters. Because of drug resistance, this policy no longer offers much benefit.

Obstacles to Targeted Chemoprophylaxis

Despite impressive results in clinical trials, targeted chemoprophylaxis has never been recommended for children residing in malaria-endemic countries, and it has rarely been implemented in pregnant women. Concerns over cost, sustainability, and safety have all contributed to its poor uptake (Greenwood, 2004). In addition, some experts are concerned that young children routinely administered chemoprophylaxis may fail to develop natural immunity. In The Gambia, children who received chemoprophylaxis for 4-5 years did experience a statistically significant increase in clinical attacks of malaria in the year after prophylaxis ended; however overall protection from death extended to age 10 following antimalarial prophylaxis during early years of life (Greenwood et al., 1995).

A final theoretical objection to chemoprophylaxis for high-risk individuals in malaria-endemic regions is its possible induction of drug resistance. Although medicated salt and the unrestricted use of chloroquine and pyrimethamine in the 1960s contributed to the initial emergence and spread of drug resistance (Payne, 1988), there is little evidence to suggest that targeted chemoprophylaxis produces the same effect to any meaningful degree. Chemoprophylaxis will inevitably lead to an increase in drug pressure, but this may be an acceptable price to pay if benefits are large. The minimal risk of drug resistance also is likely to be mitigated by the future use of combination therapy.

Intermittent Preventive Treatment

Intermittent preventive treatment (IPT) is a full therapeutic course of antimalarial treatment administered at specified times whether or not a recipient is infected. Unlike chemoprophylaxis (which aims to sustain blood levels above the mean inhibitory concentration for a prolonged period), IPT yields shorter bursts of protective drug levels separated by periods when drug levels are too low to inhibit parasite growth. In general, there are still many unknowns regarding IPT's mechanisms of action. In the case of SP (the drug most widely used for IPT in children and pregnant women), for example, it is still not clear if IPT works primarily by eliminating existing parasites, or through a long-acting prophylactic effect of the drug (Greenwood, 2004).

IPT in Pregnant Women (IPTp)

In Malawi, Schultz and others found that a full course of SP given twice during pregnancy protected against low birth weight to a significantly greater degree than weekly chloroquine chemoprophylaxis (Schultz et al., 1994). In Kenya, a controlled trial with IPTp with SP given two or three times during pregnancy also reduced severe anemia in women pregnant for the first or second time (Shulman et al., 1999). In another area of Kenya, however, HIV-infected women required more than two or three doses of IPTp to prevent placental infection (Parise et al., 1998). Since all trials were conducted when *P. falciparum* was more sensitive than it is now, it is unlikely that IPT using SP would achieve the same effects today.

WHO now recommends that IPTp with SP be given at each antenatal clinic attendance after quickening (usually between the 16th and 18th week of pregnancy), replacing chemoprophylaxis as the preferred method for the prevention of malaria in pregnancy (WHO/UNICEF, 2003). Benefits in HIV-infected women are unclear, however, as is the efficacy of IPTp in areas where malaria transmission is highly seasonal or endemicity is low (SP resistance is particularly widespread in low transmission areas). In addition, it is not yet clear what drug or combination of drugs will eventually replace SP for intermittent preventive treatment in pregnancy.

IPT in Infants (IPTi)

The IPT concept has recently been applied to the prevention of malaria in infants. In Tanzania, administration of a full dose of SP to infants concurrent with the second and third doses of diphtheria-pertussis-tetanus, and measles vaccines reduced the incidence of clinical malaria attacks and severe anemia during the first year of life by 59 and 50 percent, respectively (Schellenberg et al., 2001). Amodiaquine given in full therapeutic dose three times during the first year of life yielded similar results (Massaga et al., 2003). Also important, no rebound in malaria attacks or anemia occurred during the second year of life in children who received IPTi as infants. Trials of IPTi using SP are nearing completion in Ghana and Kenya, and further trials have recently started in Mozambique, Gabon, and Kenya. These trials will help to determine under what conditions IPTi will prove most effective, as well as the EIR threshold below which it will not be useful.

IPT in Children (IPTc)

In many areas of Africa, perhaps covering as much as 50 percent of the population at risk, the major burden of malaria is not in infants but in older children. This is especially true in countries of the Sahel and sub-Sahel where malaria transmission is intense but seasonal. A pilot study in Senegal employing SP plus artesunate at 1-month intervals throughout the transmission season is currently exploring whether the IPT principle also can be applied to older children (Greenwood, 2004).

DIAGNOSTIC METHODS

The correct and timely diagnosis of malaria is critically important to the individual patient in whom the disease may quickly progress to a life-threatening stage. Rapid diagnosis, both on an individual and a population level, also is an important tool in overall malaria control. This section reviews currently available methods of diagnosis, with emphasis on newer rapid tests that require relatively little technical expertise to perform. Such tests are now facilitating the delivery of effective treatment in a variety of low-transmission settings, and will eventually find their place in malaria case management in high-transmission settings as well.

Clinical (Presumptive) Diagnosis

Although studies reveal that health providers cannot reliably identify malaria by clinical signs and symptoms alone (Weber et al., 1997; Perkins et al., 1997; Chandramohan et al., 2002), the use of clinical diagnosis is common in endemic areas. Ease, speed, and low cost are the advantages of presumptive diagnosis; disadvantages include overdiagnosis—which contributes in turn to wasted drugs, adverse drug effects, and accelerating drug resistance—as well as underdiagnosis of malaria. Since other common diseases—acute lower respiratory tract infection in children, in particular—may mimic the signs and symptoms of malaria, clinical diagnosis also can result in missed diagnoses of other treatable conditions (Redd et al., 1992; Rey et al., 1996). In fact, the difficulty of differentiating malaria from pneumonia was one of the major factors that led to the establishment of Integrated Management of Childhood Illnesses (IMCI)—an algorithmic approach to the treatment of sick children now used in many developing countries (Personal communication, B. Greenwood, London School of Hygiene and Tropical Medicine, March 2004). Whatever the theoretical pros and cons of presumptive diagnosis, however, it often is all that is available.

Light Microscopy

The current gold standard for the routine laboratory diagnosis of malaria and monitoring of cure is the microscopic examination of thin and thick blood films stained with Giemsa's, Wright's, or Field's stain (Warhurst and Williams, 1996). In the thick film technique, a "thick" layer of blood, containing several layers of red blood cells (RBCs), is concentrated on a small area of a microscope slide. The red and white cell membranes are lysed, and the intracellular remnants examined for the presence of plasmodial forms. The thin film technique produces a monolayer of RBCs, facilitating species identification, and serial counting of parasites. Thin films are particularly helpful in severe malaria, both as a fast diagnostic test (White and Silamut, 1989), and a prognostic tool (Silamut and White, 1993; Phu and Day, 1995).

Although experienced microscopists may detect as few as 10-50 parasites/uL, and identify the species of 98 percent of parasites seen (Moody, 2002), in actuality, obtaining such results requires a high level of skill and time, as well as optimal maintenance of equipment and reagents. Such conditions almost never exist on the periphery of health care in Africa, and other poor, malaria-endemic locales worldwide.

In one African trial, malaria diagnosis by light microscopy was shown to reduce drug use (Jonkman et al., 1995). However, the current reality in many endemic settings is that clinicians question the reliability of light microscopy results, or frankly disregard them (Barat et al., 1999). Mixed infections (involving more than one plasmodial species) also are routinely underreported by light microscopy (Personal communication, N. White, Mahidol University, March 2004).

Fluorescent Microscopy

The quantitative buffy coat test (QBC, Becton Dickinson) is a modification of light microscopy which exploits the affinity of parasite nucleic acid for acridine orange, a fluorescent dye. This test was adapted for malaria diagnosis using patented microhematocrit tubes pre-coated with acridine orange and fitted with a plastic float that spreads the buffy coat (the white blood cell and parasite fraction of blood) against the edge of the tube. When centrifuged, malaria parasites and leukocytes take up dye and collect at a predictable location within the tube where they can then be seen under ultraviolet light.

In field trials, QBC was slightly more sensitive than conventional light microscopy (Rickman et al., 1989; Tharavanij, 1990). Disadvantages of QBC are its need for electricity, special equipment, and supplies; its increased cost relative to light microscopy; and its inability to differentiate *P. falciparum* from other human malaria species.

Rapid Diagnostic Tests (RDTs)

A third diagnostic approach involves "dipstick" tests, which eliminate the need for a microscope and detect parasite antigens in blood by rapid immunochromatography using various antibodies. More than 20 such tests are currently marketed, and several are made in malaria-endemic countries. The majority are based on histidine-rich protein 2 (HRP-2) found in *P. falciparum*. Compared with light microscopy and QBC, HRP-2 tests yield a rapid and highly sensitive diagnosis of falciparum infection (WHO, 1996b; Craig and Sharp, 1997). The main drawbacks of HRP-2 tests are their high per-test cost (lowest price circa 50 U.S. cents) and inability to quantify the intensity of infection. In addition, HRP-2 antigen may persist for days or weeks following successful treatment. As a result, HRP-2 tests do not distinguish cured from nonresolving (i.e., drug-resistant) infections (WHO, 1996b). Several tests using HRP-2 to detect *P. falciparum* also include a second antigen to distinguish *P. falciparum* from other malaria species, although sensitivity generally is lower for *P. vivax*, and other non-*P. falciparum* species (Murray et al., 2003).

The OptiMAL dipstick detects the parasite enzyme lactate dehydrogenase (pLDH), which is actively produced by all malaria parasites during growth in human red cells (Piper et al., 1999). Unlike HRP-2, pLDH disappears from the bloodstream along with malaria parasites following successful treatment. OptiMAL also distinguishes *P. falciparum* from the other malaria species without differing levels of sensitivity for other species of malaria. In general, performance of OptiMAL in field studies has been high, but sensitivity in some recent trials has been erratic, perhaps due to batch problems or poor test handling (Murray et al., 2003). Quality control procedures for all rapid test types need improvement.

Field Application of Rapid Diagnostic Tests

In selected tropical countries and resource-poor settings where microscopy is either unavailable or unreliable, RDTs have great potential to reduce inappropriate antimalarial chemotherapy. For one thing, it is much easier to train someone to perform an RDT reliably than to be a reliable microscopist. RDTs have been used successfully in remote tribal groups in forested areas of central India (Singh et al., 2000), in refugee camps on the Thai-Burma border (Bualombai et al., 2003), and in rural health centers in Cambodia (Rimon et al., 2003). However, none of these areas approach the transmission levels of certain highly endemic areas of sub-Saharan Africa.

The utility of antigen detection in areas of Africa hyperendemic for malaria is less clear, because the tests are not quantitative, and the mere finding of parasites may be insufficient grounds for a diagnosis of malaria. One study in Zimbabwe indicated that mistreatment was reduced by up to 81 percent when ParaSight-F was used compared to presumptive diagnosis (Mharakurwa et al., 1997). However, the improvement in diagnostic accuracy was most marked in the hypodendemic part of the study region.

In summary, *when* to introduce RDTs into areas of sub-Saharan Africa hyperendemic for falciparum malaria remains an open question. One perspective on the use of RDTs comes from Asia, where providing the means to diagnose and treat malaria on the village level has coincided with a dramatic fall in morbidity and mortality. The fact that drug pressure is a major contributor to transmission of resistant parasites is another reason why universal treatment without RDTs should not be permitted indefinitely anywhere in the world. However, in high prevalence areas of sub-Saharan Africa, universal treatment of clinically suspected cases with ACTs is the safest near-term strategy, given the desperate need for rapid, in- or near-home treatment in order to save lives. Eventually, combining RDTs and ACTs in areas of Africa of low and medium malaria prevalence could reduce the number of illnesses misdiagnosed as malaria *and* yield major savings in terms of drug cost and delayed onset of drug resistance. In the meantime, following the introduction of ACTs in Africa, pilot programs and operational research combining ACTs and RDTs in a variety of epidemiologic settings and at-risk populations should be encouraged.

Molecular Methods

When malaria patients are parasitemic, their blood also contains malaria DNA and RNA. Applying a DNA probe to a filter paper with a small spot of human blood can identify malaria genetic material, including mutations or gene amplifications conferring drug resistance (Plowe and Wellems, 1995). Today, such methods are increasingly being used to detect molecular markers of drug resistance to chloroquine and SP. As long as the filter papers are properly handled, DNA can be recovered from them months after obtaining the samples (Farnert et al., 1999).

DNA and RNA techniques for rapid malaria diagnosis are currently impractical in most endemic regions, but their role may expand in selected populations as the tests become simpler and cheaper. Sensitive PCR techniques can detect parasites at a density as low as 1 per microliter, in contrast to 10-50 parasites per microliter with expert light microscopy (Greenwood, 2002).

MALARIA VACCINES

No malaria vaccine has yet entered routine use, and a safe and effective vaccine is at least another 10 years away (Greenwood and Alonso, 2002). This fact alone supports the central argument of this report, namely that a subsidy for effective treatment is an urgent priority that cannot wait until another control measure such as a vaccine is implemented. Nonetheless, the last 2 decades have seen significant progress in malaria vaccine research (Greenwood and Alonso, 2002). Highlights are summarized below.

The malaria vaccine era launched in the 1970s when, building on earlier work in rodent models, investigators at the University of Maryland demonstrated that irradiated sporozoites of *P. falciparum* and *P. vivax* protected naïve volunteers against challenge by infective mosquitoes (Clyde, 1975). For the next 2 decades, advances came mainly in experimental models rather than in human trials (Kwiatkowski and Marsh, 1997). In 1990, the first report of a vaccine field trial in an endemic area was published: a study of pre-erythrocytic vaccine in Burkina Faso (Guiguemde et al., 1990). A recent meta-analysis of malaria vaccine trials documented 18 trials with 10,971 participants using pre-erythrocytic and blood-stage vaccines (Graves and Gelband, 2003). Table 8-2 lists vaccines in field trials as

TABLE 8-2 Candidate Malaria Vaccines in Clinical Trials

Group (field collaboration)	Vaccines (type)	Target
Apovia, USA; New York University, USA	ICC-1132 (protein)	Pre-erythrocytic
GlazoSmithKline Biologicals, Belgium; and WRAIR, USA (Medical Research Council [MRC] Laboratories, The Gambia; Centro de investigacao em Suade de Manhica [CISM], Mozambique)	RTS,S (protein)	Pre-erythrocytic
Malaria Vaccine Development Unit, National Institutes of Health, USA	Pvs25, AMA-1 (protein)	Transmission blocking, blood stage
Naval Medical Research Center (NMRC), USA; Vical USA	Pf-CS, Pf-SSP2/TRAP, Pf-LSA-1, Pf-EXP-1, Pf-LSA-3 (DNA vaccines)	Pre-erythrocytic
New York University, USA	CS (synthetic polymers, MAPs, polyoximes)	Pre-erythrocytic
Oxford University, UK (MRC Laboratories, The Gambia; Wellcome-Kenya Medical Research Institute [KEMRI] collaboration, Kilifi, Kenya)	DNA ME-TRAP, MVA ME-TRAP, FP9 ME-TRAP, MVA-CS (DNA and recombinant viral)	Pre-erythrocytic
Statens Serum Institut (SSI), Copenhagen; Institut Pasteur; Institute of Lausanne, Switzerland	GLURP, MSP-3 (synthetic peptide)	Pre-erythrocytic, blood stage
Walter and Eliza Hall Institute of Medical Research, Melbourne; Queensland Institute of Medical Research (QIMR), Brisbane; Swiss Tropical Institute; Biotech Australia Pty (Papua New Guinea Institute of Medical Research)	MSP-1, MSP-2, RESA (protein)	Blood stage
Walter Reed Army Institute of Research (WRAIR), USA (KEMRI, Kisumu, Kenya)	FMP-1 (protein)	Blood stage

EXP = exported protein. LSA = liver stage antigen. MAP = multiple antigen peptide. Pvs = *Plasmodium vivax* surface protein. AMA-1 = apical membrane antigen-1. RESA = ring infected erythrocyte surface antigen. SSP2 and TRAP are synonyms: sporozoite surface protein 2 and thrombospondin-related adhesion protein.

Only vaccines being tested in clinical trials as of May 2003 are listed. Field collaborations are listed only if field trials of the candidate had begun as of May 2003.

SOURCE: Moorthy et al. (2004).

of May 2003 (Moorthy et al., 2004). Additional single and combination antigens are currently in various stages of pre-clinical assessment.

A comprehensive discussion of all malaria vaccines is beyond the scope of this report; however, certain basic concepts and prototype vaccines are covered below. For further details of specific vaccine antigens and strategies, readers are directed to several excellent published reviews (Moore et al., 2002; Carvalho et al., 2002; Mahanty et al., 2003; Moorthy et al., 2004).

Natural Immunity to Malaria

In malaria-endemic areas, natural human infection with *P. falciparum* induces some degree of immunity which first protects against severe, then mild malaria (McGregor, 1974). Maintaining functional immunity requires repeated infective mosquito bites, however (Cohen et al., 1961; Marsh and Howard, 1986). Of the 5,300 antigens encoded by *P. falciparum*, possibly 20 trigger key protective immune responses of both major types—antibody, and T-cell dependent—that follow natural exposure (Moorthy et al., 2004).

Vaccine Strategies Based on Parasite Life Cycle Stages

Unlike natural infection, experimental vaccines have traditionally targeted one of malaria's three biologic stages in its human or mosquito host: sporozoite, merozoite, or gametocyte. The goal of pre-erythrocytic (or sporozoite) vaccines is to block the initial entry of sporozoites into human liver cells. A current candidate of this class is RTS,S—a recombinant protein vaccine which pairs hepatitis B surface antigen DNA with DNA encoding a large portion of *P. falciparum* circumsporozoite protein. In a randomized controlled trial of three-dose RTS,S in Gambian adults, vaccine efficacy was 34 percent over a 15-week surveillance period (falling from 71 percent efficacy in the first 9 weeks to 0 percent in the next 6 weeks) (Church et al., 1997). Although short-lived, this vaccine-induced defense constituted the first protection against natural *P. falciparum* infection by a pre-erythrocytic vaccine. Phase I trials of RTS,S in children aged 1-11 years in The Gambia and Mozambique have now been completed, and a trial in children 1-4 years in Mozambique is currently under way. However, it is likely to be 10 years at least before RTS,S finds a place in routine immunization programs, even if the current pediatric trials are successful (Personal communication, B. Greenwood, London School of Hygiene and Tropical Medicine, March 2004).

In contrast to the all-or-none protective action of pre-erythrocytic vaccines, merozoite (or blood stage) vaccines have two potential effects: limiting RBC invasion, and reducing disease complications. Merozoite surface protein-1 (MSP-1) is the best characterized antigen mediating RBC invasion; it forms the basis of several candidate vaccines. Although some data suggest that vaccine-induced antibodies to MSP-1 may block natural malaria-protective antibodies (Holder et al., 1999), an anti-invasion vaccine based on MSP-1 has now moved to an adult phase I study in western Kenya.

Intravascular attachment of schizonts to endothelial cells in the brain, kidneys, and placenta is the most serious consequence of falciparum malaria. PfEMP-1 antigen is the main ligand for this sequestration event. Unfortunately, this antigen's high degree of variability, rapid rate of antigenic variation, and high copy number within individual parasites complicates vaccine development. Some investigators remain hopeful that conserved regions of PfEMP-1 may yield protective responses in humans (Moorthy et al., 2004).

Sexual-stage vaccines, rather than protecting vaccinated individuals, are meant to reduce malaria transmission, especially in combination with other control methods. Their principle is as follows. Anti-gametocyte antibodies induced in vaccinated humans enter female anophelines via blood meals. These antibodies interfere with parasite development in the vector's midgut, preventing further transmission. One major drawback to sexual stage vaccine candidates is their lack of commercial appeal to major pharmaceutical companies. Unlike sporozoite vaccines in particular (which could find a sizable market in tourists, migrants, and military personnel entering malarious zones) (Hoffman, 2003), sexual-stage vaccines are unlikely to be marketed outside malaria-endemic countries. An NIH-sponsored clinical trial of a recombinant protein (Pfs25) *P. falciparum* gametocyte vaccine is currently in development.

What Is Really Needed from a Malaria Vaccine?

Modern malaria vaccine development has followed a somewhat chance course thus far, guided by discoveries of particular antigens or enthusiasms of individual investigators (Greenwood and Alonso, 2002). However, as resources increase and more potential vaccine antigens are identified, defining the primary characteristics needed in a malaria vaccine becomes essential.

A perfect malaria vaccine would induce lifelong sterilizing immunity, provide cross-species protection, protect the very young, and be compatible with routine EPI (Expanded Programme on Immunization) vaccines. Since none of these goals will be achieved quickly, vaccine researchers are faced with a choice: either to work on a safe, highly efficacious and commercially viable vaccine (such as a pre-erythrocytic vaccine) for the short-term traveler or to work on a vaccine that offers more long-lasting protection, augmenting (as opposed to replacing) natural immunity in residents of malaria-endemic areas. For example, among semi-immune recipients, a blood-stage vaccine that lowered parasite density might prove beneficial even if it had little effect on the incidence of infection. Similarly, a partially effective pre-erythrocytic vaccine might protect against death from malaria just as ITNs do. Whether or not an imperfect malaria vaccine justifies use in a particular setting will depend upon its efficacy relative to other available control tools, its acceptability, and its cost.

Pregnant women in malaria-endemic areas, especially primigravidae, have a special need for enhanced malaria protection because of malaria's damaging effects in pregnancy. In some areas, it is becoming difficult to provide this protection through any other means (e.g., chemoprophylaxis, or intermittent treatment). A vaccine that prevented sequestration of *P. falciparum* parasites in the placenta might lessen the chance of a pregnant woman giving birth to a low-birth weight baby, but would not protect her from anemia.

Single versus Combination Candidates

For various reasons, including malaria's antigenic variation and protein polymorphisms, it is unlikely that any single malaria antigen will be found that meets all of the criteria for a perfect vaccine. Thus, the most effective malaria vaccines are likely to contain a "cocktail" of antigens from the same stage of the parasite's life cycle, or different antigens from different stages. The most extensively tested combination vaccine thus far is SPf 66, which includes several erythrocytic-stage antigens originally found protective in Colombia (Pattarroyo and Armador, 1999). However, trials using SPf66 in holoendemic areas of Africa showed marginal, if any, protection (Alonso et al., 1994; D'Alessandro et al., 1995), nor did the vaccine confer protection upon Tanzanian infants when administered as part of their initial EPI vaccine package (Acosta et al., 1999). The vaccine also failed to protect Karen children in a malarious region of northwestern Thailand (Nosten et al., 1996).

The first multistage, multiantigen *P. falciparum* vaccine candidate was NYVAC-Pf7, an attenuated vaccinia virus genetically engineered to include seven *P. falciparum* genes encoding the pre-erythrocytic antigens CSP and LSA1; the asexual blood stage antigens MSP1, AMA1 and SERA; and the transmission-blocking antigen PFs25 (Tine et al., 1996). Initial studies did not demonstrate protection against *P. falciparum* in human volunteers, although detectable immune responses were elicited (Ockenhouse et al., 1998). MuStDO (Multi-Stage Malaria DNA Vaccine Operation) is an ongoing collaboration involving several scientific institutions worldwide, including the Naval Medical Research Center (NMRC), the U.S. Agency for

International Development (USAID), the Noguchi Memorial Institute of Medical Research in Accra, Ghana, and the Navrongo Health Research Centre in Navrongo, Ghana. Experimental development of the MuStDO vaccine is currently focused on 15 *P. falciparum* antigens (5 pre-erythrocytic and 10 erythrocytic proteins) (Kumar et al., 2002), although future versions also may incorporate transmission-blocking antigens.

Practical Realities of Vaccine Testing and Use

Selecting which malaria antigens should enter clinical trials was not a major problem when there were relatively few candidates to choose from. However, characterization of the *P. falciparum* genome has now identified hundreds of parasite proteins that could potentially be tested as individual vaccine components. Selecting future vaccine components should rest upon: 1) evidence that the antigen plays an important role in the survival or pathogenicity of the parasite; 2) evidence from animal experiments that the antigen induces protective immunity in vivo; and 3) evidence that immune responses to the antigen are associated with protection (Greenwood and Alonso, 2002). If a vaccine candidate passes Phase I and Phase II testing, further considerations in designing phase III trials include study site, study population, study size, and appropriate clinical end points (Table 8-3). Another important factor that will influence whether a partially effective malaria vaccine is introduced into routine use will be its cost effectiveness relative to other malaria control measures, such as ITNs (Graves, 1998; Goodman et al., 1999).

TABLE 8-3 Possible End Points for Phase-III Malaria Vaccine Trials

End Point	Advantages	Disadvantages
Death	Most important public health end point	Requires large trial
Malaria mortality rate		Difficult to measure
Severe clinical malaria	Important end point	Requires high hospital admission rate
Mild, clinical malaria	Requires relatively small trial	May miss an effect on severe disease
Parasitemia	Easy to measure	May miss an important clinical effect

SOURCE: Greenwood and Alonso (2002).

No matter when and where vaccination enters widescale use, it is unlikely to supplant the need for effective treatment of drug-resistant falciparum malaria for several decades (Personal communication, B. Greenwood, London School of Hygiene and Tropical Medicine, March 2004).

INTEGRATED CONTROL PROGRAMS AND SPECIAL SETTINGS

Past and Present Models

Over recent years, several historical examples have been cited as evidence that malaria control could be achieved in endemic areas by combining environmental and human interventions. In the 1930s and 1940s, successful multipronged approaches to control transmission by *A. gambiae* operated in Brazil, Egypt, and Zambia (Utzinger et al., 2001; Killeen et al., 2002). In the Zambian copper mines, clearing vegetation, modifying river boundaries, draining swamps, and applying oil to open bodies of water coupled with house screening, mosquito nets, and quinine treatment reduced the local incidence of malaria by 70 to 95 percent for over 30 years (Utzinger et al., 2001). Today, contemporary versions of such programs are run by Exxon-Mobil in Cameroon and Chad, British Petroleum in Angola, and Konkola copper mine in Zambia.

In addition to commercial operations with a financial incentive to protect workers or residents from malaria using various combinations of environmental and vector control measures plus chemotherapy, local health authorities in endemic and epidemic settings have sometimes mounted integrated malaria programs within the normal health structure incorporating some or all of these elements (Shiff, 2002). Needless to say, such programs require coordination and planning, cooperation of local communities, and sustainable financing. A campaign that combined IRS plus artemisinin-containing combination therapy in KwaZulu Natal province, South Africa (in response to a local epidemic of multidrug resistant *Plasmodium falciparum)* is the most recent example of a successful government-sponsored integrated control program (Muheki et al, 2003). In recent years, research studies in Sierra Leone (Marbiah et al., 1998) and The Gambia (Alonso et al., 1993) have also supported the packaging of ITNs plus targeted chemoprophylaxis as a successful control package. On the other hand, the systematic deployment of ACTs in refugee camps on the northwest border of Thailand (population 120,000) produced a sustained reduction of more than 90 percent in the incidence of falciparum malaria without any additional control intervention (Nosten et al., 2000).

Urban Malaria

Integrated approaches are especially suited to malaria control programs based in urban areas. Although urban centers traditionally experience lower rates of malaria transmission than rural areas, the rapid increase in the world's urban population has major implications for the epidemiology of malaria (Robert et al., 2003). This is particularly true in sub-Saharan Africa, the most rapidly urbanizing continent (United Nations, 1999). In 1900, 10 percent of Africans lived in an urban area, whereas today almost half of the population in sub-Saharan Africa lives in urban or suburban areas. This proportion is expected to continue to rise over the next 25 years.

In fact, many African cities have unique features that still favor the transmission of malaria. Unlike Western cities with their distinct patterns of land use, housing construction, public utilities, and social services, many African cities have no such infrastructure, and feature larval habitats such as rice fields and garden wells adjacent to residential, market, and commercial areas (Robert et al., 2003), as well as suburban slums and shantytowns. Limited data also suggest that certain anopheline vectors may be adapting to urban ecology. In Accra, Ghana, *A. gambiae* has adapted to water-filled domestic containers and polluted water habitats (Chinery, 1990). In a newly urbanized area of Kenya, *A. gambiae* also bred in temporary man-made sites during the rainy season (Khaemba et al., 1994).

Excluding large private operations, it is currently believed that reducing malaria in a sustained fashion by vector control alone is near impossible in areas of high and moderate transmission (Trape et al., 2002). On the other hand, areas with naturally low or unstable transmission—such as highlands, mountain areas, semi-arid regions and urbanized areas—are far more amenable to vector control. As urbanization progresses, anopheline breeding sites in African cities should decrease and localize, thus facilitating control by classical methods such as drainage, larviciding, and indoor spraying (Trape and Zoulani, 1987; Trape et al., 1992). In the future, the upside of sub-Saharan urbanization may be the creation of malaria-free zones harboring a significant proportion of a country's population. This success could, in turn, stimulate expanding eradication efforts using vector control and other integrated interventions.

Epidemic Malaria

Malaria epidemics generally occur in regions where transmission is low or absent most of the time and populations lack protective immunity, although epidemics also can strike higher-transmission areas when there is a breakdown in health or environmental services, increasing drug resistance, or recent immigration of nonimmune individuals (e.g., laborers coming to work in a construction or other development project). Climate change also contributes to the development of epidemics. In terms of population effect, two common features of nearly all malaria epidemics are: 1) an equal risk of clinical disease and death among children and adults, and 2) a clinical burden that outweighs and overwhelms available health services (Snow and Gilles, 2002).

Epidemics and Climate Change

On the fringes of endemic areas, climate often restricts malaria transmission—i.e., normal conditions are either too dry, too wet, or too cold for propagation of vectors or parasites. In such sites, small environmental changes can trigger an epidemic. The El Niño Southern Oscillation (a weather event that originates in the Pacific Ocean but has wide-ranging global consequences, in particular droughts and floods) has been particularly well studied in this regard (Kovats et al., 2003). For example, El Niño-related droughts have been associated with malaria outbreaks in Sri Lanka (Bouma and van der Kaay, 1996), Colombia (Poveda et al., 2001), and Irian Jaya (Bangs and Subianto, 1999). Conversely, in highland regions, elevated temperatures due to El Niño may increase malaria transmission, as occurred in Northern Pakistan in 1981-1991(Bouma et al., 1996). Higher than usual temperatures, and heavy rainfall also have contributed to short-term increases in highland malaria in Rwanda (Loevinsohn, 1994) and Uganda (Lindblade et al., 1999).

Despite the effect of climate change on highland malaria, emerging evidence suggests that drug resistance has influenced highland epidemics in east Africa to a far greater degree than any other environmental factor (Hay et al., 2002). For example, chloroquine resistance has been identified as a key factor in the resurgence of malaria on the Kericho tea estates in Kenya where climate, environment, human population, health care provision, and malaria control measures remained stable (Shanks et al., 2000). Similarly, the malaria resurgence in the Usambara mountains of Tanzania has now been linked to the rise in antimalarial drug resistance (Bodker et al., 2000) as opposed to previously postulated climate change (Matola et al., 1987).

Mass Population Movements

There are many reasons for mass migration: war and civil strife, economic resettlement, environmental and natural disasters. Under appropriate conditions, this mobility can affect malaria transmission. Among 20 countries with a high risk of malaria transmission in the Americas, 16 identified human mobility as a major cause of persistence of transmission (PAHO, 1995). Migration also has been associated with the spread of drug-resistant malaria in Africa and Southeast Asia and with a dramatic change in the local epidemiology of malaria in Pakistan (Verdrager, 1986; Thimasarn et al., 1995; Kazmi and Pandit, 2001). In Kenya, the seasonal movement of many workers from lowlands to highland tea plantations has triggered epidemics (Malakooti et al., 1998; Shanks et al., 2000). Seasonal influx of migrant farm workers from Central and South America has produced local outbreaks of malaria in the United States (Zucker, 1996).

Similar data link malaria outbreaks with political upheaval and migration. In Southeast Asia, malaria was the leading cause of morbidity and mortality among Cambodian refugees upon arrival in eastern Thailand (Glass et al., 1980) and the Karen refugees in western Thailand (Luxemburger et al., 1996). In Central Asia, civil war and the collapse of the health care infrastructure led to a reemergence of malaria in Tajikistan (Pitt et al., 1998). In East Timor and Afghanistan, recent relief efforts have been complicated by malaria (Ezard, 2001; Sharp et al., 2002b). Africa's examples are most numerous. To name just a few: malaria was the leading cause of death among Mozambican refuges in Malawi and Ethiopian refugees in eastern Sudan, whereas fever due to malaria was second only diarrheal disease as the leading cause of morbidity and mortality among Rwandan refugees entering eastern Zaire (now Democratic Republic of Congo) (Bloland and Williams, 2002).

Following a mass migration into a malarious region, added risk factors for malaria outbreaks include: substandard housing and environmental protection from nighttime anopheline bites, deliberate relocation near open water, overcrowding, proximity of livestock, low socioeconomic status, poor nutritional status, a lack of immunity to malaria, destruction or overburdening of existing infrastructure, and scarce to non-existent health care services (Bloland and Williams, 2002).

Roll Back Malaria (RBM) Goals

One pillar of Roll Back Malaria's efforts to reduce Africa's malaria burden is the application of malaria early warning systems (MEWS) to speed responses to epidemics (WHO, 2000; WHO, 2001). Specifically, the Abuja target aims to identify, and respond to 60 percent of malaria epidemics in Africa within 2 weeks of onset and detection (WHO, 2001). The main tools of MEWS are:

- Forecasting (usually refers to seasonal climate forecasts)
- Early warning (monitoring meteorological conditions such as rainfall and temperature)
- Early detection (based on routine clinical surveillance)

Although RBM reports that MEWS generally are performing well in southern Africa and programs have started in Ethiopia, Kenya, Uganda, Tanzania, and Sudan (WHO/UNICEF, 2003), a recent failure to detect epidemics in Kenya is revealing. In summer 2002, early warning based on district-level rainfall estimates had the potential to detect two epidemics in four highland districts in southwestern Kenya. District-specific warnings could have given 4 weeks notice of possible emergency conditions. In this case, not only did the early warning system fail, early detection based on outpatient surveillance also was delayed because reporting was only being performed monthly. The authors of a retrospective analysis of the 2002 Kenya experience advocate better planning based on known seasonal epidemiologic risks (Hay et al., 2003).

Antimalarial Treatment and Other Control Measures During Epidemics

A timely and effective response to a possible malaria epidemic typically requires the deployment of additional drug stocks, use of highly effective treatments, and vector control, in particular, widespread IRS (Luxemburger et al., 1998; Rowland and Nosten, 2001). Early diagnosis also is important during rapid refugee influx; rapid diagnostic tests have proved very useful in such situations (Nosten et al., 1998). In addition, drug treatment policies that take into account the immune status of victims are needed. Artemisinin-based combinations are particularly attractive during epidemics because of their clinical efficacy and independent effects on gametocyte carriage (which, in turn, reduces transmission). Since epidemics frequently involve a high proportion of the population for a relatively short period, one or more rounds of mass drug administration (MDA) along with other control measures is another option for rapidly terminating an outbreak (von Seidlein and Greenwood, 2003). If MDA is chosen, the drug selected needs to kill gametocytes. It also should be given as promptly as possible, which poses a major logistical challenge.

MALARIA CONTROL PROGRAMS AND DRUG POLICIES

Malaria control cannot be a campaign; it should be a policy, a long-term programme. It cannot be accomplished by spasmodic effort. It requires the adoption of a practical programme . . . that will be sustained for a long time.

(Boyd, 1949)

Malaria Control Programs—Recent History and Lessons Learned

The strategy for malaria control approved by the WHO in 1979 stressed the need for program flexibility—namely, the adaptation of any and all available methods to realistic aims set by national health authorities, and feasible within the limitations of human and material resources (WHO, 1979). Subsequently, Article VIII of the World Declaration on Malaria Control (WHO, 1992b) made at the WHO Ministerial Conference on Malaria in October 1992 issued this landmark avowal: "We commit ourselves and our countries to control malaria and will plan for malaria control as an essential component of national development."

In reality, however, the final decades of the twentieth century witnessed a steady decline in malaria control as countries moved from large vertically run organizations focused on IRS and malaria eradication (admittedly, many such programs were flawed) to a new common denominator: "a village health worker with a jar of chloroquine tablets" (Personal communication, B. Greenwood, London School of Hygiene and Tropical Medicine, March 2004). A few countries such as India kept their central control programs after the eradication era ended, but most African countries did not. Today, many African countries are painstakingly rebuilding their national programs in order to access new resources for malaria control available through the Global Fund and other donor agencies.

Although recommending an ideal template for country-level malaria control is not the mission of this report, some general observations are in order. A modern malaria control program should possess at least five components: a public health surveillance system, curative services, preventive interventions, a program for community involvement, and a capacity to perform special studies (operational research) as needed (Bloland and Williams, 2002). Special functions that should also be undertaken at the national level include drug resistance monitoring and pharmacovigilance to survey for adverse or unexpected effects of new antimalarial treatments such as ACTs. Rather than returning to the massive yet narrowly focused organizations of the past, resurrected programs should occupy a middle ground between a centrally directed structure and one that allows full participation at all levels of the health care system. In addition, national malaria programs should consider creative partnerships with the private sector. A few examples of modern public-private synergies might include training private practitioners in malaria treatment; government-sponsored social marketing campaigns to complement the sale (or subsidized distribution) of ITNs; or government licensing of pharmacies with personnel certified to dispense antimalarials, and other essential medicines on the periphery of health care.

Antimalarial Drug Policy—Recent Examples and Lessons Learned

Today, prompt and effective treatment is the key to reducing drug-resistant malaria's increasing morbidity and mortality. Rational antimalarial drug policies are therefore essential elements of any national malaria control program. Because many countries with growing resistance to first-, second-, and even third-line antimalarial drugs are burdened with debt and poorly financed health budgets, a change in antimalarial drug policy is economically daunting. The process of policy change can also be time consuming and involved.

A detailed analysis of Kenya's change from chloroquine to SP emphasizes the complexity of the decision-making and implementation process even when two drugs are similar in cost (Shretta et al., 2000). Chloroquine resistance was first acknowledged at a meeting organized by the Kenya Medical Research Institute in January 1989. In 1991, the Ministry of Health requested a review of the scientific evidence in support of a revision. In October 1997, draft guidelines were finally issued, reflecting more than 20 independent studies over 14 years documenting chloroquine failure.

Even after consensus has been reached, multiple factors can delay country-level implementation for another 18 months or more: political and financial support, training of health care providers, and sensitization of the general population, which is crucial for ultimate success of the antimalarial changeover (WHO/UNICEF, 2003). In the future, a culture in which changes in malaria treatment, based on sound evidence, can occur on a fairly regular basis will be crucial. This is happening to some extent now (e.g., in Kenya, and Tanzania) but far more flexibility, and rapid response is needed in most malaria endemic countries.

Current Status of National Malaria Drug Policy in Africa, Asia, and South America

In 1993, Malawi was the first sub-Saharan country to switch from chloroquine to SP as first-line therapy for *P. falciparum*. Between 1998 and 2001, Kenya, Uganda, Tanzania, Zanzibar, Rwanda, and Burundi followed suit (like Malawi, they either chose SP monotherapy or a combination of SP plus chloroquine or amodiaquine). Countries that have now adopted and (more recently) implemented ACTs include Tanzania (Zanzibar) (2001), Zambia (2001), and Burundi (2002). In South Africa, the provinces where ACTs have been fully implemented are KwaZulu Natal (Coartem), and Mpumalanga (artesunate+SP) (WHO/UNICEF, 2003). First-line antimalarial drug policies for selected countries in Africa, Asia, and South America, as of March 2003, are listed in Table 8-4.

TABLE 8-4 Countries/Regions Using ACTs as First-Line Therapy for Uncomplicated Malaria

Region/Country	First-Line Treatment
Africa Region	
Burundi	AS+AQ
Comoros	AL
South Africa (KwaZulu Natal)	AL
Zambia	AL
Zanzibar	AS+AQ
Western Pacific Region	
Cambodia	AS(3d)+MQ
China, Yunnan, Hainan	ATM/AS(5d)
Lao PDR	AS+MFQ
Viet Nam, north	ATS/AS(5d)+PQ
Viet Nam other	AS(3d)+MQ25
South-East Asia Region	
Bhutan	MQ+AS(3d)
Myanmar	AS(3d)+MQ
Thailand	MQ+AS(3d)
America Region	
Bolivia	MQ15+AS(3d)CQ+PQ
Guyana	AL
Peru (Amazon area)	AS(3d)+MQ
	AS(3d)+SP
Suriname	AL

AL=Artemether-lumefantrine
AQ=Amodiaquine
AS=Artesunate
ATM=Artemether
ATS=Artemisinin
CQ=Chloroquine
MQ=Mefloquine
MQ15=Mefloquine 15mg/kg
MQ25=Mefloquine 25mg/kg
PQ=Primaquine
Q=Quinine
SP=Sulfadoxine-pyrimethamine
T=Tetracycline

SOURCE (as of March, 2003): http://rbm.who.int/amdp/amdp_amro.htm, http://rbm. who.int/amdp/amdp_afro, http://rbm.who.int/amdp/amdp_emro.htm, http://rbm.who. int/amdp/amdp_searo

Regional Networks and Future Policy Implications

At present, most control policies are still organized at a national or subnational level (Kaul and Faust, 2001), but interest in regional approaches is increasing. For one thing, individual countries can no longer make drug policy decisions in isolation. Given the fluid nature of borders, they now realize that their and their neighbors' policies affect each other. There are increasing calls for information exchanges among neighboring countries about their respective malaria situations, malaria treatment policies, and approaches used to combat drug-resistant malaria.

Recognizing that a regional approach offers a better platform for addressing malaria control problems that influence policy, several networks and initiatives have been established, most notably, the East African Network for Monitoring Antimalarial Treatments (EANMAT), the West African Networks for Monitoring Antimalarial Treatments (WANMAT I and II), the South East African Combination Antimalarial Therapy (SEACAT) Evaluation, a Central African network (Réseau d'Afrique Centrale des Thérapeutiques Antipaludiques, or RACTAP), the Amazon Malaria Initiative (AMI), and the Asian Collaborative Training Network for Malaria (ACTMalaria). These networks focus on partnership and shared goals in malaria control with a particular focus on training, research, and operational issues.

Pending full implementation of ACTs in Africa and elsewhere, one current dilemma that many malaria-endemic countries face is the practical question of when—in the face of growing antimalarial drug resistance—a change in drug policy should be implemented. Should it be initiated early, when only a small fraction of the population is at risk, or at a later stage, when risk affects a higher proportion of the susceptible population? Until recently, WHO recommended a change to more effective treatment when clinical failure rates exceeded 25 percent 14 days following treatment; now it has lowered the ceiling to >15 percent clinical and >25 percent total failure (i.e., clinical + parasitologic [WHO/HTM/RBM/2003.50]). No matter what standard threshold is selected, uniform change points fail to take into account districts where malaria is seasonal or epidemic, and local populations are therefore more vulnerable to adverse clinical outcomes from drug resistant malaria.

In addition, many authors have noted that the original WHO categories of response (grace, alert, action, and change) were developed in response to the relatively slow rate at which chloroquine resistance emerges. In contrast to chloroquine and amodiaquine, SP resistance emerges and spreads quickly in areas of high transmission (Talisuna et al., 2002). Finally, there are technical questions regarding the WHO test itself. Since it does not provide information on treatment failure beyond 14 days, many experts believe that estimates of resistance based on these tests are significantly lower than the real rates of treatment failure, which malaria patients in east Africa are actually suffering (EANMAT, 2003). A recent analysis of a sample comprising 23 percent of all randomized trials published since 1965 suggests that the 14-day test could miss as many as 63 to 100 percent of treatment failures (Stepniewska et al., in press).

CONCLUSION

In summary, as of 2004, malaria control can be viewed either as a cup half-full or half-empty. On the positive side: more money has become available for malaria control (although not nearly enough), long-lasting ITNs are finally becoming a reality, combination therapy with artemisinins is more widely available than before (although a radical solution is still needed for ACTs to reach the vast majority of malaria sufferers, especially in sub-Saharan Africa), and vaccine research is progressing. Vector control and ITNs will never have a major effect in many areas of Asia, on the other hand, because of local vector behavior; there, the main strategy *must* be effective treatment. And despite many earnest hopes for a vaccine solution to the world's malaria problem, vaccines are far from ready and will never control malaria by themselves—in Africa especially, there will always be a role for vector control and drugs. Improved drug delivery (including home management of severe malaria with ACTs) is another practical issue that is currently under consideration but will require even more attention after effective first-line treatments reach Africa.

REFERENCES

Abdulla S, Schellenberg JA, Nathan R, Mukasa O, Marchant T, Smith T, Tanner M, Lengeler C. 2001. Impact on malaria morbidity of a programme supplying insecticide treated nets in children aged under 2 years in Tanzania: Community cross sectional study. *British Medical Journal* 322(7281):270-273.

Acosta CJ, Galindo CM, Schellenberg D, Aponte JJ, Kahigwa E, Urassa H, Schellenberg JR, Masanja H, Hayes R, Kitua AY, Lwilla F, Mshinda H, Menendez C, Tanner M, Alonso PL. 1999. Evaluation of the SPf66 vaccine for malaria control when delivered through the EPI scheme in Tanzania. *Tropical Medicine and International Health* 4(5):368-376.

Agyepong IA. 1992. Malaria: Ethnomedical perceptions and practice in an Adangbe farming community and implications for control. *Social Science and Medicine* 35(2):131-137.

Alaii JA, Hawley WA, Kolczak MS, ter Kuile FO, Gimnig JE, Vulule JM, Odhacha A, Oloo AJ, Nahlen BL, Phillips-Howard PA. 2003a. Factors affecting use of permethrin-treated bed nets during a randomized controlled trial in western Kenya. *American Journal of Tropical Medicine and Hygiene* 68(4 Suppl):137-141.

Alaii JA, van den Borne HW, Kachur SP, Mwenesi H, Vulule JM, Hawley WA, Meltzer MI, Nahlen BL, Phillips-Howard PA. 2003b. Perceptions of bed nets and malaria prevention before and after a randomized controlled trial of permethrin-treated bed nets in western Kenya. *American Journal of Tropical Medicine and Hygiene* 68(4 Suppl):142-148.

Allen SJ, Snow RW, Menon A, Greenwood BM. 1990. Compliance with malaria chemopro-phylaxis over a five-year period among children in a rural area of the Gambia. *Journal of Tropical Medicine and Hygiene* 93(5):313-322.

Alonso PL, Lindsay SW, Armstrong JR, Conteh M, Hill AG, David PH, Fegan G, de Fran-cisco A, Hall AJ, Shenton FC. 1991. The effect of insecticide-treated bed nets on mortal-ity of Gambian children. *Lancet* 337(8756):1499-1502.

Alonso PL, Lindsay SW, Armstrong Schellenberg JR, Konteh M, Keita K, Marshall C, Phillips A, Cham K, Greenwood BM. 1993. A malaria control trial using insecticide-treated bed nets and targeted chemoprophylaxis in a rural area of the Gambia, West Africa. 5: Design and implementation of the trial. *Transactions of the Royal Society of Tropical Medicine and Hygiene* 87(Suppl 2):31-36.

Alonso PL, Smith T, Armstrong-Schellenberg JR, Masanja H, Mwankusye S, Urassa H, Bastos de Azevedo I, Chongela J, Kobero S, Menendez C. 1994. Randomised trial of efficacy of SPf66 vaccine against *Plasmodium falciparum* malaria in children in southern Tanzania. *Lancet* 344(8931):1175-1181.

Attaran A, Roberts DR, Curtis CF, Kilama WL. 2000. Balancing risks on the backs of the poor. *Nature Medicine* 6(7):729-731.

Bangs M, Subianto DB. 1999. El Niño and associated outbreaks of severe malaria in highland populations in Irian Jaya, Indonesia: A review and epidemiologic perspective. *Southeast Asian Journal of Tropical Medicine and Public Health* 30:608-616.

Barat L, Chipipa J, Kolczak M, Sukwa T. 1999. Does the availability of blood slide micros-copy for malaria at health centers improve the management of persons with fever in Zambia? *American Journal of Tropical Medicine and Hygiene* 60(6):1024-1030.

Barber MA. 1929. The history of malaria in the United States. *USA Public Health Report* 44:2575-2587.

Barber MA, Rice JB, Brown JY. 1932. Malaria studies on the Firestone rubber plantation in Liberia, West Africa. *American Journal of Tropical Medicine and Hygiene* 15:601-623.

Barnes KI, Durrheim DN, Jackson A. 2003. Epidemiology of malaria following implementa-tion of artemether-lumefantrine as first-line treatment of uncomplicated disease in Kwa Zulu-Natal, South Africa. *Antibiotics and Chemotherapy* 7:8.

Beach RF, Ruebush TK II, Sexton JD, Bright PL, Hightower AW, Breman JG, Mount DL, Oloo AJ. 1993. Effectiveness of permethrin-impregnated bed nets and curtains for ma-laria control in a holoendemic area of western Kenya. *American Journal of Tropical Medicine and Hygiene* 49(3):290-300.

Beales PF, Gilles HM. 2002. Rationale and technique of malaria control. In: Warrell DA, Gilles HM, eds. *Essential Malariology*. 4th ed. London: Arnold Publishing.

Binka FN, Adongo P. 1997. Acceptability and use of insecticide impregnated bednets in northern Ghana. *Tropical Medicine and International Health* 2(5):499-507.

Binka FN, Kubaje A, Adjuik M, Williams LA, Lengeler C, Maude GH, Armah GE, Kajihara B, Adiamah JH, Smith PG. 1996. Impact of permethrin impregnated bed nets on child mortality in Kassena-Nankana district, Ghana: A randomized controlled trial. *Tropical Medicine and International Health* 1(2):147-154.

Binka FN, Indome F, Smith T. 1998. Impact of spatial distribution of permethrin-impreg-nated bed nets on child mortality in rural northern Ghana. *American Journal of Tropical Medicine and Hygiene* 59(1):80-85.

Blagoveschensky D, Bregetova N, Monchadsky A. 1945. An investigation of new repellants for the protection of man against mosquito attacks. *Transactions of the Royal Society of Tropical Medicine and Hygiene* 34:147-150.

Bloland PB, Williams H. 2002. *Malaria Control During Mass Population Movements and Disasters*. Committee on Population. National Research Council of the National Acad-emies, Roundtable on the Demography of Forced Migration. Washington, DC: The National Academies Press.

Bockarie MJ, Service MW, Barnish G, Momoh W, Salia F. 1994. The effect of woodsmoke on the feeding and resting behaviour of *Anopheles gambiae s.s. Acta Tropica* 57(4):337-340.

Bodker R, Kisinza W, Malima R, Msangeni H, Lindsay S. 2000. Resurgence of malaria in the Usambara Mountains, Tanzania, an epidemic of drug-resistant parasites. *Global Change and Human Health* 1(2):134-153.

Bouma M, Rowland M. 1995. Failure of passive zooprophylaxis: Cattle ownership in Pakistan is associated with a higher prevalence of malaria. [See Comment]. *Transactions of the Royal Society of Tropical Medicine and Hygiene* 89(4):351-353.

Bouma MJ, Dye C, van der Kaay HJ. 1996a. Falciparum malaria and climate change in the northwest frontier province of Pakistan. *American Journal of Tropical Medicine and Hygiene* 55(2):131-137.

Bouma MJ, van der Kaay HJ. 1996b. The El Niño southern oscillation and the historic malaria epidemics on the Indian subcontinent and Sri Lanka: An early warning system for future epidemics? *Tropical Medicine and International Health* 1(1):86-96.

Boyd MF. 1949. *Malariology*. Philadelphia: Saunders.

Bradley DJ. 1991. Morbidity and mortality at Pare-Taveta, Kenya and Tanzania, 1954-66: The effects of a period of malaria control. In: Feachem RG, Jamison D, eds. *Disease and Mortality in Sub-Saharan Africa*. Oxford: Oxford University Press.

Brooke BD, Kloke G, Hunt RH, Koekemoer LL, Temu EA, Taylor ME, Small G, Hemingway J, Coetzee M. 2001. Bioassay and biochemical analyses of insecticide resistance in southern African *Anopheles funestus* (Diptera: Culicidae). *Bulletin of Entomological Research* 91(4):265-272.

Browne EN, Maude GH, Binka FN. 2001. The impact of insecticide-treated bednets on malaria and anaemia in pregnancy in Kassena-Nankana district, Ghana: A randomized controlled trial. *Tropical Medicine and International Health* 6(9):667-676.

Bualombai P, Prajakwong S, Aussawatheerakul N, Congpoung K, Sudathip S, Thimasarn K, Sirichaisinthop J, Indaratna K, Kidson C, Srisuphanand M. 2003. Determining cost-effectiveness and cost component of three malaria diagnostic models being used in remote non-microscope areas. *Southeast Asian Journal of Tropical Medicine and Public Health* 34(2):322-333.

Carvalho LJM, Daniel-Ribeiro CT, Goto H. 2002. Malaria vaccine: Candidate antigens, mechanisms, constraints and prospects. *Scandinavian Journal of Immunology* 56(4):327-343.

Chandramohan D, Jaffar S, Greenwood B. 2002. Use of clinical algorithms for diagnosing malaria. *Tropical Medicine and International Health* 7(1):45-52.

Chandre F, Darrier F, Manga L, Akogbeto M, Faye O, Mouchet J, Guillet P. 1999. Status of pyrethroid resistance in *Anopheles gambiae* sensu lato. *Bulletin of the World Health Organization* 77(3):230-234.

Charlwood JD, Jolley D. 1984. The coil works (against mosquitoes in Papua New Guinea). *Transactions of the Royal Society of Tropical Medicine and Hygiene* 78(5):678.

Chavasse D, Reed C, Attawall K. 1999. *Insecticide Treated Net Projects: A Handbook for Managers*. London and Liverpool: Malaria Consortium.

Chinery WA. 1990. Variation in frequency in breeding of *Anopheles gambiae s.l.* and its relationship with in-door adult mosquito density in various localities in Accra, Ghana. *East African Medical Journal* 67(5):328-335.

Church LW, Le TP, Bryan JP, Gordon DM, Edelman R, Fries L, Davis JR, Herrington DA, Clyde DF, Shmuklarsky MJ, Schneider I, McGovern TW, Chulay JD, Ballou WR, Hoffman SL. 1997. Clinical manifestations of *Plasmodium falciparum* malaria experimentally induced by mosquito challenge. *Journal of Infectious Diseases* 175(4):915-920.

Clarke T. 2002. Mosquitoes minus malaria. *Nature* 419(6906):429-430.

Clyde DF. 1975. Immunization of man against falciparum and vivax malaria by use of attenuated sporozoites. *American Journal of Tropical Medicine and Hygiene* 24(3):397-401.

Cohen S, McGregor IA, Carrington S. 1961. Gamma-globulin and acquired immunity to human malaria. *Nauchni trudove na Visshiia meditsinski institut, Sofiia* 192:733-737.

Collins FH. 1994. Prospects for malaria control through the genetic manipulation of its vectors. *Parasitology Today* 10(10):370-371.

Craig MH, Sharp BL. 1997. Comparative evaluation of four techniques for the diagnosis of *Plasmodium falciparum* infections. *Transactions of the Royal Society of Tropical Medicine and Hygiene* 91(3):279-282.

Curtis CF. 1968. Possible use of translocations to fix desirable genes in insect pest populations. *Nature* 218(139):368-369.

Curtis CF, Lines JD. 2000. Should DDT be banned by international treaty? *Parasitology Today* 16(3):119-121.

Curtis CF, Myamba J, Wilkes TJ. 1992. Various pyrethroids on bednets and curtains. *Memorias do Instituto Oswaldo Cruz* 87(Suppl 3):363-370.

D'Alessandro U, Leach A, Drakeley CJ, Bennett S, Olaleye BO, Fegan GW, Jawara M, Langerock P, George MO, Targett GA. 1995. Efficacy trial of malaria vaccine SPf66 in Gambian infants. *Lancet* 346(8973):462-467.

D'Alessandro U, Langerock P, Bennett S, Francis N, Cham K, Greenwood BM. 1996. The impact of a national impregnated bed net programme on the outcome of pregnancy in primigravidae in the Gambia. *Transactions of the Royal Society of Tropical Medicine and Hygiene* 90(5):487-492.

Desowitz R. 1999. Milestones in the history of malaria. In: Wahlgren M, Perlmann P, eds. *Malaria*. Amsterdam: Harwood Academic.

Diallo DA, Habluetzel A, Cuzin-Ouattara N, Nebie I, Sanogo E, Cousens SN, Esposito F. 1999. Widespread distribution of insecticide-impregnated curtains reduces child mortality, prevalence and intensity of malaria infection, and malaria transmission in rural Burkina Faso. *Parassitologia* 41(1-3):377-381.

Dolan G, ter Kuile FO, Jacoutot V, White NJ, Luxemburger C, Malankirii L, Chongsuphajaisiddhi T, Nosten F. 1993. Bed nets for the prevention of malaria and anaemia in pregnancy. *Transactions of the Royal Society of Tropical Medicine and Hygiene* 87(6):620-626.

East African Network for Monitoring Antimalarial Treatment (EANMAT). 2003. The efficacy of antimalarial monotherapies, sulphadoxine-pyrimethamine and amodiaquine in east Africa: Implications for sub-regional policy. *Tropical Medicine and International Health* 8(10):860-867.

Ezard N. 2001. Research in complex emergencies. Medical emergency relief international. *Lancet* 357(9250):149.

Farnert A, Arez AP, Correia AT, Bjorkman A, Snounou G, do Rosario V. 1999. Sampling and storage of blood and the detection of malaria parasites by polymerase chain reaction. *Transactions of the Royal Society of Tropical Medicine and Hygiene* 93(1):50-53.

Garfield RM, Vermund SH. 1983. Changes in malaria incidence after mass drug administration in Nicaragua. *Lancet* 2(8348):500-503.

Garner P, Gulmezoglu AM. 2000. Prevention versus treatment for malaria in pregnant women. *Cochrane Database of Systematic Reviews* (2):CD000169.

Giglioli G, Rutten FJ, Ramjattan S. 1967. Interruption of malaria transmission by chloroquinized salt in Guyana, with observations on a chloroquine-resistant strain of *Plasmodium falciparum*. *Bulletin of the World Health Organization* 36(2):283-301.

Gimnig JE, Kolczak MS, Hightower AW, Vulule JM, Schoute E, Kamau L, Phillips-Howard PA, ter Kuile FO, Nahlen BL, Hawley WA. 2003a. Effect of permethrin-treated bed nets on the spatial distribution of malaria vectors in western Kenya. *American Journal of Tropical Medicine and Hygiene* 68(4 Suppl):115-120.

Gimnig JE, Vulule JM, Lo TQ, Kamau L, Kolczak MS, Phillips-Howard PA, Mathenge EM, ter Kuile FO, Nahlen BL, Hightower AW, Hawley WA. 2003b. Impact of permethrin-treated bed nets on entomologic indices in an area of intense year-round malaria transmission. *American Journal of Tropical Medicine and Hygiene* 68(4 Suppl):16-22.

Glass RI, Cates W Jr, Nieburg P, Davis C, Russbach R, Nothdurft H, Peel S, Turnbull R. 1980. Rapid assessment of health status and preventive-medicine needs of newly arrived Kampuchean refugees, Sa Kaeo, Thailand. *Lancet* 1(8173):868-872.

Goodman CA, Coleman PG, Mills AJ. 1999. Cost-effectiveness of malaria control in sub-Saharan Africa. *Lancet* 354(9176):378-385.

Goodman CA, Mnzava AE, Dlamini SS, Sharp BL, Mthembu DJ, Gumede JK. 2001. Comparison of the cost and cost-effectiveness of insecticide-treated bednets and residual house-spraying in Kwazulu-Natal, South Africa. *Tropical Medicine and International Health* 6(4):280-295.

Graves P, Gelband H. 2003. Vaccines for preventing malaria. *Cochrane Database of Systematic Reviews* (1):CD000129.

Graves PM. 1998. Comparison of the cost-effectiveness of vaccines and insecticide impregnation of mosquito nets for the prevention of malaria. *Annals of Tropical Medicine and Parasitology* 92(4):399-410.

Graves PM, Burkot TR, Carter R, Cattani JA, Lagog M, Parker J, Brabin BJ, Gibson FD, Bradley DJ, Alpers MP. 1988. Measurement of malarial infectivity of human populations to mosquitoes in the Madang area, Papua, New Guinea. *Parasitology* 96(Pt 2):251-263.

Greenwood B. 1999. What can the residents of malaria endemic countries do to protect themselves against malaria? *Parassitologia* 41(1-3):295-299.

Greenwood B. 2002. The molecular epidemiology of malaria. *Tropical Medicine and International Health* 7(12):1012-1021.

Greenwood B. 2004. The use of anti-malarial drugs to prevent malaria in the population of malaria-endemic areas. *American Journal of Tropical Medicine and Hygiene* 70:1-7.

Greenwood B, Alonso P. 2002. Malaria vaccine trials. *Chemical Immunology* 80:366-395.

Greenwood B, Mutabingwa T. 2002. Malaria in 2002. *Nature* 415(6872):670-672.

Greenwood BM, Greenwood AM, Bradley AK, Snow RW, Byass P, Hayes RJ, N'Jie AB. 1988. Comparison of two strategies for control of malaria within a primary health care programme in the Gambia. *Lancet* 1(8595):1121-1127.

Greenwood BM, Greenwood AM, Snow RW, Byass P, Bennett S, Hatib-N'Jie AB. 1989. The effects of malaria chemoprophylaxis given by traditional birth attendants on the course and outcome of pregnancy. *Transactions of the Royal Society of Tropical Medicine and Hygiene* 83(5):589-594.

Greenwood BM, David PH, Otoo-Forbes LN, Allen SJ, Alonso PL, Armstrong Schellenberg JR, Byass P, Hurwitz M, Menon A, Snow RW. 1995. Mortality and morbidity from malaria after stopping malaria chemoprophylaxis. *Transactions of the Royal Society of Tropical Medicine and Hygiene* 89(6):629-633.

Guerin PJ, Olliaro P, Nosten F, Druilhe P, Laxminarayan R, Binka F, Kilama WL, Ford N, White NJ. 2002. Malaria: Current status of control, diagnosis, treatment, and a proposed agenda for research and development. *The Lancet Infectious Diseases* 2(9):564-573.

Guiguemde TR, Sturchler D, Ouedraogo JB, Drabo M, Etlinger H, Douchet C, Gbary AR, Haller L, Kambou S, Fernex M. 1990. [Vaccination against malaria: Initial trial with an ant-sporozoite vaccine, (Nanp)3-Tt (Ro 40-2361) in Africa (Bobo-Dioulasso, Burkina Faso)]. [French]. *Bulletin de la Societe de Pathologie Exotique* 83(2):217-227.

Guillet P, Alnwick D, Cham MK, Neira M, Zaim M, Heymann D, Mukelabai K. 2001. Long-lasting treated mosquito nets: A breakthrough in malaria prevention. *Bulletin of the World Health Organization* 79(10):998.

Gunawardena DM, Wickremasinghe AR, Muthuwatta L, Weerasingha S, Rajakaruna J, Senanayaka T, Kotta PK, Attanayake N, Carter R, Mendis KN. 1998. Malaria risk factors in an endemic region of Sri Lanka, and the impact and cost implications of risk factor-based interventions. *American Journal of Tropical Medicine and Hygiene* 58(5): 533-542.

Gyapong M, Gyapong JO, Amankwa J, Asedem J, Sory E. 1996. Introducing insecticide impregnated bednets in an area of low bednet usage: An exploratory study in North-east Ghana. *Tropical Medicine and International Health* 1(3):328-333.

Habluetzel A, Diallo DA, Esposito F, Lamizana L, Pagnoni F, Lengeler C, Traore C, Cousens SN. 1997. Do insecticide-treated curtains reduce all-cause child mortality in Burkina Faso? *Tropical Medicine and International Health* 2(9):855-862.

Hargreaves K, Koekemoer LL, Brooke BD, Hunt RH, Mthembu J, Coetzee M. 2000. *Anopheles funestus* resistant to pyrethroid insecticides in South Africa. *Medical and Veterinary Entomology* 14(2):181-189.

Harper PA, Lisansky ET, Sasse BE. 1947. Malaria and other insect-borne diseases in the South Pacific campaign. *American Journal of Tropical Medicine and Hygiene* 27(1 Suppl):1942-1945.

Harrison, G. 1978. *Mosquitoes, Malaria and Man: A History of the Hostilities Since 1880.* New York: Dutton.

Hawley WA, Phillips-Howard PA, ter Kuile FO, Terlouw DJ, Vulule JM, Ombok M, Nahlen BL, Gimnig JE, Kariuki SK, Kolczak MS, Hightower AW. 2003a. Community-wide effects of permethrin-treated bed nets on child mortality and malaria morbidity in Western Kenya. *American Journal of Tropical Medicine and Hygiene* 68(4 Suppl):121-127.

Hawley WA, ter Kuile FO, Steketee RS, Nahlen BL, Terlouw DJ, Gimnig JE, Shi YP, Vulule JM, Alaii JA, Hightower AW, Kolczak MS, Kariuki SK, Phillips-Howard PA. 2003b. Implications of the Western Kenya permethrin-treated bed net study for policy, program implementation, and future research. *American Journal of Tropical Medicine and Hygiene* 68(4 Suppl):168-173.

Hay S, Renshaw M, Ochola SA, Noor AM, Snow RW. 2003. Performance of forecasting, warning and detection of malaria epidemics in the highlands of Western Kenya. *Trends in Parasitology* 19(9):394-399.

Hay SI, Rogers DJ, Randolph SE, Stern DI, Cox J, Shanks GD, Snow RW. 2002. Hot topic or hot air? Climate change and malaria resurgence in East African Highlands. *Trends in Parasitology* 18(12):530-534.

Hemingway J, Bates I. 2003. Malaria: Past problems and future prospects. After more than a decade of neglect, malaria is finally back on the agenda for both biomedical research and public health politics. *EMBO Reports* 4(SPEC. ISS.):S29-S31.

Hewitt S, Kamal M, Muhammad N, Rowland M. 1994. An entomological investigation of the likely impact of cattle ownership on malaria in an Afghan refugee camp in the North West Frontier Province of Pakistan. *Medical and Veterinary Entomology* 8(2):160-164.

Hii JL, Smith T, Mai A, Mellor S, Lewis D, Alexander N, Alpers MP. 1997. Spatial and temporal variation in abundance of anopheles (Diptera: Culicidae) in a malaria endemic area in Papua New Guinea. *Journal of Medical Entomology* 34(2):193-205.

Hii JL, Smith T, Mai A, Ibam E, Alpers MP. 2000. Comparison between anopheline mosquitoes (Diptera: Culicidae) caught using different methods in a malaria endemic area of Papua New Guinea. *Bulletin of Entomological Research* 90(3):211-219.

Hoffman SL. 2003. Current status of malaria vaccine development efforts. Paper commissioned by the Institute of Medicine, Washington, DC.

Holder AA, Guevara Patino JA, Uthaipibull C, Syed SE, Ling IT, Scott-Finnigan T, Blackman MJ. 1999. Merozoite surface protein 1, immune evasion, and vaccines against asexual blood stage malaria. *Parassitologia* 41(1-3):409-414.

Howard SC, Omumbo J, Nevill C, Some ES, Donnelly CA, Snow RW. 2000. Evidence for a mass community effect of insecticide-treated bednets on the incidence of malaria on the Kenyan coast. *Transactions of the Royal Society of Tropical Medicine and Hygiene* 94(4):357-360.

Hung LQ, De Vries PJ, Giao PT, Nam NV, Binh TQ, Chong MT, Quoc NTTA, Thanh TN, Hung LN, Kager PA. 2002. Control of malaria: A successful experience from Viet Nam. *Bulletin of the World Health Organization* 80(8):660-666.

Ito J, Ghosh A, Moreira LA, Wimmer EA, Jacobs-Lorena M. 2002. Transgenic anopheline mosquitoes impaired in transmission of a malaria parasite. *Nature* 417(6887):452-455.

James AA, Beerntsen BT, Capurro Mde L, Coates CJ, Coleman J, Jasinskiene N, Krettli AU. 1999. Controlling malaria transmission with genetically-engineered, plasmodium-resistant mosquitoes: Milestones in a model system. *Parassitologia* 41(1-3):461-471.

Jonkman A, Chibwe RA, Khoromana CO, Liabunya UL, Chaponda ME, Kandiero GE, Molyneux ME, Taylor TE. 1995. Cost-saving through microscopy-based versus presumptive diagnosis of malaria in adult outpatients in Malawi. *Bulletin of the World Health Organization* 73(2):223-227.

Kaneko A, Taleo G, Kalkoa M, Yamar S, Kobayakawa T, Bjorkman A. 2000. Malaria Eradication on Islands. [See Comment]. *Lancet* 356(9241):1560-1564.

Karch S, Asidi N, Manzambi ZM, Salaun JJ. 1992. Efficacy of *Bacillus sphaericus* against the malaria vector *Anopheles gambiae* and other mosquitoes in swamps and rice fields in Zaire. *Journal of the American Mosquito Control Association* 8(4):376-380.

Karch S, Garin B, Asidi N, Manzambi Z, Salaun JJ, Mouchet J. 1993. [Mosquito nets impregnated against malaria in Zaire]. [French]. *Annales de la Societe Belge de Medecine Tropicale* 73(1):37-53.

Kaul I, Faust M. 2001. Global public goods and health: Taking the agenda forward. *Bulletin of the World Health Organization* 79(9):869-874.

Kazmi JH, Pandit K. 2001. Disease and dislocation: The impact of refugee movements on the geography of malaria in NWFP, Pakistan. *Social Science and Medicine* 52(7):1043-1055.

Khaemba BM, Mutani A, Bett MK. 1994. Studies of anopheline mosquitoes transmitting malaria in a newly developed highland urban area: A case study of Moi University and its environs. *East African Medical Journal* 71(3):159-164.

Killeen GF, Fillinger U, Kiche I, Gouagna LC, Knols BG. 2002. Eradication of *Anopheles gambiae* from Brazil: Lessons for malaria control in Africa? *The Lancet Infectious Diseases* 2(10):618-627.

Kovats RS, Bouma MJ, Hajat S, Worrall E, Haines A. 2003. El Niño and health. *Lancet* 362(9394):1481-1489.

Kumar S, Epstein JE, Richie TL, Nkrumah FK, Soisson L, Carucci DJ, Hoffman SL. 2002. A multilateral effort to develop DNA vaccines against falciparum malaria. *Trends in Parasitology* 18(3):129-135.

Kwiatkowski D, Marsh K. 1997. Development of a malaria vaccine. *Lancet* 350(9092):1696-1701.

Lengeler C. 2001. Comparison of malaria control interventions. *Bulletin of the World Health Organization* 79(1):77.

Lindblade KA, Walker ED, Onapa AW, Katungu J, Wilson ML. 1999. Highland malaria in Uganda: Prospective analysis of an epidemic associated with El Niño. *Transactions of the Royal Society of Tropical Medicine and Hygiene* 93(5):480-487.

Lindsay SW, Gibson ME. 1988. Bednets revisited—old idea, new angle. *Parasitology Today* 4(10):270-272.

Lindsay SW, Snow RW. 1988. The trouble with eaves: House entry by vectors of malaria. *Transactions of the Royal Society of Tropical Medicine and Hygiene* 82(4):645-646.

Lindsay SW, Ewald JA, Samung Y, Apiwathnasorn C, Nosten F. 1998. Thanaka (Limonia acidissima) and deet (di-methyl benzamide) mixture as a mosquito repellent for use by Karen women. *Medical and Veterinary Entomology* 12(3):295-301.

Loevinsohn ME. 1994. Climatic warming and increased malaria incidence in Rwanda. *Lancet* 343(8899):714-718.

Luxemburger C, Thwai KL, White NJ, Webster HK, Kyle DE, Maelankirri L, Chongsuphajaisiddhi T, Nosten F. 1996. The epidemiology of malaria in a Karen population on the western border of Thailand. *Transactions of the Royal Society of Tropical Medicine and Hygiene* 90(2):105-111.

Luxemburger C, Rigal J, Nosten F. 1998. Health care in refugee camps. *Transactions of the Royal Society of Tropical Medicine and Hygiene* 92(2):129-130.

Magesa SM, Wilkes TJ, Mnzava AE, Njunwa KJ, Myamba J, Kivuyo MD, Hill N, Lines JD, Curtis CF. 1991. Trial of pyrethroid impregnated bed nets in an area of Tanzania holoendemic for malaria. Part 2. Effects on the malaria vector population. *Acta Tropica* 49(2):97-108.

Mahanty S, Saul A, Miller LH. 2003. Progress in the development of recombinant and synthetic blood-stage malaria vaccines. *Journal of Experimental Biology* 206:3781-3788.

Makemba AM, Winch PJ, Makame VM, Mehl GL, Premji Z, Minjas JN, Shiff CJ. 1996. Treatment practices for degedege, a locally recognized febrile illness, and implications for strategies to decrease mortality from severe malaria in Bagamoyo district, Tanzania. *Tropical Medicine and International Health* 1(3):305-313.

Malakooti MA, Biomndo K, Shanks GD. 1998. Reemergence of epidemic malaria in the highlands of western Kenya. *Emerging Infectious Diseases* 4(4):671-676.

Marbiah NT, Petersen E, David K, Magbity E, Lines J, Bradley DJ. 1998. A controlled trial of lambda-cyhalothrin-impregnated bed nets and/or dapsone/pyrimethamine for malaria control in Sierra Leone. *American Journal of Tropical Medicine and Hygiene* 58(1):1-6.

Marsh K, Howard RJ. 1986. Antigens induced on erythrocytes by *P. falciparum*: Expression of diverse and conserved determinants. *Science* 231(4734):150-153.

Massaga JJ, Kitua AY, Lemnge MM, Akida JA, Malle LN, Ronn AM, Theander TG, Bygbjerg IC. 2003. Effect of intermittent treatment with amodiaquine on anaemia and malarial fevers in infants in Tanzania: a randomised placebo-controlled trial. *Lancet* 361(9372): 1853-1860.

Matola YG, White GB, Magayuka SA. 1987. The changed pattern of malaria endemicity and transmission at Amani in the eastern Usambara mountains, north-eastern Tanzania. *American Journal of Tropical Medicine and Hygiene* 90(3):127-134.

Maxwell CA, Msuya E, Sudi M, Njunwa KJ, Carneiro IA, Curtis CF. 2002. Effect of community-wide use of insecticide-treated nets for 3-4 years on malarial morbidity in Tanzania. *Tropical Medicine and International Health* 7(12):1003-1008.

McGregor IA. 1974. Mechanisms of acquired immunity and epidemiological patterns of antibody responses in malaria in man. *Bulletin of the World Health Organization* 50(3-4):259-266.

McGregor IA, Gilles HM, Walter JH, Davies AH, Pearson FA. 1956. Effects of heavy and repeated malaria infection on Gambian infants and children. Effects of erythrocytic parasitization. *British Medical Journal* ii:686-692.

Menendez C, Kahigwa E, Hirt R, Vounatsou P, Aponte JJ, Font F, Acosta CJ, Schellenberg DM, Galindo CM, Kimario J, Urassa H, Brabin B, Smith TA, Kitua AY, Tanner M, Alonso PL. 1997. Randomised placebo-controlled trial of iron supplementation and malaria chemoprophylaxis for prevention of severe anaemia and malaria in Tanzanian infants. *Lancet* 350(9081):844-850.

Meuwissen JHET. 1964. The use of medicated salt in an antimalaria campaign in west New Guinea. *Tropical and Geographical Medicine* 16:245-255.

Mharakurwa S, Manyame B, Shiff CJ. 1997. Trial of the ParaSight-F test for malaria diagnosis in the primary health care system, Zimbabwe. *Tropical Medicine and International Health* 2(6):544-550.

Mnzava AE, Sharp BL, Mthembu DJ, le Sueur D, Dlamini SS, Gumede JK, Kleinschmidt I. 2001. Malaria control—two years' use of insecticide-treated bednets compared with insecticide house spraying in Kwazulu-Natal. *South African Medical Journal* 91(11):978-983.

Moerman F, Lengeler C, Chimumbwa J, Talisuna A, Erhart A, Coosemans M, D'Alessandro U. 2003. The contribution of health-care services to a sound and sustainable malaria-control policy. *The Lancet Infectious Diseases* 3(2):99-102.

Molineaux L. 1985. The impact of parasitic diseases and their control, with an emphasis on malaria and Africa. In: Vallin J, Lopez AD, eds. *Health Policy, Social Policy and Mortality Prospects*. Paris: IUSSP.

Moody A. 2002. Rapid diagnostic tests for malaria parasites. *Clinical Microbiology Reviews* 15(1):66-78.

Moore SA, Surgey EG, Cadwgan AM. 2002. Malaria vaccines: Where are we and where are we going? *The Lancet Infectious Diseases* 2(12):737-743.

Moorthy VS, Good MF, Hill AVS. 2004. Malaria vaccine developments. *Lancet* 363(9403):150-156.

Morley D, Woodland M, Cuthbertson WF. 1964. Controlled trial of pyrimethamine in pregnant women in an African village. *British Medical Journal* i(5384):667-668.

Mouchet J. 1998. [Origin of malaria epidemics on the plateaus of Madagascar and the mountains of east and south Africa]. [French]. *Bulletin de la Societe de Pathologie Exotique* 91(1):64-66.

Muheki C, Barnes K, McIntyre D. 2003. *Economic Evaluation of Recent Malaria Control Interventions in KwaZulu, Natal, South Africa: SEACAT Evaluation*. Cape Town: SEACAT.

Muller O, Ido K, Traore C. 2002. Evaluation of a prototype long-lasting insecticide-treated mosquito net under field conditions in rural Burkina Faso. *Transactions of the Royal Society of Tropical Medicine and Hygiene* 96(5):483-484.

Murray CK, Bell D, Gasser RA, Wongsrichanalai C. 2003. Rapid diagnostic testing for malaria. *Tropical Medicine and International Health* 8(10):876-883.

Nahlen BL, Clark JP, Alnwick D. 2003. Insecticide-treated bed nets. *American Journal of Tropical Medicine and Hygiene* 68(4 Suppl):1-2.

Nevill CG, Some ES, Mung'ala VO, Mutemi W, New L, Marsh K, Lengeler C, Snow RW. 1996. Insecticide-treated bednets reduce mortality and severe morbidity from malaria among children on the Kenyan coast. *Tropical Medicine and International Health* 1(2):139-146.

Nosten F, Luxemburger C, Kyle DE, Ballou WR, Wittes J, Wah E, Chongsuphajaisiddhi T, Gordon DM, White NJ, Sadoff JC, Heppner DG, Bathe K, Blood J, Brockman A, Cobley UT, Hacking D, Hogg D, Kyaw HU, Maelankiri L. 1996. Randomised double-blind placebo-controlled trial of SPf66 malaria vaccine in children in northwestern Thailand. *Lancet* 348(9029):701-707.

Nosten F, Hien TT, White NJ. 1998. Use of artemisinin derivatives for the control of malaria. [Erratum appears in Medecine Tropicale (Mars 1998) 58(4):368]. *Medecine Tropicale* 58(3 Suppl):45-49.

Nosten F, van Vugt M, Price R, Luxemburger C, Thway KL, Brockman A, McGready R, ter Kuile F, Looareesuwan S, White NJ. 2000. Effects of artesunate-mefloquine combination on incidence of *Plasmodium falciparum* malaria and mefloquine resistance in western Thailand: A prospective study. *Lancet* 356(9226):297-302.

Ockenhouse CF, Sun PF, Lanar DE, Wellde BT, Hall BT, Kester K, Stoute JA, Magill A, Krzych U, Farley L, Wirtz RA, Sadoff JC, Kaslow DC, Kumar S, Church LW, Crutcher JM, Wizel B, Hoffman S, Lalvani A, Hill AV, Tine JA, Guito KP, de Taisne C, Anders R, Ballou WR. 1998. Phase I/IIa safety, immunogenicity, and efficacy trial of NYVAC-Pf7, a pox-vectored, multiantigen, multistage vaccine candidate for *Plasmodium falciparum* malaria. *Journal of Infectious Diseases* 177(6):1664-1673.

PAHO. 1995. Regional status of malaria in the Americas. *Epidemiologic Bulletin* 16:10-14.

Parise ME, Ayisi JG, Nahlen BL, Schultz LJ, Roberts JM, Misore A, Muga R, Oloo AJ, Steketee RW. 1998. Efficacy of sulfadoxine-pyrimethamine for prevention of placental malaria in an area of Kenya with a high prevalence of malaria and human immunodeficiency virus infection. *American Journal of Tropical Medicine and Hygiene* 59(5):813-822.

Patarroyo ME, Armador R. 1999. The first and toward the second generation of malaria vaccines. In: Wahlgren M, Perlmann P, eds. *Malaria*. Amsterdam: Harwood Academic Publishers.

Payne D. 1988. Did medicated salt hasten the spread of chloroquine resistance in Plasmodium falciparum? *Parasitology Today* 4(4):112-115.

Payne D, Grab B, Fontaine RE, Hempel JH. 1976. Impact of control measures on malaria transmission and general mortality. *Bulletin of the World Health Organization* 54(4):369-377.

Perkins BA, Zucker JR, Otieno J, Jafari HS, Paxton L, Redd SC, Nahlen BL, Schwartz B, Oloo AJ, Olango C, Gove S, Campbell CC. 1997. Evaluation of an algorithm for integrated management of childhood illness in an area of Kenya with high malaria transmission. *Bulletin of the World Health Organization* 75(1 Suppl):33-42.

Phillips-Howard PA, Nahlen BL, Kolczak MS, Hightower AW, Ter Kuile FO, Alaii JA, Gimnig JE, Arudo J, Vulule JM, Odhacha A, Kachur SP, Schoute E, Rosen DH, Sexton JD, Oloo AJ, Hawley WA. 2003. Efficacy of permethrin-treated bed nets in the prevention of mortality in young children in an area of high perennial malaria transmission in western Kenya. *American Journal of Tropical Medicine and Hygiene* 68(4 Suppl):23-29.

Phu NH, Day NPJ. 1995. Intraleukocytic malaria pigment and prognosis in severe malaria. *Transactions of the Royal Society of Tropical Medicine and Hygiene* 89:197-199.

Pinotti M. 1954. Chemoprophylaxis of malaria by the association of an antimalarial drug to the sodium chloride used daily in the preparation of meals. In: *Fifth International Congress of Tropical Medicine and Malaria, 1953*, Vol. 2. Istanbul, Turkey.

Piper R, Lebras J, Wentworth L, Hunt-Cooke A, Houze S, Chiodini P, Makler M. 1999. Immunocapture diagnostic assays for malaria using plasmodium lactate dehydrogenase (pLDH). *American Journal of Tropical Medicine and Hygiene* 60(1):109-118.

Pitt S, Pearcy BE, Stevens RH, Sharipov A, Satarov K, Banatvala N. 1998. War in Tajikistan and re-emergence of *Plasmodium falciparum*. *Lancet* 352(9136):1279.

Plowe CV, Wellems TE. 1995. Molecular approaches to the spreading problem of drug resistant malaria. *Advances in Experimental Medicine and Biology* 390:197-209.

Poveda G, Rojas W, Quinones ML, Velez ID, Mantilla RI, Ruiz D, Zuluaga JS, Rua GL. 2001. Coupling between annual and ENSO timescales in the malaria-climate association in Colombia. *Environmental Health Perspectives* 109(5):489-493.

Pringle G. 1969. Experimental malaria control and demography in a rural East African community: A retrospect. *Transactions of the Royal Society of Tropical Medicine and Hygiene* 63:2-18.

Prinsen Geerligs PD, Brabin BJ, Eggelte TA. 2003. Analysis of the effects of malaria chemoprophylaxis in children on haematological responses, morbidity and mortality. *Bulletin of the World Health Organization* 81(3):205-216.

Ranson H, Claudianos C, Ortelli F, Abgrall C, Hemingway J, Sharakhova MV, Unger MF, Collins FH, Feyereisen R. 2002. Evolution of supergene families associated with insecticide resistance. *Science* 298(5591):179-181.

Redd SC, Bloland PB, Kazembe PN, Patrick E, Tembenu R, Campbell CC. 1992. Usefulness of clinical case-definitions in guiding therapy for African children with malaria or pneumonia. *Lancet* 340(8828):1140-1143.

Rey JL, Cavallo JD, Milleliri JM, L'Hoest S, Soares JL, Piny N, Coue JC, Jouan A. 1996. [Fever of unknown origin (FUO) in the camps of Rwandan refugees in the Goma region of in Zaire (September 1994)]. [French]. *Bulletin de la Societe de Pathologie Exotique* 89(3):204-208.

Rickman LS, Long GW, Oberst R, Cabanban A, Sangalang R, Smith JI, Chulay JD, Hoffman SL. 1989. Rapid diagnosis of malaria by acridine orange staining of centrifuged parasites. *Lancet* 1(8629):68-71.

Rimon MM, Kheng S, Hoyer S, Thach V, Ly S, Permin AE, Pieche S. 2003. Malaria dipsticks beneficial for IMCI in Cambodia. *Tropical Medicine and International Health* 8(6):536-543.

Robert V, Carnevale P. 1991. Influence of deltamethrin treatment of bed nets on malaria transmission in the Kou Valley, Burkina Faso. *Bulletin of the World Health Organization* 69(6):735-740.

Robert V, Macintyre K, Keating J, Trape JF, Duchemin JB, Warren M, Beier JC. 2003. Malaria transmission in urban sub-Saharan Africa. *American Journal of Tropical Medicine and Hygiene* 68(2):169-176.

Roberts DR, Manguin S, Mouchet J. 2000. DDT house spraying and re-emerging malaria. *Lancet* 356(9226):330-332.

Rogerson SJ, Chaluluka E, Kanjala M, Mkundika P, Mhango C, Molyneux ME. 2000. Intermittent sulfadoxine-pyrimethamine in pregnancy: Effectiveness against malaria morbidity in Blantyre, Malawi, in 1997-99. *Transactions of the Royal Society of Tropical Medicine and Hygiene* 94(5):549-553.

Romi R, Ravoniharimelina B, Ramiakajato M, Majori G. 1993. Field trials of *Bacillus thuringiensis* H-14 and *Bacillus sphaericus* (Strain 2362) formulations against *Anopheles arabiensis* in the central highlands of Madagascar. *Journal of the American Mosquito Control Association* 9(3):325-329.

Rowland M, Nosten F. 2001. Malaria epidemiology and control in refugee camps and complex emergencies. *Annals of Tropical Medicine and Parasitology* 95(8):741-754.

Rowley J, Cham B, Pinder M. 1999. Availability and affordability of insecticide of treating bednets in The Gambia. Presentation at the meeting of the 48th Annual Meeting of the American Society of Tropical Medicine and Hygiene. Washington, DC: American Society of Tropical Medicine and Hygiene.

Russell PF. 1952. Nation-wide malaria eradication projects. *Anais do Instituto de Higiene e Medicina Tropical (Lisbon)* 9(2):331-338.

Schellenberg D, Menendez C, Kahigwa E, Aponte J, Vidal J, Tanner M, Mshinda H, Alonso P. 2001. Intermittent treatment for malaria and anaemia control at time of routine vaccinations in Tanzanian infants: A randomised, placebo-controlled trial. *Lancet* 357(9267):1471-1477.

Schofield CJ, White GB. 1984. House design and domestic vectors of disease. *Transactions of the Royal Society of Tropical Medicine and Hygiene* 78(3):285-292.

Schultz LJ, Steketee RW, Macheso A, Kazembe P, Chitsulo L, Wirima JJ. 1994. The efficacy of antimalarial regimens containing sulfadoxine-pyrimethamine and/or chloroquine in preventing peripheral and placental *Plasmodium falciparum* infection among pregnant women in Malawi. *American Journal of Tropical Medicine and Hygiene* 51(5):515-522.

Shanks GD, Biomndo K, Hay SI, Snow RW. 2000. Changing patterns of clinical malaria since 1965 among a tea estate population located in the Kenyan highlands. *Transactions of the Royal Society of Tropical Medicine and Hygiene* 94(3):253-255.

Sharp B, van Wyk P, Sikasote JB, Banda P, Kleinschmidt I. 2002a. Malaria control by residual insecticide spraying in Chingola and Chililabombwe, Copperbelt Province, Zambia. *Tropical Medicine and International Health* 7(9):732-736.

Sharp TW, Burkle FM Jr, Vaughn AF, Chotani R, Brennan RJ. 2002b. Challenges and opportunities for humanitarian relief in Afghanistan. *Clinical Infectious Diseases* 34(Suppl 5):S215-S228.

Shiff C. 2002. Integrated approach to malaria control. *Clinical Microbiology Reviews* 15(2):278-293.

Shretta R, Omumbo J, Rapuoda B, Snow RW. 2000. Using evidence to change antimalarial drug policy in Kenya. *Tropical Medicine and International Health* 5(11):755-764.

Shulman CE, Dorman EK, Talisuna AO, Lowe BS, Nevill C, Snow RW, Jilo H, Peshu N, Bulmer JN, Graham S, Marsh K. 1998. A community randomized controlled trial of insecticide-treated bed nets for the prevention of malaria and anaemia among primigravid women on the Kenyan coast. *Tropical Medicine and International Health* 3(3):197-204.

Shulman CE, Dorman EK, Cutts F, Kawuondo K, Bulmer JN, Peshu N, Marsh K. 1999. Intermittent sulphadoxine-pyrimethamine to prevent severe anaemia secondary to malaria in pregnancy: A randomised placebo-controlled trial. *Lancet* 353(9153):632-636.

Silamut K, White NJ. 1993. Relation of the stage of parasite development in the peripheral blood to prognosis in severe falciparum malaria. *Transactions of the Royal Society of Tropical Medicine and Hygiene* 87(4):436-443.

Sina BJ, Aultman K. 2001. Resisting resistance. *Trends in Parasitology* 17(7):305-306.

Singh N, Saxena A, Valecha N. 2000. Field evaluation of the ICT Malaria P.f/P.v immunochromatographic test for diagnosis of *Plasmodium falciparum* and *P. vivax* infection in forest villages of Chhindwara, central India. *Tropical Medicine and International Health* 5(11):765-770.

Snow RW, Gilles HM. 2002. The epidemiology of malaria. In: Warrell DA, Gilles HM, eds. *Essential Malariology*. 4th ed. London: Arnold Publishing.

Snow RW, Bradley AK, Hayes R, Byass P, Greenwood BM. 1987. Does woodsmoke protect against malaria? *Annals of Tropical Medicine and Parasitology* 81(4):449-451.

Snow RW, McCabe E, Mbogo CN, Molyneux CS, Some ES, Mung'ala VO, Nevill CG. 1999. The effect of delivery mechanisms on the uptake of bed net re-impregnation in Kilifi district, Kenya. *Health Policy and Planning* 14(1):18-25.

Soderlund DM, Bloomquist JR. 1989. Neurotoxic actions of pyrethroid insecticides. *Annual Review of Entomology* 34:77-96.

Stepniewska K, Taylor WRJ, Mayxay M, Smithuis F, Guthmann J-P, Barnes K, Myint H, Price R, Olliaro P, Pukrittayakamee S, Hien TT, Farrar J, Nosten F, Day NPJ, White NJ. In press. The *in vivo* assessment of antimalarial drug efficacy in falciparum malaria; the duration of follow-up. *Antimicrobial Agents and Chemotherapy*.

Strickland GT, Zafar-Latif A, Fox E, Khaliq AA, Chowdhry MA. 1987. Endemic malaria in four villages of the Pakistani province of Punjab. *Transactions of the Royal Society of Tropical Medicine and Hygiene* 81(1):36-41.

Tabashnik BE. 1989. Managing resistance with multiple pesticide tactics: Theory, evidence, and recommendations. *Journal of Economic Entomology* 82(5):1263-1269.

Takken W. 2002. Do insecticide-treated bed nets have an effect on malaria vectors? *Tropical Medicine and International Health* 7(12):1022-1030.

Talisuna AO, Langi P, Bakyaita N, Egwang T, Mutabingwa TK, Watkins W, Van Marck E, D'Alessandro U. 2002. Intensity of malaria transmission, antimalarial-drug use and resistance in Uganda: What is the relationship between these three factors? *Transactions of the Royal Society of Tropical Medicine and Hygiene* 96(3):310-317.

Taverne J. 1999. DDT—to ban or not to ban? *Parasitology Today* 15(5):180-181.

ter Kuile FO, Terlouw DJ, Kariuki SK, Phillips-Howard PA, Mirel LB, Hawley WA, Friedman JF, Shi YP, Kolczak MS, Lal AA, Vulule JM, Nahlen BL. 2003a. Impact of permethrin-treated bed nets on malaria, anemia, and growth in infants in an area of intense perennial malaria transmission in western Kenya. *American Journal of Tropical Medicine and Hygiene* 68(4 Suppl):68-77.

ter Kuile FO, Terlouw DJ, Phillips-Howard PA, Hawley WA, Friedman JF, Kariuki SK, Shi YP, Kolczak MS, Lal AA, Vulule JM, Nahlen BL. 2003b. Reduction of malaria during pregnancy by permethrin-treated bed nets in an area of intense perennial malaria transmission in Western Kenya. *American Journal of Tropical Medicine and Hygiene* 68(4 Suppl):50-60.

Tharavanij S. 1990. New developments in malaria diagnostic techniques. *Southeast Asian Journal of Tropical Medicine and Public Health* 21(1):3-16.

Thimasarn K, Sirichaisinthop J, Vijaykadga S, Tansophalaks S, Yamokgul P, Laomiphol A, Palananth C, Thamewat U, Thaithong S, Rooney W. 1995. In vivo study of the response of *Plasmodium falciparum* to standard mefloquine/sulfadoxine/ pyrimethamine (MSP) treatment among gem miners returning from Cambodia. *Southeast Asian Journal of Tropical Medicine and Public Health* 26(2):204-212.

Tine JA, Lanar DE, Smith DM, Wellde BT, Schultheiss P, Ware LA, Kauffman EB, Wirtz RA, De Taisne C, Hui GS, Chang SP, Church P, Hollingdale MR, Kaslow DC, Hoffman S, Guito KP, Ballou WR, Sadoff JC, Paoletti E. 1996. NYVAC-Pf7: A poxvirus-vectored, multiantigen, multistage vaccine candidate for *Plasmodium falciparum* malaria. *Infection and Immunity* 64(9):3833-3844.

Trape JF, Zoulani A. 1987. Malaria and urbanization in central Africa: The example of Brazzaville. Part III: Relationships between urbanization and the intensity of malaria transmission. *Transactions of the Royal Society of Tropical Medicine and Hygiene* 81(Suppl 2):19-25.

Trape JF, Lefebvre-Zante E, Legros F, Ndiaye G, Bouganali H, Druilhe P, Salem G. 1992. Vector density gradients and the epidemiology of urban malaria in Dakar, Senegal. *American Journal of Tropical Medicine and Hygiene* 47(2):181-189.

Trape JF, Pison G, Spiegel A, Enel C, Rogier C. 2002. Combating malaria in Africa. *Trends in Parasitology* 18(5):224-230.

United Nations. 1999. *World Urbanization Prospects: The 1999 Revision, Key Findings.* New York: United Nations Population Division.

Utzinger J, Tozan Y, Singer BH. 2001. Efficacy and cost-effectiveness of environmental management for malaria control. *Tropical Medicine and International Health* 6(9):677-687.

Van der Hoek W, Konradsen F, Dijkstra DS, Amerasinghe PH, Amerasinghe FP. 1998. Risk factors for malaria: A microepidemiological study in a village in Sri Lanka. *Transactions of the Royal Society of Tropical Medicine and Hygiene* 92(3):265-269.

Verdrager J. 1986. Epidemiology of the emergence and spread of drug-resistant falciparum malaria in south-east Asia and Australasia. *Journal of Tropical Medicine and Hygiene* 89(6):277-289.

Von Seidlein L, Greenwood BM. 2003. Mass administrations of antimalarial drugs. *Trends in Parasitology* 19(10):452-460.

Von Seidlein L, Clarke S, Alexander N, Manneh F, Doherty T, Pinder M, Walraven G, Greenwood B. 2002. Treatment uptake by individuals infected with *Plasmodium falciparum* in rural Gambia, West Africa. *Bulletin of the World Health Organization* 80(10):790-796.

Warhurst DC, Williams JE. 1996. Laboratory diagnosis of malaria. *Journal of Clinical Pathology* 49(7):533-538.

Weber MW, Mulholland EK, Jaffar S, Troedsson H, Gove S, Greenwood BM. 1997. Evaluation of an algorithm for the Integrated Management of Childhood Illness in an area with seasonal malaria in the Gambia. *Bulletin of the World Health Organization* 75(Suppl 1):25-32.

White NJ. 1999. Delaying antimalarial drug resistance with combination chemotherapy. *Parassitologia* 41(1-3):301-308.

White NJ, Silamut K. 1989. Rapid diagnosis of malaria. *Lancet* 1(8635):435.

WHO. 1979. *Seventeenth Report of the Expert Committee on Malaria.* Geneva: World Health Organization.

WHO. 1992a. *Fifteenth Report of the Expert Committee on Vector Biology and Control. Technical Report Series No. 818. Vector Resistance to Pesticides.* Geneva: World Health Organization.

WHO. 1992b. Presentation at the meeting of the World Declaration on the Control of Malaria, Ministerial Conference on Malaria. Geneva: World Health Organization.

WHO. 1993. *WHO Technical Report Series. Plan of Action for Malaria Control 1993-2000.* Geneva: World Health Organization.

WHO. 1996a. *Report of the WHO Informal Consultation WHO/HQ, Geneva 7-11 October 1996. Evaluation and Testing of Insecticides.* Geneva: World Health Organization.

WHO. 1996b. A rapid dipstick antigen capture assay for the diagnosis of falciparum malaria. *Bulletin of the World Health Organization* 74(1):47-54.

WHO. 1999. *Report of the WHO Informal Cosultation, April 28-30, 1999. Draft Guideline Specifications for Bacterial Larvicides for Public Health Use.* Geneva: World Health Organization.

WHO. 2000. *WHO Expert Committee Report on Malaria: 20th Report.* World Health Organization Technical Report Series 892.

WHO. 2001. *Malaria Early Warning System, Concepts, Indicators, and Partners, A Framework for Field Research in Africa.* WHO/CDS/RBM.

WHO Expert Committee on Insecticides. 1970. *Insecticide Resistance and Vector Control.* Geneva: World Health Organization.

WHO/UNICEF. 2003. *The Africa Malaria Report 2003.* Geneva: World Health Organization.

Zucker JR. 1996. Changing patterns of autochthonous malaria transmission in the United States: A review of recent outbreaks. *Emerging Infectious Diseases* 2(1):37-43.

9

Antimalarial Drugs and Drug Resistance

This chapter describes antimalarial drugs currently in use, with an emphasis on the artemisinins. It also reviews the way drug resistance develops and spreads, methods used to assess the presence and level of drug resistance, and the extent to which chloroquine and sulfadoxine/pyrimethamine (SP)—the two most widely used antimalarial drugs in the world today—have now lost efficacy.

CLINICAL MALARIA AND THE AIMS OF ANTIMALARIAL DRUG TREATMENT

Malaria sickens and kills people through several pathological mechanisms, understood to varying degrees. In addition to first- and second-line antimalarial drug treatments, adjunctive and supportive care measures (e.g., intravenous fluids, blood transfusions, supplemental oxygen, antiseizure medications) may be needed for severe manifestations. The aims of treatment are to prevent death or long-term deficits from malaria, to cut short the morbidity of an acute episode of illness, and to clear the infection entirely so that it does not recur.

Fever, sweating, and chills (or, in some cases, merely fever) triggered by the release of plasmodia into the bloodstream from mature blood schizonts, are the most common symptoms heralding the onset of a clinical case of uncomplicated falciparum malaria (see Chapter 6 for a description of the evolution of clinical symptoms). Without treatment—or an active immune response primed by repeated previous malaria infections—the number of parasites will increase with every 2-day cycle of reproduction. A mature infection may involve up to 10^{12} circulating plasmodia.

At any time after the infection is established, the vast majority of plasmodia will be in some stage of asexual maturation leading to another round of multiplication within the patient's bloodstream. However, a few parasites will have transformed into sexual stages (gametocytes) that, once ingested by mosquitoes, can perpetuate the transmission cycle. Because each stage of the malarial life cycle exhibits distinct biochemical and other characteristics (i.e., it expresses different proteins or locates in different sites within the body), a drug may kill one stage but have little effect on another. In other words, in each life-cycle stage the parasite manifests unique biological properties that can offer a target for the action of one or more antimalarial drugs.

ANTIMALARIAL DRUG CLASSES

Currently available antimalarials fall into three broad categories according to their chemical structure and mode of action (Appendix 9-A):

1. Aryl aminoalcohol compounds: quinine, quinidine, chloroquine, amodiaquine, mefloquine, halofantrine, lumefantrine, piperaquine, tafenoquine
2. Antifolate compounds ("antifols"): pyrimethamine, proguanil, chlorproguanil, trimethoprim
3. Artemisinin compounds (artemisinin, dihydroartemisinin, artemether, artesunate)

Atovaquone is an antimalarial in its own class with a unique mode of action; combined with proguanil it is sold under the trade name Malarone®. Several antibacterial drugs (e.g., tetracycline, clindamycin) also have antiplasmodial activity, although in general their action is slow for malaria treatment (as opposed to prophylaxis); they are recommended only in combination with other antimalarial drugs. Drugs active against *Plasmodium falciparum* also are active against the other three malaria species that affect humans—*P. vivax, P. malariae,* and *P. ovale*—with the exception of antifols, which work poorly against *P. vivax*.

Current treatment protocols for uncomplicated malaria and severe malaria are given in Tables 9-1 and 9-2.

TABLE 9-1 Treatment of Uncomplicated Malaria[a]

Malaria	Drug Treatment
P. vivax, P. malariae, P. ovale, known chloroquine-sensitive *P. falciparum*[a]	Chloroquine 10 mg base/kg stat. Followed by: a. 5 mg/kg at 12, 24 and 36 h; or b. 10 mg/kg at 24 h, 5 mg/kg at 48 h or Amodiaquine 10 mg base/kg/day for 3 days[1]
Chloroquine-resistant *P. falciparum*[a] known to be sensitive to sulfadoxine-pyrimethamine (SP)	Pyrimethamine 1.25 mg/kg + sulfadoxine 25 mg/kg (single dose; 3 tablets in an adult) or Amodiaquine 10 mg base/kg/day for 3 days
Chloroquine-resistant *P. vivax*[b] and multidrug resistant *P. falciparum*[a]	a. Oral Artesunate 4 mg/kg daily for 3 days + mefloquine 25 mg base/kg (15 mg/kg on day 2, 10 mg/kg on day 3) b. Artemether-lumefantrine 1.5/9 mg/kg twice daily for 3 days with food c. Quinine 10 mg salt/kg three times daily plus tetracycline 4 mg/kg four times daily or doxycycline 3 mg/kg once daily or clindamycin 10 mg/kg twice daily for 7 days[2]

[a]For acute treatment of falciparum malaria combinations containing an artemisinin-derivative are preferred. Artesunate (4 mg/kg/day for 3 days) has been combined successfully with chloroquine, amodiaquine, SP, mefloquine, and atovaquone-proguanil.

[b]This refers to truly resistant *P. vivax* infections, which are a significant problem only in Oceania and Indonesia and should not be confused with relapses. Amodiaquine is more effective than chloroquine for resistant *P. vivax.*

Basic Properties of Antimalarials: Pharmacokinetics and Pharmacodynamics

Pharmacokinetics

The interactions of drugs with people who take them—how the compounds are absorbed, metabolized, distributed, and excreted—is referred to as pharmacokinetics. Antimalarial drugs differ considerably in their pharmacokinetics, which affect how well they work, how they are dosed, and how long they must be taken. People also vary in how they respond to drugs. Some of these responses are genetically determined, others by health status, others by dietary factors. In general, the pharmacokinetic properties of the antimalarials are similar in children and adults, although the metabo-

General points
A. There are now few places in the world where chloroquine can be relied upon for
    falciparum malaria, and SP resistance is spreading rapidly—so recent information
    on drug susceptibility is required if these drugs are used. Amodiaquine is more
    effective than chloroquine against chloroquine-resistant *P. falciparum*, but highly
    amodiaquine-resistant parasites are prevalent in East Asia.
B. Pregnancy: There are insufficient data on the safety of most antimalarial drugs in
    pregnancy. Artemisinin and its derivatives should not be given in the first
    trimester. Halofantrine, primaquine, and tetracycline should not be used at any
    time in pregnancy. There are theoretical concerns over inducing kernicterus when
    long-acting sulfonamides are used near term, but no evidence that this is a
    significant problem in practice. There are uncertainties over the safety of
    mefloquine in pregnancy. Quinine, chloroquine, proguanil, SP, and clindamycin
    are regarded as safe in the first trimester. Quinine may cause hypoglycemia,
    particularly in late pregnancy.
C. Vomiting is less likely if the patient's temperature is lowered before oral drug
    administration.
D. Where possible, artesunate or quinine should be combined with a tetracycline or
    clindamycin. Short courses for artesunate or quinine (< 7 days) alone are not
    recommended.
E. In renal failure. the dose of quinine should be reduced by one-third to one-half
    after 48 hours, and doxycycline but *not* tetracycline should be prescribed.
F. The doses of all drugs are unchanged in children: however, several drugs
    including atovaquone, proguanil and artesunate have significantly altered kinetics
    in pregnancy.

Specific points
1. Patients with *P. vivax* and *P. ovale* infections also should be given primaquine
    0.25 mg base/kg daily (0.375-0.5 mg base/kg in Oceania) for 14 days to prevent
    relapse. In mild G6PD deficiency 0.75 mg base/kg should be given once weekly
    for 6 weeks. In severe G6PD deficiency, primaquine should not be used.
2. None of the tetracyclines should be given to pregnant women or children under 8
    years of age.

lism of several drugs is altered in pregnancy (e.g., atovaquone, mefloquine,
cycloguanil).

A key pharmacokinetic property of antimalarials is how long they
remain in the body. Artemisinin and its derivatives are absorbed and eliminated the most rapidly (half-life = 1 hour or less). Quinine also is absorbed
and eliminated within one parasite life cycle (11 hours in healthy subjects to
18 hours in those with severe malaria). Other antimalarials are eliminated
very slowly, remaining in significant concentrations for several days (pyrimethamine, halofantrine, lumefantrine, atovaquone), or even weeks
(mefloquine, chloroquine, and piperaquine). In general, rapidly eliminated
drugs (artemisinin, and quinine) must be taken over four asexual cycles (7
days) to ensure cure in nonimmune patients. In contrast, drugs that are

TABLE 9-2 Treatment of Severe Malaria

| | Health Clinic: | | Rural Health Clinic: |
	Hospital Intensive Care Unit (Icu)	No Intravenous Infusions Possible	No Injection Facilities
Chloroquine-resistant *P. falciparum*	*Quinine* Quinine dihydrochloride 7 mg salt/kg infused over 30 minutes followed by immediately 10 mg/kg over 4 hours; or 20 mg salt/kg infused over 4 hours. Maintenance dose: 10 mg salt/kg infused over 2-8 hours at 8-hour intervals[a] *Quindine* 10 mg base/kg infused over 1-2 hours followed by 1.2 mg base/kg per hour[b] Electrocardiographic monitoring advisable	Quinine dihydrochloride 20 mg salt/kg diluted 1:2 with sterile water given by split injection into both anterior thighs. Maintenance dose: 10 mg/kg 8-hourly[a]	

Artemisinin derivatives	As for hospital ICU: artesunate can also be given by i.m. injection	Artesunate rectocap: 10 mg/kg daily Artemisinin suppository 20 mg/kg at 0 and 4 hrs. then daily
a) Artemether 3.2 mg/kg stat. by i.m. injection followed by 1.6 mg/kg daily:		
b) Artesunate 2.4 mg/kg stat. by i.v. injection followed by 1.2 mg/kd daily		
Known chloroquine-sensitive *P. falciparum*		
Chloroquine 10 mg base/kg infused intravenously at constant rate over 8 hours followed by 15 mg base/kg over 24 hours	Chloroquine 3.5 mg base/kg 6-hourly or 2.5 mg base/kg 4-hourly by i.m. or s.c. injection. Total dose 25 mg base/kg	10 mg/kg daily or nasogastric chloroquine as for oral regimen

[a]The preferred dosage interval for parenteral quinine in African children is 12 hours.

[b]Some authorities recommend a lower dose of 6.2 mg base/kg initially over 1 hour followed by 0.012 mg base/kg per hour. There are insufficient data for confident dosage recommendations.

General points

A. If in doubt, consider the infection as chloroquine-resistant. There are very few places where chloroquine can now be relied upon.
B. Infusions can be given in 0.9% saline, 5% or 10% dextrose/water.
C. Infusion rates for the quinoline antimalarials should be carefully controlled.
D. Oral treatment should start as soon as patient can swallow reliably enough to complete a full course of treatment.

eliminated slowly require fewer doses over shorter periods because they remain active in the body.

Halofantrine, lumefantrine, atovaquone and, to a much lesser extent, mefloquine, are hydrophobic and lipophilic (i.e., insoluble in water and capable of dissolving in fat); as a result, their absorption also varies according to the amount of dietary fat consumed. For this reason, blood concentrations of these drugs may vary considerably from one individual to another following the same dose.

Pharmacodynamics

The way drugs act on their target—in this case, plasmodia—is called pharmacodynamics. The principal effect of antimalarial drugs in uncomplicated malaria is to inhibit parasite multiplication by killing parasites. If an untreated infection progressed at maximum efficiency, with each life cycle, the total body parasite load would increase by a multiplication factor approximating the average number of viable parasites in a mature schizont (18-36) (White, 1997). Proliferation of parasites in nonimmune individuals often proceeds at multiplication rates of 6 to 20 per 2-day cycle (30-80 percent efficiency). Antimalarial drugs exerting maximum effect (Emax), on the other hand, reduce total parasite numbers 10- to 10,000-fold per cycle.

Individual antimalarial drugs differ in their Emax (i.e., the proportion of total plasmodia killed per treatment); for example, artemisinins often yield a 10,000-fold reduction per asexual cycle, whereas antimalarial antibiotics such as tetracycline or clindamycin may only achieve a 10-fold parasite reduction per cycle. The lowest blood or plasma concentration of an antimalarial drug that results in Emax can be considered a "minimum parasiticidal concentration" (MPC). Parasite reduction appears to be a first-order process throughout (Day et al., 1996), which means that a fixed fraction of the infecting malaria parasite population is removed with each successive cycle as long as the MPC is exceeded.

Clinical Pharmacodynamics

Patients with acute malaria may have up to 10^{12} parasites circulating in their blood. Even with killing rates of 99.99 percent per cycle, complete eradication of the parasite load requires at least three life cycles (6 days); therefore, therapeutic drug concentrations should be present for 4 cycles to effect a cure (White, 1997, 1998). Simply put, patients taking rapidly eliminated drugs must continue treatment for a full week. Treatment responses are always better in patients with some immunity (York and Macfie, 1924) because the immune response kills parasites in much the same way that a drug does. In endemic areas, the worst treatment results are seen in young children who have little immunity. In contrast, although their degree of immune protection cannot be quantitated or assumed, older children or adults in high-transmission areas may do surprisingly well with failing drugs because much of their therapeutic response stems from immunity rather than antimalarial drug action.

In severe falciparum malaria, the stage at which an antimalarial drug acts is especially important since the ultimate goal of treatment is to halt parasite maturation to late-stage, cytoadherent parasites (i.e., mature schizonts that attach to endothelial cells lining small blood vessels), which are primarily responsible for life-threatening complications. The artemisinin derivatives are advantageous because they prevent parasites from maturing to these more pathological stages, whereas quinine and quinidine do not affect parasites until they have already cytoadhered. The antifols act even later in the cycle, and are not recommended for severe malaria (Yayon et al., 1983; ter Kuile et al., 1993). None of the drugs will prevent rupture of infected erythrocytes and reinvasion once a schizont has formed. Young ring forms (i.e., early asexual parasites) also are relatively drug resistant, especially to quinine and pyrimethamine.

Artemesinin derivatives offer the broadest antimalarial action against the range of developmental stages, and the most rapid in vivo activity (ter Kuile et al., 1993; White, 1997). These compounds (and, to a lesser extent, chloroquine) prevent ring stages from maturing, hastening their clearance, and preventing end-organ pathology that would otherwise occur if cytoadherence progressed unchecked (Chotivanich et al., 2000).

MECHANISMS OF ACTION AND DRUG RESISTANCE

Antifolate Drugs

Pyrimethamine, and biguanides such as cycloguanil interfere with folic acid synthesis, inhibiting the parasite enzyme known as dihydrofolate reductase-thymidilate synthase (DHFR). Sulfonamides act at the previous step in the folic acid pathway, inhibiting the parasite enzyme dihydropteroate synthase (DHPS). There is marked synergy between these two classes of drugs when they are taken together. However, resistance to pyrimethamine in *P. falciparum* developed within a few years of its introduction (Peters, 1987) due to point mutations in the DHFR gene, which cause 100- to 1,000-fold reduced affinity of the enzyme complex to the drug. Progressive mutations in the DHFR gene of *P. falciparum* further decreased efficacy. Triple mutant infections are relatively resistant to antifolate treatment; with a fourth mutation within the malaria parasite, antifolate drugs become completely ineffective.

Quadruple mutant *P. falciparum* strains are now prevalent in parts of Southeast Asia, and South America (Imwong et al., 2001). Resistance to partner antifols sulfonamide and sulfone results from progressive acquisition of mutations in the *P. falciparum* gene encoding the target enzyme DHPS.

Chloroquine

One of chloroquine's most dramatic characteristics is its ability to concentrate itself from nanomolar (10^{-9}) levels outside the parasite to levels one million times higher (millimolar levels, 10^{-3}) in the acid food vacuole of the parasite inside a red blood cell (Krogstad and Schlesinger, 1987). This action in itself does not explain chloroquine's antimalarial activity, however. Chloroquine works by interfering with heme dimerization, the detoxifying biochemical process within the malaria parasite that normally yields malaria pigment (hemozoin).

Reduced intracellular drug concentrations accompany chloroquine resistance because resistant parasites expel chloroquine from their acid food vacuoles 40-50 times faster than do drug-sensitive parasites (Bray et al., 1998). Such accumulation deficits were once attributed to changes in pH gradient, or to altered membrane permeability, or both (Le Bras and Durand, 2003). However, chloroquine resistance was then found to be reversible by verapamil, a drug which also modulates resistance in multidrug resistant (MDR) mammalian cancer cells. This discovery led to the identification of the protein Pgh1 (an analog to overexpressed glycoproteins that expel cytotoxic drugs in cancer cells) in the digestive vacuole membrane of *P. falciparum*. Genes encoding MDR proteins have been identified in *P. falciparum* (*pfmdr1*); amplification of these "wild type" MDR genes has recently been shown to cause mefloquine resistance (Price et al., 1999b).

Point mutations in the gene encoding a food vacuole transporter protein (*pfcrt*) have been linked to chloroquine resistance (Durand et al., 2001; Warhurst, 2001) and correlate with reduced in vivo chloroquine efficacy (Djimde et al., 2001). In the presence of *pfcrt* mutations, mutations in the second transport genes (*Pfmdr1*) further modulate resistance in vitro although the role of *Pfmdr1* mutations in determining in vivo responses to chloroquine treatment is still unclear. Additional unlinked mutations are probably involved in the development of chloroquine resistance, some of which have not yet been discovered.

In the laboratory, the efflux mechanism seen in chloroquine-resistant *P. falciparum* parasites can be inhibited by several unrelated drugs (calcium channel blockers such as verapamil as well as tricyclic antidepressants, phenothiazines, and antihistamines), whereas mefloquine resistance can be reversed by penfluridol (Martin et al., 1987; Oduola et al., 1993). Clinical applications of these findings are few to date, although chloroquine plus high doses of chlorpheniramine (an antihistamine) did show improved efficacy against chloroquine-resistant *P. falciparum* in Nigerian children (Sowunmi et al., 1997). Whether general use of resistance reversers will be safe and feasible in the future remains an open question (Personal communication, N. White, Mahidol University, March 2004).

Other Antimalarial Drugs

In general, antimalarial drug resistance to mefloquine, quinine, lumefantrine, and halofantrine is linked, whereas chloroquine, and mefloquine resistance are not. Cross-resistance between antimalarials is related to common aspects of their modes of action as well as their resistance mechanisms. Parasites with high-level chloroquine resistance (present in Southeast Asia), are generally resistant to amodiaquine as well; in residents of Southeast Asia, amodiaquine may thus fail as a back-up treatment (Le Bras and Durand, 2003). The same relationship holds true for halofantrine, and mefloquine. On the other hand, there may be an inverse correlation between chloroquine and mefloquine sensitivity: in Africa, for example, chloroquine-sensitive strains are substantially less sensitive to mefloquine or halofantrine, and vice versa (Oduola et al., 1987; Simon et al., 1988).

Atovaquone is a component of Malarone®, a new combination drug (consisting of atovaquone and proguanil) used for treatment and prevention of chloroquine-resistant *P. falciparum*. Atovaquone interferes with mitochondrial electron transport, and also blocks cellular respiration (Srivastava et al., 1997). High levels of atovaquone resistance result from single-point mutations in a gene encoding cytochrome *b* found on a small, extrachromosomal DNA-containing element in the parasite (Korsinczky et al., 2000).

ARTEMISININS

Of the available antimalarials, the artemisinins are effective at killing the broadest range of asexual stages of the parasite, ranging from medium-sized rings to early schizonts; they also produce the most rapid therapeutic responses by accelerating clearance of circulating ring-stage parasites (ter Kuile et al., 1993).

Qinghaosu, or artemisinin, is a sesquiterpene lactone peroxide extracted from the leaves of the shrub *Artemisia annua* (qinghao). Three derivatives are widely used: the oil-soluble methyl ether, artemether (artemotil [arteether] is a closely related compound); the water soluble hemi-succinate derivative, artesunate; and dihydroartemisinin (DHA).

Artesunate, artemether, and arteether are all synthesized from DHA, and they are converted back to it within the body. Artemisinin itself is available in a few countries in Asia. It is 5-10 times less active than the derivatives, and it is not metabolized to DHA.

Artemisinin is available as capsules of powder, or as suppositories. Artemether is formulated in peanut oil, and arteether in sesame seed oil, for intramuscular injection, and in capsules or tablets for oral use. Artesunate is formulated either as tablets, in a gel enclosed in gelatin for rectal administration (called a rectocap™), or as dry powder of artesunic acid for injection, supplied with an ampoule of 5 percent sodium bicarbonate. The powder is dissolved in the sodium bicarbonate to form sodium artesunate, and then diluted in 5 percent dextrose or normal saline for intravenous or intramuscular injection. Artelinic acid is a water-soluble second-generation compound under long-term development. It has not yet been used in treatment. The majority of clinical data pertain to the most widely used derivative, artesunate.

Botanical Properties

Artemisinin was first isolated from the stems, leaves, and flowers of *Artemisia annua* by Chinese scientists (Anonymous, 1982; Klayman et al., 1984), but details of the process were not released. Researchers at the Walter Reed Army Institute of Medical Research (WRAIR) successfully isolated artemisinin derivatives from air-dried parts of plants growing in the wild near Washington, D.C., using petroleum ether extraction (Klayman, 1985). The plant grows easily in temperate areas, and has become naturalized in many countries. It can attain a height of two meters or more, appearing as an erect specimen with a woody stem. Artemisinin accumulates in all parts of *A. annua* except for the roots (Abdin et al., 2003). Artemisinin content in flowers is 4-5 times higher than in leaves. Plant age correlates with artemisinin yield, presumably due to a progressive increase in leaf yield and artemisinin content with plant growth. In agricultural settings in Asia, artesunate production has varied from 5 kg/hectare to 50 kg/hectare (Personal communication, J-M. Kindermans, Médecins Sans Frontières, February 2004).

Mechanism of Action

Artemisinin's chemical structure is unlike any other known antimalarial. It includes an endoperoxide bridge necessary for its antimalarial action (Brossi et al., 1988). Artemisinin treatment of membranes, especially in the presence of heme, causes lipid peroxidation (Scott et al., 1989;

Wei and Sadrzadeh, 1994; Berman and Adams, 1997); this event may occur as a result of the drug's interaction with intracellular heme or iron (Meshnick et al., 1991). With respect to artemisinin's direct effect on the malaria parasite, recent work suggests that artemisinin specifically inhibits PfATP6, the SERCA orthologue of *Plasmodium falciparum*, a calcium ATPase (Eckstein-Ludwig et al., 2003).

In vivo, artemisinins kill malaria parasites within host erythrocytes, after which dead parasites are culled by the spleen, leaving formerly infected red blood cells intact and circulating (Chotivanich et al., 2000). It is not yet clear which asexual parasite life-cycle stages are most sensitive to artemisinin derivatives: late rings and early trophozoites (ter Kuile et al., 1993) versus trophozoites (Geary et al., 1989). There is clear consensus, however, that artemisinin derivatives kill early-stage gametocytes and are more active over a broader range of the parasite life cycle than any other antimalarial drug currently in use.

General Clinical Experience with Artemisinins and ACTs

More randomized clinical trials have been published regarding the effects of artemisinins than any other individual or class of antimalarial drug (Myint et al., 2004). The artemisinins' pharmacodynamic effects are due to their rapid absorption and activity against many stages of the malaria life cycle, from young asexual forms (rings) to early sexual forms (gametocytes) (Kumar and Zheng, 1990). Their half-lives are short (<1 hour for artesunate) which protects them from resistance. They reduce gametocyte carriage, thus decreasing infectiousness following treatment as witnessed by the dramatic fall in malaria transmission on the Thai-Burma border (Price et al., 1996; Nosten et al., 2000). Tolerability of the drugs is excellent (White and Olliaro, 1998).

Administered alone, artemisinin derivatives require at least 7 days of treatment. When combined with other drugs, however, artemisinin combination therapies (ACTs) given in 3-day regimens can eradicate parasites quickly and protect against the development of resistance to both drugs. In addition, artemisinin derivatives are the only first-line malaria treatments to act on gametocytes (early-stage).

On February 20, 2002, the World Health Organization (WHO) released a statement recommending that "Governments . . . rapidly adopt more effective treatments [for malaria]. The aim is to provide effective treatment against malaria and to slow the spread of drug resistance. . . . In particular, WHO recommends the use of artemisinin-based combination therapy" (WHO, 2001).

Current Evidence Base for ACTs[1]

Through the largest randomized controlled trials ever conducted on antimalarials in Africa, a considerable body of evidence has now been collected showing that artemisinin-based combinations improve cure rates, decrease gametocyte carriage, and are well tolerated with few serious adverse effects. In the first of these multicenter trials to be published, 941 children who had uncomplicated *P. falciparum* malaria were randomly assigned 3 days treatment with amodiaquine plus artesunate, or amodiaquine plus placebo. Both regimens were well tolerated. The combination of artesunate and amodiaquine significantly improved treatment efficacy in Gabon (85 versus 71 percent, p=0.02) and in Kenya (68 vs. 41 percent, p<0.0001). In Senegal, however, the two regimens were equivalent: day-28 cure rates for amodiaquine-artesunate versus amodiaquine were 82 versus 79 percent (p=0.5) (Adjuik et al., 2002).

The efficacy and safety of artesunate in combination with sulfadoxine-pyrimethamine (SP) has been evaluated in randomized controlled trials involving 2,865 patients in sub-Saharan Africa. Results from the first study published from The Gambia (von Seidlein et al., 2000) (where the cure rate with SP monotherapy was then 93 percent), showed that both cure rate and parasite clearance were significantly higher in patients who received 3 days of artesunate plus a single dose of SP compared with those who received SP alone. Gametocyte carriage was 68 percent following solo SP treatment in comparison with 21 percent following the artesunate-SP combination (p=0.001).

In contrast, underlying SP resistance in Uganda led to unacceptable rates of late recrudescence when artesunate-SP was used there (Dorsey et al., 2002). This finding underscores that combining an artemisinin with a longer-acting drug without any underlying resistance may prove the optimal regimen in many areas. On the other hand, in Thailand, where drug resistance is particularly severe, artesunate plus mefloquine was highly effective, even in areas where mefloquine resistance was previously quite common (Price et al., 1997). In the largest-ever series of therapeutic efficacy studies with ACTs, artesunate plus mefloquine produced a sustained, increased cure rate (almost 100 percent from 1998 onward) despite established resistance to high-dose mefloquine alone seen between 1990 and 1994 (Nosten et al., 2000). Cure rates with other ACTs (atovaquone-proguanil-artesunate, artemether-lumefantrine) in Asia have also been consistently above 90 percent (van Vugt et al., 1998, 1999).

Coartem (artemether-lumefantrine) is the first fixed-dose ACT whose

---

[1]This section draws heavily from Barnes and Folb (2003) with permission of the authors.

two antimalarial components were not widely used prior to marketing. When given in a six-dose regimen over 3 days, Coartem is effective against all *P. falciparum* and extremely well tolerated. Coartem's principal drawback is its twice daily dosing and lumefantrine's variable absorption linked to dietary fat intake (if patients are unable to eat, or consume a very low fat diet while taking the drug, low cure rates can result).

In randomized trials comparing a six-dose regimen of orally administered artemether-lumefantrine with mefloquine-artesunate for multidrug-resistant *P. falciparum* malaria, artemether-lumefantrine was as effective (94-100 percent) and overall better tolerated than mefloquine-artesunate (van Vugt et al., 1999, 2000; Lefevre et al., 2001).

Artesunate

Artesunate can be administered as a tablet, an injection, or as a rectal suppository. A comparison of intravenous artesunate and quinine in 113 adults with severe malaria reported mortality of 12 percent with artesunate, and 22 percent with quinine (p=0.22) (Newton et al., 2003). In patients with hyperparasitemia who had no other features of severe malaria but were at an increased risk of developing severe malaria, oral artesunate was found to be superior to intravenous quinine in reducing both the clinical symptoms and parasites (Luxemburger et al., 1995).

Rectally administered artesunate has been shown to be safe and highly effective in children and adults with uncomplicated or moderately severe falciparum malaria (Sabchareon et al., 1998; Karunajeewa et al., 2003; Barnes et al., 2004). A number of recent randomized controlled and open-label studies of rectal artesunate in Africa and Asia have demonstrated the rapid antimalarial efficacy of a single dose of rectal artesunate (10 mg/kg) in moderately severe falciparum malaria in both children and adults prior to referral for definitive treatment. All patients had evidence of adequate absorption of the drug. Clearance of malaria parasites from the peripheral blood was consistently more rapid with rectal artesunate than with quinine injection. There also are a number of small open label studies, some of which were randomized, demonstrating the clinical and parasitological efficacy of rectal artesunate in adults with severe *P. falciparum* infections (Awad et al., 2003) where rectal artesunate was administered repeatedly, and combined with a second oral antimalarial to prevent recrudescence.

These clinical and parasitological responses suggest that rectal artesunate could prove highly beneficial in the initial management of acute malaria in patients who cannot take medication by mouth (and for whom parenteral medication is not immediately available due to limited local resources). In Ghana, artesunate suppositories have already been given by trained village volunteers; in the future, traditional healers also could be trained to use them as an emergency treatment for febrile seizures in malaria-endemic areas (Personal communication, B. Greenwood, London School of Hygiene and Tropical Medicine, April 2004). If used widely enough, rectal artesunate could have a major effect on malaria deaths in Africa.

Toxicity of Artemisinins[2]

In the early 1970s, Chinese scientists characterized the antimalarial properties of artemisinins and their excellent tolerability and safety (Anonymous, 1982; Luo and Shen, 1987). A subsequent review of published and unpublished studies of the arteminisinin derivatives confirmed the earlier Chinese findings (Pukrittayakamee et al., 2000). Those adverse events that were reported were not specifically associated with a single form of artemisinin or route of administration. Neutropenia (but not agranulocytosis) and asymptomatic ECG abnormalities occurred in 1.3 percent of patients; reduced reticulocyte count, anemia, eosinophilia, and elevated aspartate aminotransferase (a liver enzyme) occurred in ≤ 1.0 percent (Taylor and White, 2004).

In western Thailand, Price and colleagues (1999a) conducted a detailed study of oral artesunate or artemether used as monotherapy or in combination with mefloquine. The artemisinin derivatives were associated with substantially fewer adverse effects than the mefloquine-containing regimens: acute nausea (16 vs. 31 percent), vomiting (11 vs. 24 percent), anorexia (34 vs. 52 percent), and dizziness (15 vs. 47 percent). Oral artesunate or artemether alone were well tolerated. Since these data were published two cases of acute hives and anaphylaxis developed in the same population following artesunate monotherapy, raising the total number of allergic reactions to 6 patients out of roughly 17,000, or 1 in 2,833 (Leonardi et al., 2001).

Artemether-Lumefantrine (Coartem)

Experience with Coartem is increasing rapidly. In large-scale clinical trials the combination was very well tolerated, whether taken as a four- or six-dose regimen. Coartem has been better tolerated than either mefloquine alone or artesunate plus mefloquine (van Vugt et al., 1998; Looareesuwan et al., 1999). Reported adverse effects have generally been mild, including

---

[2]This section is drawn largely from Taylor and White (2004). Sections of the text are taken verbatim, with permission of the authors.

gastrointestinal upset, headache, dizziness, fatigue, sleep disturbance, palpitations, maylgia, arthralgia, and rash (Bakshi et al., 2000). Detailed prospective studies have not demonstrated any cardiotoxicity (van Vugt et al., 1999; Bindschedler et al., 2000). Twenty severe adverse effects in 1,869 patients include 19 that could be explained on the basis of the malarial episode or a concurrent illness; artemether-lumefantrine may have contributed to the development of hemolytic anemia in one 35-year-old patient 13 days following discontinuation of the drug (Bakshi et al., 2000).

Neurotoxicity: Animal Studies

Dogs receiving high doses of intramuscular artemether or arteether have developed a peculiar selective pattern of brain stem damage, in particular involving the reticular formation, the vestibular system nuclei, and nuclei related to the auditory system. Clinical features included gait disturbances; loss of spinal and pain response reflexes; prominent loss of brain stem and eye reflexes; cardiorespiratory depression; and death. ECG changes included prolongation of QTc interval and bizarre ST-T segment changes (Brewer et al., 1994). A similar selective pattern of brain stem pathology also was found in mice, rats, and Rhesus monkeys given arteether or arthemether (Genovese et al., 1998; Petras et al., 2000). In mice, parenteral artemether was more neurotoxic than artesunate, resulting in escalating, irreversible neurological deficits involving balance, and death with increasing doses (Nontprasert et al., 1998). Recent studies have shown that neurotoxicity is determined by the pharmacokinetic properties of the drugs. Sustained CNS exposure from slowly absorbed or eliminated artemisinins is considerably more neurotoxic than intermittent brief exposure. Thus intramuscular artemether and arteether are more neurotoxic in experimental animals than the same drugs given orally, or artesunate given by any route.

Neurotoxicity in Humans

One case report to date has described acute cerebellar dysfunction including slurred speech, ataxia, impaired heel to shin movement, and dysdiadochokinesis after treatment of falciparum malaria with oral artesunate (Miller and Panosian, 1997). Detailed neurologic data from Price and colleagues (1999a) include neurological examinations conducted in nearly 2,000 children older than 5 at baseline, and on days 2, 7, and 28 posttreatment, with artemether alone, artesunate alone, or artesunate plus mefloquine. Short-course therapy with the artemisinins either alone or in combination with mefloquine was associated with self-limited, minor neurological deficits in a minority (<1 percent) of patients during the first few days of falciparum malaria.

In a recent case control study of 150 patients with uncomplicated malaria who received artemether-lumefantrine, a slight reduction in auditory acuity was noted compared with age-matched healthy controls (Toovey and Jamieson, 2004). In contrast, no differences in audiometry or auditory-evoked potentials were noted in 242 Vietnamese patients who received up to 21 treatment doses of artemisinin or artesunate compared with 108 age- and location-matched controls (Kissinger et al., 2000), or in 79 Karen patients who received two or more treatment doses of artemether or artesunate compared with 79 age- and location-matched controls (van Vugt et al., 2000).

Most recently, neuropathologic assessments of the brain stems of patients who died from severe falciparum malaria following treatment with high dose intramuscular artemether (the doses were higher than generally recommended) were performed (Hien et al., 2003), revealing no evidence for damage similar to that seen in experimental animals. Taken together with the cumulative body of negative clinical data—including detailed studies of audiometry, and auditory-evoked potentials in patients who received multiple courses of artemisinin derivatives in uncomplicated malaria as well as high dose artemether in severe malaria (Hien et al., 1996)—the weight of evidence suggests that neurotoxicity observed in animals does not occur in humans receiving current recommended treatment doses. The widespread use of water-soluble compounds (which are far less neurotoxic in animal models) as opposed to injected oil-based derivatives adds a further margin of safety.

Safety of Artemisinins During Pregnancy

Observations in Pregnant Women

Published data on treating malaria during pregnancy with artemisinin derivatives have come from China (Li et al., 1990), the Thai-Burmese border (where use has been greatest) (McGready et al., 1998, 2000, 2001), and The Gambia (Deen et al., 2001). The data from China describe 23 women treated with artemether or artemisinin between 17 and 38 weeks of gestation who developed no evidence of fetal or maternal toxicity. The published experience of artemisinin use during pregnancy in Thailand includes observational data on 461 women treated with artesunate (n=528) or artemether (n=11) for 539 episodes of acute *P. falciparum* malaria, including 44 episodes during the first trimester. Birth outcomes in the artemisinin-treated Thai women were comparable to community rates for abortion, stillbirth, congenital abnormality, and/or mean gestation at delivery. All newborns who were followed for 1 year developed normally, including those who had been exposed to an artemisinin in the first trimester of pregnancy

(McGready et al., 2001). Another study of 287 pregnant Gambian women inadvertently treated (during a mass drug administration) with a single dose of artesunate plus SP during their first, second, or third trimesters of pregnancy found no evidence of obstetric or fetal toxicity compared with women who were not exposed to artesunate plus SP (Deen et al., 2001). There are no published data on the use of artemether-lumefantrine in pregnant or breast-feeding women.

Evidence from Experimental Animals

Studies investigating the possible risks of artemisinins in during the first trimester of pregnancy (when birth defects are most likely to occur), also have been conducted in laboratory animals. In 2001, a WHO report concluded: "Preclinical studies have consistently shown that artemisinin and its derivatives do not exhibit mutagenic or teratogenic activity, but all of these drugs caused fetal resorption in rodents at relatively low doses" (WHO, 2001). More recently, in some experiments in rats and rabbits, but not in others, cardiovascular and limb abnormalities occurred when pregnant animals were given artemisinin doses similar to those used in man. For this reason, in 2002, WHO convened two further meetings of experts who reviewed the animal and human evidence relevant to the use of artemisinins by pregnant women, concluding:

> Presently, artemisinin compounds cannot be recommended for treatment of malaria in the first trimester. However, they should not be withheld if treatment is considered to be lifesaving for the mother and other antimalarials are considered to be unsuitable. Because the safety data are limited, artemisinin compounds should only be used in the second and third trimesters when other treatments are considered unsuitable.

> There is a need for further evidence of the safety of artemisinin compounds in pregnancy. All pregnant women treated with artemisinin compounds should be carefully followed up to document the pregnancy outcomes and subsequent development of the child and reported to the appropriate authorities. (WHO/RBM/UNDP/World Bank, 2003).

In summary, current data are encouraging but more safety data for the artemisinin derivatives are needed to support use in pregnant women with uncomplicated malaria. In contrast, although there are no published data regarding the treatment of *severe* malaria in pregnancy with artesunate or artemether, these drugs have been used widely and found effective. In particular, artesunate and artemether are often preferred over quinine and quinidine during pregnancy because they do not induce hypoglycemia, and they are easier to administer (Tran et al., 1996). Nonetheless, if ACTs are widely introduced, tens of thousands of pregnant African women—including some of whom do not have malaria at all—will receive them. The use of artemisinins by pregnant women, especially during the first trimester, is an issue that is, appropriately, receiving continued attention by international monitoring bodies. On the country level, pharmacovigilance programs will be needed to track a variety of effects caused by artemisinins as well as new ACT partner drugs throughout pregnancy. For example, mefloquine given at any stage of pregnancy in Thailand has been associated with a fourfold increase in stillbirth (Nosten et al., 1999), whereas the same effect was not observed in pregnant women treated with mefloquine in Malawi (Steketee et al., 1996). This finding also requires further follow-up.

ANTIMALARIAL DRUG RESISTANCE

Although not every factor responsible for the emergence and spread of parasite resistance is fully known, what is clear is that antimalarial drug resistance can develop to *any* antimalarial drug, and that drug pressure is a key prerequisite. Other important contributors include drug elimination half-life, parasite biomass, and malaria transmission intensity (Talisuna et al., 2004).

How Resistance to Antimalarial Drugs Arises

The emergence of drug-resistant organisms can be considered in two discrete phases: the initial de novo event (a rare genetic occurrence) that first produces the resistant mutant, and the subsequent selection process that leads to its preferential transmission and spread. Resistance *arises* from spontaneous mutations or gene duplications, which are independent of drug pressure. Once formed, however, resistant mutants have a survival advantage in the presence of antimalarial drugs and, conversely, a survival disadvantage in the absence of at least certain antimalarial drugs. The resulting fitness cost may lead to a declining prevalence of resistance once drug pressure is removed (this pattern has been demonstrated for chloroquine resistance in Malawi [Kublin et al., 2003] although its operational significance is still uncertain).

Factors affecting the development of resistance include: the parasite mutation rate, the degree of resistance conferred by the genetic change, the fitness cost of the resistance mechanism, the proportion of all transmissible infection exposed to the drug, the drug concentration profile, the individual (e.g., dosing, duration, adherence) and community (e.g., quality, availability, distribution) patterns of drug use, and the immunity profile of the community (White, 1999).

The possible role of mass drug administration in accelerating the emergence of antimalarial drug resistance was first highlighted by Payne (Payne,

1988), who observed that chloroquine resistance in different sites had one common denominator: the long-term, local use of chloroquine for treatment. Later studies in coastal Kenya, Malawi, Mali and Bolivia found a positive correlation between patterns of drug use and in vitro parasite resistance or the prevalence of mutations linked to resistance (Diourte et al., 1999; Nzila et al., 2000). A recent study in Uganda observed that the prevalence of chloroquine resistance was higher in sites with high-frequency chloroquine use as reflected in detectable chloroquine metabolites in urine (Talisuna et al., 2002b). However, SP resistance was highest in high-transmission sites with relatively low SP use, suggesting that factors in addition to drug pressure influence the spread of SP drug resistance.

The role of drug elimination half-life in the development of parasite resistance has recently been reviewed, and modeled (Hastings et al., 2002). Drugs with long elimination phases are, in essence, "selective filters," allowing infection by resistant parasites to flourish while the residual drug levels suppress infection by sensitive parasites (Watkins and Mosobo, 1993). Slowly eliminated drugs such as mefloquine (T $^1/_2$=3 weeks) provide such a filter for months after drug administration. The resulting selection pressure can be enormous.

In Kenya, a potent selective pressure for SP resistance was found to operate even under conditions of supervised drug administration and optimal SP dosing (Watkins and Mosobo, 1993). *Plasmodium falciparum* infections appearing between days 15 and 52 after SP treatment were more likely to exhibit pyrimethamine resistance in vitro. The selective pressure of home-based use of SP (per the WHO strategy of home-based management of fevers) could accelerate the emergence of SP resistance to an even greater degree (Talisuna et al., 2004).

Finally, drug resistant mutant parasites are statistically more likely to emerge from infections involving large numbers of parasites. Such large parasite biomass infections are more common in nonimmune individuals, as demonstrated by the higher prevalence of chloroquine-resistant infections, and chloroquine treatment failures seen in African children compared to adults (Dorsey et al., 2000; Djimde et al., 2001; Talisuna et al., 2002a). Nonimmune patients infected with large numbers of parasites who receive inadequate treatment (either because of poor drug quality, adherence, vomiting of an oral treatment, etc.) are another potent source of resistance. This emphasizes the importance of correct prescribing and good adherence to prescribed drug regimens in slowing the emergence of resistance.

The Relationship between Resistance and Transmission Intensity

Recrudescence and onward transmission of a de novo resistant malaria parasite are essential for the propagation of resistance. Killing the transmis-

SAVING LIVES, BUYING TIME

sible sexual stages (gametocytes) during the primary infection does *not* lessen resistance because these gametocytes derive from drug sensitive parasites. Gametocytes carrying the resistance genes will not reach transmission intensities until the resistant biomass has expanded to numbers close to those producing illness (>10^7 parasites) (Jeffery and Eyles, 1955). In order to decrease the spread of resistance, gametocyte production from the *recrudescent* resistant infection must be prevented.

One way to look at the relationship between resistance and transmission intensity is as follows. In low-transmission areas the majority of malaria is symptomatic, and selection therefore takes place at a time when relatively large numbers of parasites in a given individual encounter antimalarial drugs. In higher transmission areas, however, symptomatic disease usually occurs during the first years of life. Later on, malaria becomes less symptomatic due to imperfect immunity (sometimes called premunition), which holds the infection in check at levels below the symptom threshold.

Despite premunition, many residents of high-transmission areas still receive antimalarial treatments throughout their lives, often inappropriately. Fortunately, most "treatments" are largely unrelated to the peaks of parasitemia, thereby minimizing the selection of resistant strains. Immunity also reduces the emergence of resistance considerably (White and Pongtavornpinyo, 2003). Even if a resistant mutant does survive and multiply, the likelihood that it will produce sufficient gametocytes for transmission is reduced by the presence of other competing parasite genotypes (Dye and Williams, 1997).

Since significant symptoms generally are confined to young children in high-transmission areas, the fact that children comprise only 20 percent of the population, roughly speaking, and their blood volumes are much lower than adults' (therefore containing fewer total parasites) are final curbs on the emergence of drug resistance in such areas. The net result overall is considerable reduction in the probability of de novo selection and subsequent transmission of a resistant parasite in high- versus low-transmission areas, as borne out by the historical emergence of chloroquine resistance and more rapid increase of antifol resistance in low transmission areas.[3]

---

[3]The situation is probably even more complex than described above. For instance, certain individuals with low-level parasitemia may still go on producing gametocytes, particularly in response to chronic anemia (Nacher, 2002). Recent studies also suggest that exposure to a drug can select for resistant gametocytes (Sutherland et al., 2002). Therefore, in certain highly endemic communities where drugs are widely available and misused, there may still be some selection of drug resistant mutants in asymptomatic subjects who vastly outnumber those who are acutely ill.

Global Overview of Current Antimalarial Drug Resistance to *P. falciparum*

The historical emergence of drug-resistant *P. falciparum* is reviewed elsewhere in this report (see Chapter 5). The following is a brief summary of current levels of global drug resistance to chloroquine and SP based on in vivo assessment of therapeutic treatment failure (TTF). Data showing in vivo resistance to chloroquine and SP in Africa also are presented in maps (Figures 9-1, and 9-2).

In Africa, median chloroquine (CQ)-TTF among children younger than 5 years was above the critical value (TTF=25 percent) in all the countries in the eastern/great lakes (seven of seven), and central/southern (four of four) regions. However, in West Africa, only one of five countries had a median CQ-TTF above the critical value. The median CQ parasitologic failure (CQ-PF) varied from 38 to 91 percent in Southeast Asia, from 23 to 38

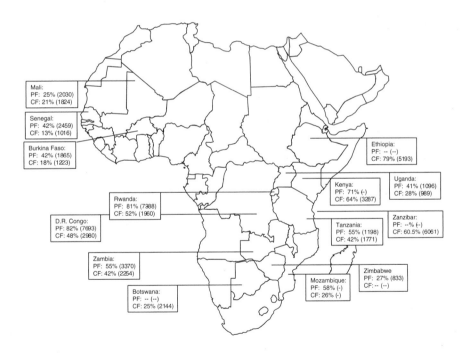

FIGURE 9-1 In vivo chloroquine resistance in selected countries, sub-Saharan Africa, 1996-2002 (median range).
PF = parasitologic failure; CF = clinical failure.
SOURCE: From Talisuna et al. (2004); Kazadi et al. (2003).

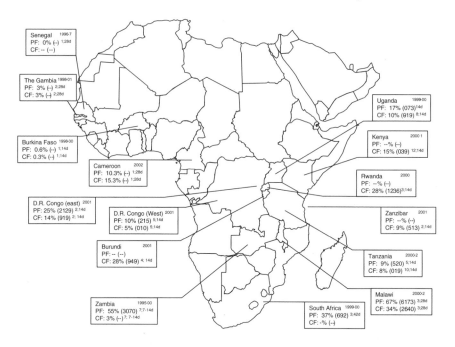

FIGURE 9-2 In vivo sulfadoxine-pyrimethamine resistance in selected countries, sub-Saharan Africa.
Dates of studies in upper right corner; PF = parasitologic failure; CF = clinical failure. Median (range) given. Superscript numbers following range = number of studies contributing to data; duration of follow-up in days.
SOURCE: From Talisuna et al. (2004); Kazadi et al. (2003); Plowe et al. (2004); CDC unpublished data.

percent in the Pacific region, from 46 to 77 percent in the Indian subcontinent, and from 12 to 69 percent in the Middle East. In South America, the lowest median CQ-PF was 33 percent, and the highest was 50 percent, while the corresponding lowest and highest estimates for CQ-TTF were 44 and 100 percent, respectively.

In Africa, the median SP-TTF varied from 0 to 35 percent and the median SP parasitologic failure (SP-PF) ranged from 0 to 76 percent. In Asia, the SP-TTF varied from 9 to 35 percent, and in South America it varied from 3 to 32 percent. The SP-PF was higher, and varied between 5 and 67 percent in Asia, and between 6 and 20 percent in South America.

In summary, these recent data indicate a high prevalence of CQ resistance (TTF>25 percent) in the eastern/great lakes and central/southern regions of Africa, where SP resistance is emerging. Such a situation could quickly lead to multidrug resistance, particularly if SP is adopted widely as first-line treatment.

Resistance to Artemisinins

At present, although artemisinin-resistant strains of *P. falciparum* (Inselburg, 1985) and *Plasmodium yoelii* (Peters and Robinson, 1999) have been produced in the laboratory, there is no evidence for clinically relevant artemisinin resistance. Clinical and laboratory strains of *P. falciparum* also can vary in their artemisinin sensitivity in vitro (Le Bras and Durand, 2003) without clinical effects. Two *P. falciparum*-infected patients who failed artesunate therapy had parasites that were later shown to be sensitive to artemisinin in vitro (Luxemburger et al., 1998). In general, recrudescence after artemisinin monotherapy is due to host factors (such as drug metabolism) as opposed to failure due to parasite resistance.

In the absence of a functioning spleen, dead intraerythrocytic malaria parasites are not removed. The persistence of these parasites on blood smears—implying delayed clearance—may be misinterpreted as artemisinin resistance (Chotivanich et al., 2002). However, even when 7-day courses of artemisinin derivatives are given, cure rates generally do not exceed 90-95 percent. This failure to cure all patients with artemisinin does not reflect resistance per se but a curious phenomenon in which a subpopulation of very young parasites remain in an arrested state of development for over a week following treatment (Personal communication, D. Kyle, 1997). These parasites may later multiply and cause a recrudescence. However, the recrudescent parasites are no more resistant to artemisinin than the primary infection (White, 1998).

Multidrug resistant *P. falciparum* (with MDR amplification) are more resistant to artemisinin than non-MDR parasites but the differences do not influence therapeutic outcomes. They have, however, led to incorrect suppositions about the selection of resistance (Wongsrichanalai et al., 1999). For example, on the western border of Thailand, as mefloquine resistance worsened, in vitro susceptibility to dihydroartemisinin (the major metabolite of artesunate and artemether) also fell. However, full artemisinin efficacy along with mefloquine efficacy restored following the systematic use of mefloquine-artesunate in the region (Brockman et al., 2000).

Plasmodium vivax

Chloroquine Resistance

It was not until 1989—30 years after chloroquine resistance first emerged in *P. falciparum*—that a chloroquine-resistant strain of *P. vivax* was first detected in Papua New Guinea (Rieckmann et al., 1989). Chloroquine-resistant *P. vivax* (CRPV) infections were subsequently reported from Indonesian New Guinea (Baird et al., 1996; Fryauff et al., 1998), Burma (Marlar-Than et al., 1995), India (Garg et al., 1995), and Guyana (Phillips et al., 1996). Sporadic CRPV infections have now surfaced in many geographic regions of the world but do not appear to be a growing problem in most areas (Mendis et al., 2001). One exception is eastern Indonesia, where the risk of therapeutic failure following chloroquine approached 80 percent 28 days after treatment (Baird et al., 1997). Fortunately, drug-sensitive parasites of *P. vivax* are at little disadvantage vis-à-vis drug resistant strains, largely because *P. vivax* gametocytes develop quickly in the blood of infected individuals, and they have less drug exposure than *P. falciparum* prior to transmission.

Primaquine Tolerance

Among the species of *Plasmodium* that infect humans, only *P. vivax* and *P. ovale* have latent liver hypnozoites that can trigger a clinical relapse of malaria after successful eradication of bloodstream parasites. Although primaquine, an 8-aminoquinoline drug, has been used for several decades to prevent relapse, some *P. vivax* and *P. ovale* infections acquired in Southeast Asia and the Southwest Pacific area are now tolerant to its effects. As a result, the new recommended adult dose of primaquine is 30 mg base drug daily for 14 days (420 mg total dose) as opposed to the previous 15 mg daily dose over the same time period. An alternative regimen for primaquine-tolerant infections is the weekly administration of 45 mg PQ for 8 weeks. This approach lessens primaquine's likelihood of producing hemolysis in patients with mild G6PD deficiency while enhancing its efficacy against tolerant strains. In patients with severe G6PD deficiency, primaquine should be strictly avoided.

ASSESSING ANTIMALARIAL DRUG EFFICACY AND RESISTANCE

Four methods are currently available to study or measure antimalarial drug efficacy vis-à-vis drug resistance: in vivo, in vitro, animal model studies, and molecular markers (Bloland, 2001).

In Vivo Testing

Of all available methods, in vivo tests most closely predict the likelihood that parasites infecting a target human population will respond to a particular treatment regimen. The process of in vivo testing involves monitoring a malaria-infected subject following administration of known doses of an antimalarial drug. In 1973, the World Health Organization defined criteria for the evaluation of chloroquine and amodiaquine and recommended a 28-day follow-up period. These protocols stipulated that patients remain in screened quarters for 28 days to avoid reinfection during the period of evaluation. The original WHO definitions of in vivo drug sensitivity (sensitive [S], and progressively worsening degrees of resistance [R1, R2 and R3]) are shown in Table 9-3.

The original protocols were generally used until the 1990s when shorter durations of follow-up (usually 14 days) were recommended—particularly in areas of high transmission—whereas some research groups adopted longer periods of follow-up (up to 63 days) when evaluating slowly eliminated antimalarial drugs. Shorter periods of follow-up in assessing antimalarial treatment often underestimate drug-resistant recrudescent infections, which, even in areas of high stable transmission, cause significant morbidity, especially anemia.

WHO's modified protocol, with a shortened follow-up period (WHO, 1996), emphasized clinical over parasitologic outcomes, recognizing that clinical parameters are equally important indicators of treatment response. The most recent 2003 protocol was developed with the specific goal of unifying testing around the world under a single methodology and classification scheme. In this scheme, parasitologic failure was brought back into the classification scheme in recognition that even outwardly asymptomatic parasitemia has adverse health consequences (Price et al., 2001). In all areas, regardless of the intensity of malaria transmission, the evaluation of

TABLE 9-3 Original WHO Classification of in Vivo Antimalarial Drug Sensitivity

S (sensitive)	Reduction to <25% of initial parasitemia on day 2 with smears negative for malaria from day 7 to end of follow-up (28 days, or longer for drugs with long half-lives, such as mefloquine)
R1 response	Initial clearance of parasitemia, a negative smear on day 7, followed by recrudescence 8 days or more after treatment
R2 response	Initial clearance or substantial reduction of parasitemia (<25% of the initial count on day 2) but with persistence or recrudescence of parasitemia days 4-7
R3 Response	No significant reduction of parasitemia

SOURCE: Bruce-Chwatt et al. (1985).

antimalarials for uncomplicated malaria now emphasizes treatment efficacy in children under five years with clinically apparent malaria. The rationale for this requirement is that, even in populations with little acquired immunity (as in areas of low or highly seasonal malaria transmission), younger children typically have a less favorable therapeutic response to antimalarials than do older children and adults (ter Kuile et al., 1995).

The range of initial parasite densities appropriate for inclusion in vivo testing is between 1,000 and 100,000 asexual parasites/uL in areas of low to moderate transmission, and between 2,000 and 200,000 asexual parasites/uL in areas of high transmission, as supported by the currently accepted definition of hyperparasitemia (WHO, 2000) (Box 9-1).

In vivo methods tend to underestimate the number of true treatment failures and therefore underestimate the level of antimalarial drug resistance. The reasons for this are:

1. In areas of intermediate and high transmission, older children and adults have significant antiparasitic immunity. This leads to a high probability of self-cure giving a false impression of drug efficacy.

2. Short-term (<14 days) follow-up assessments miss treatment failures. In a recent review of more than 16,000 patients followed for 28 days in treatment arms of randomized trials conducted between 1990 and 2003, the widely used day 14 assessment missed between 63 and 100 percent of all treatment failures, and had no predictive value of the true failure rate; the 28 day assessment also missed one-third of treatment failures but did have predictive value for overall treatment rates (Stepniewska et al., in press).

In Vitro Testing

In vitro assays of antimalarial drug resistance are analogous to antibiotic susceptibility assays performed in hospital and commercial microbiology laboratories. In brief, malaria parasites obtained from venous blood samples are co-cultured in microtiter wells with known concentrations of antimalarial drugs. The drug effect is then quantified according a given agent's ability to inhibit the growth of parasites or their maturation into schizonts (Rieckmann et al., 1978).

In vitro assays are useful because they allow multiple tests (including panels of new and experimental drugs) to be performed on single blood isolates. However, their results frequently differ from those of in vivo tests because the latter are influenced by multiple host factors, chiefly immunity. At present, in vitro tests are only used to test *P. falciparum* drug susceptibility. Their relative expense plus the technical demands of culturing fresh blood samples limit their wide-scale use under routine field conditions.

BOX 9-1
In Vivo Drug Efficacy Testing, Drug Choice, and Formulation
of Malaria Treatment Policy–2003

In vivo assessments of malaria drug efficacy are designed to estimate treatment success or failure rates among malaria patients who are representative of the larger population at risk in a given area. In these assessments, a relatively small number of patients (a minimum of 50 is recommended) with slide-confirmed malaria are recruited, treated with the drug or drug combination, and monitored over time. All treatments are observed to ensure adherence. Patients are monitored for recurrence or persistence of malaria parasitemia for 14 or 28 days (occasionally longer). Recurrence of parasitemia with or without accompanying clinical symptoms is noted.

Patients' responses to treatment are classified into early treatment failures ("ETF"—failure occurring within 3 days of initiation of treatment), late clinical failures ("LCF"—recurrence of parasitemia accompanied by fever between 4 and 14 or 28 days), late parasitologic failure ("LPF"—recurrence of parasitemia not accompanied by fever between 4 and 14 or 28 days), and adequate clinical and parasitologic response ("ACPR"—no recurrence of parasites for the duration of monitoring).

Ideally, a system of sentinel sites (typically between four and eight sites) chosen to represent the epidemiologic, ecologic, and geographic variation within the country is used to characterize treatment efficacy within the country. Data from these sentinel sites are used to inform the development of malaria drug policy, and/or national malaria treatment guidelines.

These data define when a specific malaria treatment can no longer be considered efficacious, and consequently should no longer be used within a national malaria treatment policy. For areas of high transmission intensity in sub-Saharan Africa, WHO recommends a cut-off of greater than 15% total clinical failure (ETF + LCF), and greater than 25% parasitologic failure (LPF) over 14 days (WHO, 2003). There are no clear recommendations, however, on how to reconcile conflicting data from different sentinel sites (i.e., should policy be changed when one of eight sites demonstrates high failure rates, when all eight do, or some time in between?). In any case, because changing and implementing a new treatment policy takes time, the process of policy revision needs to be initiated *before* these levels are reached. In many cases, programs have waited too long to initiate change, and resistance levels are much higher by the time new drugs are in use.

Molecular Markers of Resistance

Recent advances in molecular biology—in particular, the use of polymerase chain reaction (PCR)—have allowed the characterization of several genetic markers of drug resistance in *P. falciparum* (Greenwood, 2002; Wongsrichanalai et al., 2002). At present, attention is focused on four drug resistance genes (Wernsdorfer and Noedl, 2003). The key genes determining resistance to the antifolate drugs pyrimethamine and sulfadoxine are the dihydrofolate reductase gene (*pfdhfr*) and the dihyropteroate synthase gene *(pfdhps)*. High-level pyrimethamine resistance results from the accumulation of mutations in the *dhfr* gene, principally at codons 108, 59, 51, and 164 (Plowe et al., 1997; Wang et al., 1997); quadruple mutants combining all four point mutations confer the most severe resistance (Wongsrichanalai et al., 2002). Point mutations in *dhps* have been associated with decreased susceptibility to sulfadoxine in vitro (Wang et al., 1995). Although the precise relation between mutations in the *dhfr* and *dhps* genes and clinical SP resistance is unclear, current data indicate that a sensitive *dhfr* allele is predictive of SP treatment success independent of the *dhps* allele (Sibley et al., 2001).

The principal determinant of chloroquine resistance is polymorphism in the *P. falciparum* chloroquine resistance transporter gene *(pfcrt)* which is located on chromosome 7 and encodes the digestive vacuole transmembrane protein PfCRT (Wellems et al., 1991; Djimde et al., 2001). Although many polymorphisms associated with chloroquine resistance have been identified, the substitution of threonine for lysine in codon 76 has now been shown to correlate unequivocally with in vitro resistance in *P. falciparum* isolates from Africa, South America, Asia, and Papua New Guinea (Fidock et al., 2000; Djimde et al., 2001). The same finding has been corroborated by an additional in vitro study of isolates of various geographic origins (Durand et al., 2001) as well as clinical studies conducted in Mali (Djimde et al., 2001), Cameroon (Basco and Ringwald, 2001), Sudan (Babiker et al., 2001), Mozambique (Mayor et al., 2001), Laos (Pillai et al., 2001), Thailand (Chen et al., 2001), and Brazil (Vieira et al., 2001). Paradoxically, although cumulative data indicate that the Thr76 mutation is necessary for expression of the resistant phenotype, Thr76 also has been found to lesser degrees in chloroquine-sensitive *P. falciparum* strains, suggesting that other polymorphisms or genes contribute to resistance (Wongsrichanalai et al., 2002). Conversely, because of the added contribution of host immunity, individuals from malaria-endemic areas harboring parasites with the Thr76 mutation also have had successful treatment outcomes following chloroquine (Djimde et al., 2001).

A fourth gene, known as the *P. falciparum* multi-drug resistance gene *(pfmdr)*, encodes the transmemebrane protein P-glycoprotein homologue 1 (Pgh1), and modulates the resistance phenotype in some if not all PfCRT mutant parasites. (Wongsrichanalai et al., 2002). The aspartic acid to tyrosine point mutation in codon 86 has been positively associated with chloroquine resistance in Mali (Djimde et al., 2001), The Gambia (von Seidlein et al., 1997), Sudan (Babiker et al., 2001), Uganda (Flueck et al., 2000), Thailand (Price et al., 1999b), and Brazil (Zalis et al., 1998); however, the same mutation was not associated with chloroquine resistance in other studies conducted in Uganda (Dorsey et al., 2001), Laos (Pillai et al., 2001), Thailand (Chaiyaroj et al., 1999), and Brazil (Povoa et al., 1998).

The relationship between mefloquine sensitivity and *pfmdr1* gene mutations and/or overexpression also was ambiguous until studies in Thailand identified amplification (increased copy number) of *Pfmdr1* to be the main determinant of mefloquine resistance (Price et al., 1999b).

In summary, while molecular markers allow drug resistance testing of multiple samples in a relatively short time, a continuing difficulty of this approach—particularly for chloroquine and mefloquine—has been to identify the specific mutations conferring resistance. The problem becomes even more challenging when drug resistance stems from multiple mutations on one or more genes.

REFERENCES

Abdin MZ, Israr M, Rehman RU, Jain SK. 2003. Artemisinin, a novel antimalarial drug: Biochemical and molecular approaches for enhanced production. *Planta Medica* 69(4): 289-299.

Adjuik M, Agnamey P, Babiker A, Borrmann S, Brasseur P, Cisse M, Cobelens F, Diallo S, Faucher JF, Garner P, Gikunda S, Kremsner PG, Krishna S, Lell B, Loolpapit M, Matsiegui PB, Missinou MA, Mwanza J, Ntoumi F, Olliaro P, Osimbo P, Rezbach P, Some E, Taylor WR. 2002. Amodiaquine-artesunate versus amodiaquine for uncomplicated *Plasmodium falciparum* malaria in African children: A randomised, multicentre trial. *Lancet* 359(9315):1365-1372.

Alving AS, Johnson CF, Tarlov AR, Brewer GJ, Kellermeyer RW, Carson PE. 1960. Mitigation of the haemolytic effect of primaquine and enhancement of its action against exoerythrocytic forms of the Chesson strain of *Plasmodium vivax* by intermittent regimens of drug administration: A preliminary report. *Bulletin of the World Health Organization* 22:621-631.

Anonymous. 1982. Clinical studies on the treatment of malaria with qinghaosu and its derivatives. China cooperative research group on qinghaosu and its derivatives as antimalarials. *Journal of Traditional Chinese Medicine* 2(1):45-50.

Awad MI, Alkadru AM, Behrens RH, Baraka OZ, Eltayeb IB. 2003. Descriptive study on the efficacy and safety of artesunate suppository in combination with other antimalarials in the treatment of severe malaria in Sudan. *American Journal of Tropical Medicine and Hygiene* 68(2):153-158.

Babiker HA, Pringle SJ, Abdel-Muhsin A, Mackinnon M, Hunt P, Walliker D. 2001. High-level chloroquine resistance in Sudanese isolates of *Plasmodium falciparum* is associated with mutations in the chloroquine resistance transporter gene pfcrt and the multidrug resistance gene pfmdr1. *Journal of Infectious Diseases* 183(10):1535-1538.

Baird JK, Sustriayu Nalim MF, Basri H, Masbar S, Leksana B, Tjitra E, Dewi RM, Khairani M, Wignall FS. 1996. Survey of resistance to chloroquine by *Plasmodium vivax* in Indonesia. *Transactions of the Royal Society of Tropical Medicine and Hygiene* 90(4):409-411.

Baird JK, Wiady I, Fryauff DJ, Sutanihardja MA, Leksana B, Widjaya H, Kysdarmanto, Subianto B. 1997. In vivo resistance to chloroquine by *Plasmodium vivax* and *Plasmodium falciparum* at Nabire, Irian Jaya, Indonesia. *American Journal of Tropical Medicine and Hygiene* 56(6):627-631.

Bakshi R, Hermeling-Fritz I, Gathmann I, Alteri E. 2000. An integrated assessment of the clinical safety of artemether-lumefantrine: A new oral fixed-dose combination antimalarial drug. *Transactions of the Royal Society of Tropical Medicine and Hygiene* 94(4):419-424.

Barnes K, Folb P. 2003. *Reducing Malaria's Burden: Evidence of Effectiveness for Decision Makers (Technical Report). The Role of Artemisinin-Based Combination Therapy in Malaria Management.* Washington, DC: Global Health Council.

Barnes KI, Mwenechanya J, Tembo M, McIlleron H, Folb PI, Ribeiro I, Little F, Gomes M, Molyneux ME. 2004. Efficacy of rectal artesunate compared with parenteral quinine in initial treatment of moderately severe malaria in African children and adults: A randomised study. *Lancet* 363(9421):1598-1605.

Basco LK, Ringwald P. 2001. Analysis of the key pfcrt point mutation and *in vitro* and *in vivo* response to chloroquine in Yaounde, Cameroon. *Journal of Infectious Diseases* 183(12):1828-1831.

Berman PA, Adams PA. 1997. Artemisinin enhances heme-catalysed oxidation of lipid membranes. *Free Radical Biology and Medicine* 22(7):1283-1288.

Bindschedler M, Lefevre G, Ezzet F, Schaeffer N, Meyer I, Thomsen MS. 2000. Cardiac effects of co-artemether (artemether/lumefantrine) and mefloquine given alone or in combination to healthy volunteers. *European Journal of Clinical Pharmacology* 56(5):375-381.

Bloland PB. 2001. *Drug Resistance in Malaria.* Geneva: World Health Organization.

Bray PG, Mungthin M, Ridley RG, Ward SA. 1998. Access to hematin: The basis of chloroquine resistance. *Molecular Pharmacology* 54(1):170-179.

Brewer TG, Grate SJ, Peggins JO, Weina PJ, Petras JM, Levine BS, Heiffer MH, Schuster BG. 1994. Fatal neurotoxicity of arteether and artemether. *American Journal of Tropical Medicine and Hygiene* 51(3):251-259.

Brockman A, Price RN, van Vugt M, Heppner DG, Walsh D, Sookto P, Wimonwattrawatee T, Looareesuwan S, White NJ, Nosten F. 2000. *Plasmodium falciparum* antimalarial drug susceptibility on the north-western border of Thailand during five years of extensive use of artesunate-mefloquine. *Transactions of the Royal Society of Tropical Medicine and Hygiene* 94(5):537-544.

Brossi A, Venugopalan B, Dominguez Gerpe L, Yeh HJ, Flippen-Anderson JL, Buchs P, Luo XD, Milhous W, Peters W. 1988. Arteether, a new antimalarial drug: Synthesis and antimalarial properties. *Journal of Medicinal Chemistry* 31(3):645-650.

Bruce-Chwatt, LJ. 1985. *Essential Malariology.* 2nd ed. New York: John Wiley and Sons.

Chaiyaroj SC, Buranakiti A, Angkasekwinai P, Looareesuwan S, Cowman AF. 1999. Analysis of mefloquine resistance and amplification of pfmdr1 in multidrug-resistant *Plasmodium falciparum* isolates from Thailand. *American Journal of Tropical Medicine and Hygiene* 61(5):780-783.

Chen N, Russell B, Staley J, Kotecka B, Nasveld P, Cheng Q. 2001. Sequence polymorphisms in pfcrt are strongly associated with chloroquine resistance in *Plasmodium falciparum*. *Journal of Infectious Diseases* 183(10):1543-1545.

Chotivanich K, Udomsangpetch R, Dondorp A, Williams T, Angus B, Simpson JA, Pukrittayakamee S, Looareesuwan S, Newbold CI, White NJ. 2000. The mechanisms of parasite clearance after antimalarial treatment of *Plasmodium falciparum* malaria. *Journal of Infectious Diseases* 182(2):629-633.

Chotivanich K, Udomsangpetch R, McGready R, Proux S, Newton P, Pukrittayakamee S, Looareesuwan S, White NJ. 2002. Central role of the spleen in malaria parasite clearance. *Journal of Infectious Diseases* 185(10):1538-1541.

Day NP, Pham TD, Phan TL, Dinh XS, Pham PL, Ly VC, Tran TH, Nguyen TH, Bethell DB, Nguyan HP, Tran TH, White NJ. 1996. Clearance kinetics of parasites and pigment-containing leukocytes in severe malaria. *Blood* 88(12):4694-4700.

Deen JL, von Seidlein L, Pinder M, Walraven GE, Greenwood BM. 2001. The safety of the combination artesunate and pyrimethamine-sulfadoxine given during pregnancy. *Transactions of the Royal Society of Tropical Medicine and Hygiene* 95(4):424-428.

Diourte Y, Djimde A, Doumbo OK, Sagara I, Coulibaly Y, Dicko A, Diallo M, Diakite M, Cortese JF, Plowe CV. 1999. Pyrimethamine-sulfadoxine efficacy and selection for mutations in *Plasmodium falciparum* dihydrofolate reductase and dihydropteroate synthase in Mali. *American Journal of Tropical Medicine and Hygiene* 60(3):475-478.

Djimde A, Doumbo OK, Cortese JF, Kayentao K, Doumbo S, Diourte Y, Dicko A, Su XZ, Nomura T, Fidock DA, Wellems TE, Plowe CV, Coulibaly D. 2001. A molecular marker for chloroquine-resistant falciparum malaria. *New England Journal of Medicine* 344(4): 257-263.

Dorsey G, Kamya MR, Ndeezi G, Babirye JN, Phares CR, Olson JE, Katabira ET, Rosenthal PJ. 2000. Predictors of chloroquine treatment failure in children and adults with falciparum malaria in Kampala, Uganda. *American Journal of Tropical Medicine and Hygiene* 62(6):686-692.

Dorsey G, Kamya MR, Singh A, Rosenthal PJ. 2001. Polymorphisms in the *Plasmodium falciparum* pfcrt and pfmdr-1 genes and clinical response to chloroquine in Kampala, Uganda. *Journal of Infectious Diseases* 183(9):1417-1420.

Dorsey G, Njama D, Kamya MR, Cattamanchi A, Kyabayinze D, Staedke SG, Gasasira A, Rosenthal PJ. 2002. Sulfadoxine/pyrimethamine alone or with amodiaquine or artesunate for treatment of uncomplicated malaria: a longitudinal randomised trial. *Lancet* 360(9350):2031-2038.

Durand R, Jafari S, Vauzelle J, Delabre JF, Jesic Z, Le Bras J. 2001. Analysis of pfcrt point mutations and chloroquine susceptibility in isolates of *Plasmodium falciparum*. *Molecular and Biochemical Parasitology* 114(1):95-102.

Dye C, Williams BG. 1997. Multigenic drug resistance among inbred malaria parasites. *Proceedings of the Royal Society of London—Series B: Biological Sciences* 264(1378):61-67.

Eckstein-Ludwig U, Webb RJ, Van Goethem ID, East JM, Lee AG, Kimura M, O'Neill PM, Bray PG, Ward SA, Krishna S. 2003. Artemisinins target the serca of *Plasmodium falciparum*. [See Comment]. *Nature* 424(6951):957-961.

Fidock DA, Nomura T, Talley AK, Cooper RA, Dzekunov SM, Ferdig MT, Ursos LM, Sidhu AB, Naude B, Deitsch KW, Su XZ, Wootton JC, Roepe PD, Wellems TE. 2000. Mutations in the *P. falciparum* digestive vacuole transmembrane protein pfcrt and evidence for their role in chloroquine resistance. *Molecular Cell* 6(4):861-871.

Flueck TP, Jelinek T, Kilian AH, Adagu IS, Kabagambe G, Sonnenburg F, Warhurst DC. 2000. Correlation of in vivo-resistance to chloroquine and allelic polymorphisms in *Plasmodium falciparum* isolates from Uganda. *Tropical Medicine and International Health* 5(3):174-178.

Fryauff DJ, Tuti S, Mardi A, Masbar S, Patipelohi R, Leksana B, Kain KC, Bangs MJ, Richie TL, Baird JK. 1998. Chloroquine-resistant *Plasmodium vivax* in transmigration settlements of west Kalimantan, Indonesia. *American Journal of Tropical Medicine and Hygiene* 59(4):513-518.

Garg M, Gopinathan N, Bodhe P, Kshirsagar NA. 1995. Vivax malaria resistant to chloroquine: Case reports from Bombay. *Transactions of the Royal Society of Tropical Medicine and Hygiene* 89(6):656-657.

Geary TG, Divo AA, Jensen JB. 1989. Stage specific actions of antimalarial drugs on *Plasmodium falciparum* in culture. *American Journal of Tropical Medicine and Hygiene* 40(3): 240-244.

Genovese RF, Newman DB, Petras JM, Brewer TG. 1998. Behavioral and neural toxicity of arteether in rats. *Pharmacology, Biochemistry and Behavior* 60(2):449-458.

Greenwood B. 2002. The molecular epidemiology of malaria. *Tropical Medicine and International Health* 7(12):1012-1021.

Hastings IM, Watkins WM, White NJ. 2002. The evolution of drug-resistant malaria: The role of drug elimination half-life. *Philosophical Transactions of the Royal Society of London—Series B: Biological Sciences* 357(1420):505-519.

Hien TT, Day NPJ, Phu NH, Mai NTH, Chau TTH, Loc PP, Sinh DX, Chuong LV, Vinh H, Waller D, Peto TEA, White NJ. 1996. A controlled trial of artemether or quinine in Vietnamese adults with severe falciparum malaria. *New England Journal of Medicine* 335(2):76-83.

Hien TT, Turner GD, Mai NT, Phu NH, Bethell D, Blakemore WF, Cavanagh JB, Dayan A, Medana I, Weller RO, Day NP, White NJ. 2003. Neuropathological assessment of artemether-treated severe malaria. *Lancet* 362(9380):295-296.

Imwong M, Pukrittakayamee S, Looareesuwan S, Pasvol G, Poirreiz J, White NJ, Snounou G. 2001. Association of genetic mutations in *Plasmodium vivax* dhfr with resistance to sulfadoxine-pyrimethamine: Geographical and clinical correlates. *Antimicrobial Agents and Chemotherapy* 45(11):3122-3127.

Inselburg J. 1985. Induction and isolation of artemisinin-resistant mutants of *Plasmodium falciparum*. *American Journal of Tropical Medicine and Hygiene* 34(3):417-418.

Jeffery GM, Eyles D. 1955. Infectivity to mosquitoes of *Plasmodium falciparum* as related to gametocyte density and duration of infection. *American Journal of Tropical Medicine and Hygiene* 4:781-789.

Karunajeewa HA, Kemiki A, Alpers MP, Lorry K, Batty KT, Ilett KF, Davis TM. 2003. Safety and therapeutic efficacy of artesunate suppositories for treatment of malaria in children in Papua New Guinea. *Pediatric Infectious Disease Journal* 22(3):251-256.

Kazadi WM, Vong S, Makina BN, Mantshumba JC, Kabuya W, Kebela BI, Ngimbi NP. 2003. Assessing the Efficacy of chloroquine and sulfadoxine-pyrimethamine for treatment of uncomplicated *Plasmodium falciparum* malaria in the Democratic Republic of Congo. *Tropical Medicine and International Health* 8(10):868-75.

Kissinger E, Hien TT, Hung NT, Nam ND, Tuyen NL, Dinh BV, Mann C, Phu NH, Loc PP, Simpson JA, White NJ, Farrar JJ. 2000. Clinical and neurophysiological study of the effects of multiple doses of artemisinin on brain-stem function in Vietnamese patients. *American Journal of Tropical Medicine and Hygiene* 63(1-2):48-55.

Klayman DL. 1985. Qinghaosu (artemisinin): An antimalarial drug from China. *Science* 228(4703):1049-1055.

Klayman DL, Lin AJ, Acton N, Scovill JP, Hoch JM, Milhous WK, Theoharides AD, Dobek AS. 1984. Isolation of artemisinin (qinghaosu) from *Artemisia annua* growing in the United States. *Journal of Natural Products* 47(4):715-717.

Korsinczky M, Chen N, Kotecka B, Saul A, Rieckmann K, Cheng Q. 2000. Mutations in *Plasmodium falciparum* cytochrome-b that are associated with atovaquone resistance are located at a putative drug-binding site. *Antimicrobial Agents and Chemotherapy* 44(8):2100-2108.

Krogstad DJ, Schlesinger PH. 1987. Acid-vesicle function, intracellular pathogens, and the action of chloroquine against *Plasmodium falciparum*. *New England Journal of Medicine* 317(9):542-549.

Kublin JG, Cortese JF, Njunju EM, Mukadam RA, Wirima JJ, Kazembe PN, Djimde AA, Kouriba B, Taylor TE, Plowe CV. 2003. Reemergence of chloroquine-sensitive *Plasmodium falciparum* malaria after cessation of chloroquine use in Malawi. *Journal of Infectious Diseases* 187(12):1870-1875.

Kumar N, Zheng H. 1990. Stage-specific gametocytocidal effect in vitro of the antimalaria drug qinghaosu on *Plasmodium falciparum*. *Parasitology Research* 76(3):214-218.

Le Bras J, Durand R. 2003. The mechanisms of resistance to antimalarial drugs in *Plasmodium falciparum*. *Fundamental and Clinical Pharmacology* 17(2):147-153.

Lefevre G, Looareesuwan S, Treeprasertsuk S, Krudsood S, Silachamroon U, Gathmann I, Mull R, Bakshi R. 2001. A clinical and pharmacokinetic trial of six doses of artemether-lumefantrine for multidrug-resistant *Plasmodium falciparum* malaria in Thailand. *American Journal of Tropical Medicine and Hygiene* 64(5):247-256.

Leonardi E, Gilvary G, White NJ, Nosten F. 2001. Severe allergic reactions to oral artesunate: A report of two cases. *Transactions of the Royal Society of Tropical Medicine and Hygiene* 95(2):182-183.

Li GQ, Guo XB, Yang F. 1990. *Clinical Trials on Qinghaosu and Its Derivatives.* China. Guangzhou Medicine Institute. Vol. 1.

Looareesuwan S, Wilairatana P, Chokejindachai W, Chalermrut K, Wernsdorfer W, Gemperli B, Gathmann I, Royce C. 1999. A randomized, double-blind, comparative trial of a new oral combination of artemether and benflumetol (Cgp 56697) with mefloquine in the treatment of acute *Plasmodium falciparum* malaria in Thailand. *American Journal of Tropical Medicine and Hygiene* 60(2):238-243.

Luo XD, Shen CC. 1987. The chemistry, pharmacology, and clinical applications of qinghaosu (artemisinin) and its derivatives. *Medicinal Research Reviews* 7(1):29-52.

Luxemburger C, Nosten F, Raimond SD, Chongsuphajaisiddhi T, White NJ. 1995. Oral artesunate in the treatment of uncomplicated hyperparasitemic falciparum malaria. *American Journal of Tropical Medicine and Hygiene* 53(5):522-525.

Luxemburger C, Brockman A, Silamut K, Nosten F, van Vugt M, Gimenez F, Chongsuphajaisiddhi T, White NJ. 1998. Two patients with falciparum malaria and poor in vivo responses to artesunate. *Transactions of the Royal Society of Tropical Medicine and Hygiene* 92(6):668-669.

Marlar-Than, Myat-Phone-Kyaw, Aye-Yu-Soe, Khaing-Khaing-Gyi, Ma-Sabai, Myint-Oo. 1995. Development of resistance to chloroquine by *Plasmodium vivax* in Myanmar. *Transactions of the Royal Society of Tropical Medicine and Hygiene* 89(3):307-308.

Martin SK, Oduola AM, Milhous WK. 1987. Reversal of chloroquine resistance in *Plasmodium falciparum* by verapamil. *Science* 235(4791):899-901.

Mayor AG, Gomez-Olive X, Aponte JJ, Casimiro S, Mabunda S, Dgedge M, Barreto A, Alonso PL. 2001. Prevalence of the k76t mutation in the putative *Plasmodium falciparum* chloroquine resistance transporter (pfcrt) gene and its relation to chloroquine resistance in Mozambique. *Journal of Infectious Diseases* 183(9):1413-1416.

McGready R, Cho T, Cho JJ, Simpson JA, Luxemburger C, Dubowitz L, Looareesuwan S, White NJ, Nosten F. 1998. Artemisinin derivatives in the treatment of falciparum malaria in pregnancy. *Transactions of the Royal Society of Tropical Medicine and Hygiene* 92(4):430-433.

McGready R, Brockman A, Cho T, Cho D, van Vugt M, Luxemburger C, Chongsuphajaisiddhi T, White NJ, Nosten F. 2000. Randomized comparison of mefloquine-artesunate versus quinine in the treatment of multidrug-resistant falciparum malaria in pregnancy. *Transactions of the Royal Society of Tropical Medicine and Hygiene* 94(6):689-693.

McGready R, Cho T, Keo NK, Thwai KL, Villegas L, Looareesuwan S, White NJ, Nosten F. 2001. Artemisinin antimalarials in pregnancy: A prospective treatment study of 539 episodes of multidrug-resistant *Plasmodium falciparum*. *Clinical Infectious Diseases* 33(12):2009-2016.

Mendis K, Sina BJ, Marchesini P, Carter R. 2001. The neglected burden of *Plasmodium vivax* malaria. *American Journal of Tropical Medicine and Hygiene* 64(1-2 Suppl):97-106.

Meshnick SR, Thomas A, Ranz A, Xu CM, Pan HZ. 1991. Artemisinin (Qinghaosu): The role of intracellular hemin in its mechanism of antimalarial action. *Molecular and Biochemical Parasitology* 49(2):181-189.

Miller LG, Panosian CB. 1997. Ataxia and slurred speech after artesunate treatment for falciparum malaria. *New England Journal of Medicine* 336(18):1328.

Myint HY, Tipmanee P, Nosten F, Day NPJ, Pukrittayakamee S, Looareesuwan S, White NJ. 2004. A systematic overview of published antimalarial drug trials. *Transactions of the Royal Society of Tropical Medicine and Hygiene* 98(2):73-81.

Nacher M. 2002. Malarial anaemia: A crossroad? *Medical Hypotheses* 59(3):363-365.

Newton PN, Angus BJ, Chierakul W, Dondorp A, Ruangveerayuth R, Silamut K, Teerapong P, Suputtamongkol Y, Looareesuwan S, White NJ. 2003. Randomized comparison of artesunate and quinine in the treatment of severe falciparum malaria. *Clinical Infectious Diseases* 37(1):7-16.

Nontprasert A, Nosten-Bertrand M, Pukrittayakamee S, Vanijanonta S, Angus BJ, White NJ. 1998. Assessment of the neurotoxicity of parenteral artemisinin derivatives in mice. *American Journal of Tropical Medicine and Hygiene* 59(4):519-522.

Nosten F, McGready R, Simpson JA, Thwai KL, Balkan S, Cho T, Hkirijaroen L, Looareesuwan S, White NJ. 1999. Effects of *Plasmodium vivax* malaria in pregnancy. *Lancet* 354(9178):546-549.

Nosten F, van Vugt M, Price R, Luxemburger C, Thway KL, Brockman A, McGready R, ter Kuile F, Looareesuwan S, White NJ. 2000. Effects of artesunate-mefloquine combination on incidence of *Plasmodium falciparum* malaria and mefloquine resistance in Western Thailand: A prospective study. *Lancet* 356(9226):297-302.

Nzila AM, Nduati E, Mberu EK, Hopkins Sibley C, Monks SA, Winstanley PA, Watkins WM. 2000. Molecular evidence of greater selective pressure for drug resistance exerted by the long-acting antifolate pyrimethamine/sulfadoxine compared with the shorter-acting chlorproguanil/dapsone on Kenyan *Plasmodium falciparum*. *Journal of Infectious Diseases* 181(6):2023-2028.

Oduola AM, Milhous WK, Salako LA, Walker O, Desjardins RE. 1987. Reduced in-vitro susceptibility to mefloquine in West African isolates of *Plasmodium falciparum*. *Lancet* 2(8571):1304-1305.

Oduola AMJ, Omitowoju GO, Gerena L, Kyle DE, Milhous WK, Sowunmi A, Salako LA. 1993. Reversal of mefloquine resistance with penfluridol in isolates of *Plasmodium falciparum* from South-west Nigeria. *Transactions of the Royal Society of Tropical Medicine and Hygiene* 87(1):81-83.

Omari AA, Preston C, Garner P. 2003. Artemether-lumefantrine for treating uncomplicated falciparum malaria. *Cochrane Database of Systematic Reviews* (2):CD003125.

Payne D. 1988. Did medicated salt hasten the spread of chloroquine resistance in Plasmodium falciparum? *Parasitology Today* 4(4):112-115.

Peters W. 1987. *Chemotherapy and Drug Resistance in Malaria.* 2nd ed. London: Academic Press.

Peters W, Robinson BL. 1999. The chemotherapy of rodent malaria. LVI: Studies on the development of resistance to natural and synthetic endoperoxides. *Annals of Tropical Medicine and Parasitology* 93(4):325-329.

Petras JM, Young GD, Bauman RA, Kyle DE, Gettayacamin M, Webster HK, Corcoran KD, Peggins JO, Vane MA, Brewer TG. 2000. Arteether-induced brain injury in *Macaca mulatta*. I. The precerebellar nuclei: The lateral reticular nuclei, paramedian reticular nuclei, and perihypoglossal nuclei. *Anatomy and Embryology* 201(5):383-397.

Phillips EJ, Keystone JS, Kain KC. 1996. Failure of combined chloroquine and high-dose primaquine therapy for *Plasmodium vivax* malaria acquired in Guyana, South America. *Clinical Infectious Diseases* 23(5):1171-1173.

Pillai DR, Labbe AC, Vanisaveth V, Hongvangthong B, Pomphida S, Inkathone S, Zhong K, Kain KC. 2001. *Plasmodium falciparum* malaria in Laos: Chloroquine treatment outcome and predictive value of molecular markers. *Journal of Infectious Diseases* 183(5):789-795.

Plowe CV, Cortese JF, Djimde A, Nwanyanwu OC, Watkins WM, Winstanley PA, Estrada-Franco JG, Mollinedo RE, Avila JC, Cespedes JL, Carter D, Doumbo OK. 1997. Mutations in *Plasmodium falciparum* dihydrofolate reductase and dihydropteroate synthase and epidemiologic patterns of pyrimethamine-sulfadoxine use and resistance. *Journal of Infectious Diseases* 176(6):1590-1596.

Plowe CV, Kublin JG, Dzinjalamala FK, Kamwendo DS, Mukadam RAG, Chimpeni P, Molyneux ME, Taylor TE. 2004. Sustained clinical efficacy of sulfadoxine-pyrimethamine for uncomplicated falciparum malaria in Malawi after 10 years as first line treatment: Five year prospective study. *British Medical Journal* 328(7439):545-548.

Povoa MM, Adagu IS, Oliveira SG, Machado RL, Miles MA, Warhurst DC. 1998. Pfmdr1 Asn1042asp and Asp1246tyr polymorphisms, thought to be associated with chloroquine resistance, are present in chloroquine-resistant and -sensitive Brazilian field isolates of *Plasmodium falciparum*. *Experimental Parasitology* 88(1):64-68.

Price RN, Nosten F, Luxemburger C, ter Kuile FO, Paiphun L, Chongsuphajaisiddhi T, White NJ. 1996. Effects of artemisinin derivatives on malaria transmissibility. *Lancet* 347(9016):1654-1658.

Price RN, Nosten F, Luxemburger C, van Vugt M, Phaipun L, Chongsuphajaisiddhi T, White NJ. 1997. Artesunate/mefloquine treatment of multi-drug resistant falciparum malaria. *Transactions of the Royal Society of Tropical Medicine and Hygiene* 91(5):574-577.

Price R, van Vugt M, Phaipun L, Luxemburger C, Simpson J, McGready R, ter Kuile F, Kham A, Chongsuphajaisiddhi T, White NJ, Nosten F. 1999a. Adverse effects in patients with acute falciparum malaria treated with artemisinin derivatives. *American Journal of Tropical Medicine and Hygiene* 60(4):547-555.

Price RN, Cassar C, Brockman A, Duraisingh M, van Vugt M, White NJ, Nosten F, Krishna S. 1999b. The pfmdr1 gene is associated with a multidrug-resistant phenotype in *Plasmodium falciparum* from the western border of Thailand. *Antimicrobial Agents and Chemotherapy* 43(12):2943-2949.

Price RN, Simpson JA, Nosten F, Luxemburger C, Hkirjaroen L, ter Kuile F, Chongsuphajaisiddhi T, White NJ. 2001. Factors contributing to anemia after uncomplicated falciparum malaria. *American Journal of Tropical Medicine and Hygiene* 65(5):614-622.

Pukrittayakamee S, Chantra A, Simpson JA, Vanijanonta S, Clemens R, Looareesuwan S, White NJ. 2000. Therapeutic responses to different antimalarial drugs in vivax malaria. *Antimicrobial Agents and Chemotherapy* 44(6):1680-1685.

Rieckmann KH, Campbell GH, Sax LJ, Mrema JE. 1978. Drug sensitivity of *Plasmodium falciparum*: An in-vitro microtechnique. *Lancet* 1(8054):22-23.

Rieckmann KH, Davis DR, Hutton DC. 1989. *Plasmodium vivax* resistance to chloroquine? *Lancet* 2(8673):1183-1184.

Sabchareon A, Attanath P, Chanthavanich P, Phanuaksook P, Prarinyanupharb V, Poonpanich Y, Mookmanee D, Teja-Isavadharm P, Heppner DG, Brewer TG, Chongsuphajaisiddhi T. 1998. Comparative clinical trial of artesunate suppositories and oral artesunate in combination with mefloquine in the treatment of children with acute falciparum malaria. *American Journal of Tropical Medicine and Hygiene* 58(1):11-16.

Scott MD, Meshnick SR, Williams RA, Chiu DT, Pan HC, Lubin BH, Kuypers FA. 1989. Qinghaosu-mediated oxidation in normal and abnormal erythrocytes. *Journal of Laboratory and Clinical Medicine* 114(4):401-406.

Sibley CH, Hyde JE, Sims PF, Plowe CV, Kublin JG, Mberu EK, Cowman AF, Winstanley PA, Watkins WM, Nzila AM. 2001. Pyrimethamine-sulfadoxine resistance in *Plasmodium falciparum*: What next? *Trends in Parasitology* 17(12):582-588.

Simon F, Le Bras J, Gaudebout C, Girard PM. 1988. Reduced sensitivity of *Plasmodium falciparum* to mefloquine in West Africa. *Lancet* 1(8583):467-468.

Sowunmi A, Oduola AM, Ogundahunsi OA, Falade CO, Gbotosho GO, Salako LA. 1997. Enhanced efficacy of chloroquine-chlorpheniramine combination in acute uncomplicated falciparum malaria in children. *Transactions of the Royal Society of Tropical Medicine and Hygiene* 91(1):63-67.

Srivastava IK, Rottenberg H, Vaidya AB. 1997. Atovaquone, a broad spectrum antiparasitic drug, collapses mitochondrial membrane potential in a malarial parasite. *Journal of Biological Chemistry* 272(7):3961-3966.

Steketee RW, Wirima JJ, Slutsker L, Khoromana CO, Breman JG, Heymann DL. 1996. Objectives and methodology in a study of malaria treatment and prevention in pregnancy in rural Malawi: The Mangochi Malaria Research Project. *American Journal of Tropical Medicine and Hygiene* 55(1 Suppl):8-16.

Stepniewska K, Taylor WRJ, Mayxay M, Smithuis F, Guthmann J-P, Barnes K, Myint H, Price R, Olliaro P, Pukrittayakamee S, Hien TT, Farrar J, Nosten F, Day NPJ, White NJ. In press. The *in vivo* assessment of antimalarial drug efficacy in falciparum malaria; the duration of follow-up. *Antimicrobial Agents and Chemotherapy*

Sutherland CJ, Alloueche A, Curtis J, Drakeley CJ, Ord R, Durasingh M, Greenwood BM, Pinder M, Warhurst D, Targett GAI. 2002. Gambian children successfully treated with chloroquine can harbor and transmit *Plasmodium falciparum* gametocytes carrying resistance genes. *American Journal of Tropical Medicine and Hygiene* 67:578-585.

Talisuna AO, Kyosiimire-Lugemwa J, Langi P, Mutabingwa TK, Watkins W, Van Marck E, Egwang T, D'Alessandro U. 2002a. Role of the pfcrt codon 76 mutation as a molecular marker for population-based surveillance of chloroquine (Cq)-resistant *Plasmodium falciparum* malaria in Ugandan sentinel sites with high Cq resistance. *Transactions of the Royal Society of Tropical Medicine and Hygiene* 96(5):551-556.

Talisuna AO, Langi P, Bakyaita N, Egwang T, Mutabingwa TK, Watkins W, Van Marck E, D'Alessandro U. 2002b. Intensity of malaria transmission, antimalarial-drug use and resistance in Uganda: What is the relationship between these three factors? *Transactions of the Royal Society of Tropical Medicine and Hygiene* 96(3):310-317.

Talisuna AO, Bloland P, D'Alessandro U. 2004. History, dynamics, and public health importance of malaria parasite resistance. *Clinical Microbiology Reviews* 17:235-254.

Targett G, Drakeley C, Jawara M, von Seidlein L, Coleman R, Deen J, Pinder M, Doherty T, Sutherland C, Walraven G, Milligan P. 2001. Artesunate reduces but does not prevent posttreatment transmission of *Plasmodium falciparum* to *Anopheles gambiae*. *Journal of Infectious Diseases* 183(8):1254-1259.

Taylor WRJ, White NJ. 2004. Antimalarial drug toxicity: A review. *Drug Safety* 27(1):25-61.

ter Kuile FO, Luxemburger C, Nosten F, Thai KL, Chongsuphajaisiddhi T, White NJ. 1995. Predictors of mefloquine treatment failure: A prospective study of 1590 patients with uncomplicated falciparum malaria. *Transactions of the Royal Society of Tropical Medicine and Hygiene* 89(6):660-664.

ter Kuile F, White NJ, Holloway P, Pasvol G, Krishna S. 1993. *Plasmodium falciparum*: In vitro studies of the pharmacodynamic properties of drugs used for the treatment of severe malaria. *Experimental Parasitology* 76(1):85-95.

Toovey S, Jamieson A. 2004. Audiometric changes associated with the treatment of uncomplicated falciparum malaria with co-artemether. *Transactions of the Royal Society of Tropical Medicine and Hygiene* 98(5):261-267 [discussion 268-269].

Tran TH, Day NP, Nguyen HP, Nguyen TH, Tran TH, Pham PL, Dinh XS, Ly VC, Ha V, Waller D, Peto TE, White NJ. 1996. A controlled trial of artemether or quinine in Vietnamese adults with severe falciparum malaria. *New England Journal of Medicine* 335(2):76-83.

Van Vugt M, Brockman A, Gemperli B, Luxemburger C, Gathmann I, Royce C, Slight T, Looareesuwan S, White NJ, Nosten F. 1998. Randomized comparison of artemether-benflumetol and artesunate-mefloquine in treatment of multidrug-resistant falciparum malaria. *Antimicrobial Agents and Chemotherapy* 42(1):135-139.

Van Vugt M, Ezzet F, Nosten F, Gathmann I, Wilairatana P, Looareesuwan S, White NJ. 1999. No evidence of cardiotoxicity during antimalarial treatment with artemether-lumefantrine. *American Journal of Tropical Medicine and Hygiene* 61(6):964-967.

Van Vugt M, Angus BJ, Price RN, Mann C, Simpson JA, Poletto C, Htoo SE, Looareesuwan S, White NJ, Nosten F. 2000. A case-control auditory evaluation of patients treated with artemisinin derivatives for multidrug-resistant *Plasmodium falciparum* malaria. *American Journal of Tropical Medicine and Hygiene* 62(1):65-69.

Vieira PP, das Gracas Alecrim M, da Silva LH, Gonzalez-Jimenez I, Zalis MG. 2001. Analysis of the pfcrt K76t mutation in *Plasmodium falciparum* isolates from the Amazon region of Brazil. *Journal of Infectious Diseases* 183(12):1832-1833.

von Seidlein L, Duraisingh MT, Drakeley CJ, Bailey R, Greenwood BM, Pinder M. 1997. Polymorphism of the pfmdr1 gene and chloroquine resistance in *Plasmodium falciparum* in the Gambia. *Transactions of the Royal Society of Tropical Medicine and Hygiene* 91(4):450-453.

von Seidlein L, Milligan P, Pinder M, Bojang K, Anyalebechi C, Gosling R, Coleman R, Ude JI, Sadiq A, Duraisingh M, Warhurst D, Alloueche A, Targett G, McAdam K, Greenwood B, Walraven G, Olliaro P, Doherty T. 2000. Efficacy of artesunate plus pyrimethamine-sulphadoxine for uncomplicated malaria in Gambian children: A double-blind, randomised, controlled trial. *Lancet* 355(9201):352-357.

Wang P, Brooks DR, Sims PF, Hyde JE. 1995. A mutation-specific PCR system to detect sequence variation in the dihydropteroate synthetase gene of *Plasmodium falciparum*. *Molecular and Biochemical Parasitology* 71(1):115-125.

Wang P, Lee CS, Bayoumi R, Djimde A, Doumbo O, Swedberg G, Dao LD, Mshinda H, Tanner M, Watkins WM, Sims PF, Hyde JE. 1997. Resistance to antifolates in *Plasmodium falciparum* monitored by sequence analysis of dihydropteroate synthetase and dihydrofolate reductase alleles in a large number of field samples of diverse origins. *Molecular and Biochemical Parasitology* 89(2):161-177.

Warhurst DC. 2001. A molecular marker for chloroquine-resistant falciparum malaria. *New England Journal of Medicine* 344(4):299-302.

Watkins WM, Mosobo M. 1993. Treatment of plasmodium falciparum malaria with pyrimethamine-sulfadoxine: Selective pressure for resistance is a function of long elimination half-life. *Transactions of the Royal Society of Tropical Medicine and Hygiene* 87(1):75-78.

Wei N, Sadrzadeh SM. 1994. Enhancement of hemin-induced membrane damage by artemisinin. *Biochemical Pharmacology* 48(4):737-741.

Wellems TE, Walker-Jonah A, Panton LJ. 1991. Genetic mapping of the chloroquine-resistance locus on *Plasmodium falciparum* chromosome 7. *Proceedings of the National Academy of Sciences of the United States of America* 88(8):3382-3386.

Wernsdorfer WH, Noedl H. 2003. Molecular markers for drug resistance in malaria: Use in treatment, diagnosis and epidemiology. *Current Opinion in Infectious Diseases* 16(6):553-558.

White NJ. 1997. Assessment of the pharmacodynamic properties of antimalarial drugs in vivo. *Antimicrobial Agents and Chemotherapy* 41(7):1413-1422.

White NJ. 1998. Why is it that antimalarial drug treatments do not always work? *Annals of Tropical Medicine and Parasitology* 92(4):449-458.

White NJ. 1999. Delaying antimalarial drug resistance with combination chemotherapy. *Parassitologia* 41(1-3):301-308.

White NJ, Olliaro P. 1998. Artemisinin and derivatives in the treatment of uncomplicated malaria. *Medecine Tropicale* 58(3 Suppl):54-56.

White NJ, Pongtavornpinyo W. 2003. The de novo selection of drug-resistant malaria parasites. *Proceedings of the Royal Society of London—Series B: Biological Sciences* 270(1514):545-554.

WHO. 1996. *Assessment of Therapeutic Efficacy of Antimalarial Drugs for Uncomplicated Falciparum Malaria in Areas With Intense Transmission.* Geneva: World Health Organization.

WHO. 2000. Severe falciparum malaria. *Transactions of the Royal Society of Tropical Medicine and Hygiene* 94(Suppl 1):S1-S90.

WHO. 2001. Presentation at the meeting of the Antimalarial Drug Combination Therapy: Report of a WHO Technical Consultation. Geneva: World Health Organization.

WHO. 2003. *Assessment and Monitoring of Antimalarial Drug Efficacy for the Treatment of Uncomplicated Falciparum Malaria.* Geneva: World Health Organization. WHO/HTM/ RBM/2003.50.

WHO/RBM/UNDP/World Bank. 2003. *Assessment of the Safety of Artemisinin Compounds in Pregnancy.* Report of the two informal consultations convened by WHO in 2002. Geneva: World Health Organization.

Wongsrichanalai C, Wimonwattrawatee T, Sookto P, Laoboonchai A, Heppner DG, Kyle DE, Wernsdorfer WH. 1999. In vitro sensitivity of *Plasmodium falciparum* to artesunate in Thailand. *Bulletin of the World Health Organization* 77(5):392-398.

Wongsrichanalai C, Pickard AL, Wernsdorfer WH, Meshnick SR. 2002. Epidemiology of drug-resistant malaria. *The Lancet Infectious Diseases* 2(4):209-218.

Yayon A, Vande Waa JA, Yayon M, Geary TG, Jensen JB. 1983. Stage-dependent effects of chloroquine on *Plasmodium falciparum* in vitro. *Journal of Protozoology* 30(4):642-647.

York W, Macfie JWS. 1924. Observations on malaria made during treatment of general paralysis. *Transactions of the Royal Society of Tropical Medicine and Hygiene* 18(1&2):12-44.

Zalis MG, Pang L, Silveira MS, Milhous WK, Wirth DF. 1998. Characterization of *Plasmodium falciparum* isolated from the Amazon region of Brazil: Evidence for quinine resistance. *American Journal of Tropical Medicine and Hygiene* 58(5):630-637.

APPENDIX 9-A
Descriptions of Specific Antimalarial Drugs[1]

QUININE, first isolated from cinchona bark in 1820, remains a fundamental tool for treating malaria, especially severe disease. Quinine acts rapidly, targeting the bloodborne asexual stages of all malaria species. It is available in oral and injectable preparations and can be used in infants and pregnant women. Side effects—nausea, mood change, blurred vision, and ringing in the ears—are common but typically resolve after treatment ends.

Since *P. falciparum* parasites from most areas of the world respond well to quinine, short courses of the drug are often sufficient when paired with a second drug. In Southeast Asia, however, full course quinine treatment is necessary, usually given in combination with a second drug such as tetracycline.

CHLOROQUINE is a 4-aminoquinoline derivative of quinine first synthesized in 1934. It is safe in infants and pregnant women, and was the historical drug of choice for treatment of nonsevere or uncomplicated malaria and to prevent malaria in travelers. Chloroquine acts primarily against bloodborne asexual stages, although it also works against the bloodstream stage infective to mosquitoes. Because of widespread resistance to this drug, its usefulness is increasingly limited. Side effects are uncommon and generally mild.

AMODIAQUINE, which is closely related to chloroquine, fell out of favor because it caused adverse effects on bone marrow and liver when used for prophylaxis. Amodiaquine is currently being reevaluated as a co-formulation partner with artesunate. Concerns over toxicity remain.

ANTIFOL COMBINATION DRUGS include various combinations of dihydrofolate reductase inhibitors (proguanil, chlorproguanil, pyrimethamine, and trimethoprim) and sulfa drugs (dapsone, sulfalene, sulfamethoxazole, sulfadoxine, and others). The partner drugs in antifol combinations have similar mechanisms of action; consequently, they do not protect each other from resistance to the same degree as unrelated drugs. Current combinations include sulfadoxine-pyrimethamine (SP; Fansidar), sulfalene/pyrimethamine (Metakelfin), and sulfamethoxazole/trimethoprim (cotrimoxazole). Proguanil has also been used in combination with chloroquine for prophylaxis in areas of moderate chloroquine resistance, although it confers only minimal added benefit, especially with prolonged exposure

---

[1]Adapted from Bloland and Williams (2003).

(Steffen et al., 1993). When used for prophylaxis, Fansidar can produce severe allergic reactions: in American travelers, Fansidar was linked to severe skin reactions (1 per 5,000 to 8,000 users) and mortality (1 per 11,000 to 25,000 users) (Miller et al., 1986). These adverse outcomes are not as frequent when a single dose of Fansidar is used for treatment. Concerns about sulfa drug use during pregnancy are outweighed by the known risks to mother and fetus of untreated malaria.

The latest antifol combination is chlorproguanil and dapsone, also known as Lapdap. This particular combination is inherently more effective than Fansidar (even in areas where resistance is present) and has a far shorter elimination time, which may decrease the likelihood of resistance (Watkins et al., 1997; Mutabingwa et al., 2001). On the other hand, its shorter half-life requires that Lapdap be given over 3 days rather than as SP's one single dose.

TETRACYCLINE and derivatives such as doxycycline may be paired with other drugs for treatment or used as single agents for prophylaxis. In areas where quinine efficacy is diminished, tetracyclines are often added to quinine to improve cure rates. Tetracyclines are also used with shortened courses of quinine to decrease quinine-associated side effects. Tetracyclines are contraindicated in pregnant or breastfeeding women, or in children under age 8. Common side effects include nausea, vomiting, diarrhea, secondary yeast infections, and photosensitivity.

PRIMAQUINE, an 8-aminoquinoline, acts against malaria parasites in the liver, thereby reducing the likelihood of *P. vivax* or *P. ovale* relapse. Primaquine is also reasonably efficacious (74% efficacy against *P. falciparum*; 90 percent efficacy against *P. vivax*) when used for prophylaxis (Baird et al., 1995). Although it also has activity against blood-stage asexual parasites, drug concentrations that kill fully mature blood parasites are toxic. Primaquine is also a potent gametocidal drug, i.e., it kills the sexual stage of the malaria parasite infective to mosquitoes.

Primaquine can produce severe and potentially fatal hemolytic anemia in people with glucose-6-phosphate dehydrogenase (G6PD) enzyme deficiencies. The most severe Mediterranean B variant and related Asian variants of G6PD deficiency occur at high rates among several groups and regions: Kurdish Jews (62 percent), Saudia Arabia (13 percent), Burma (20 percent), and southern China (6 percent) and have now spread through migration and intermarriage. Primaquine should not be used in pregnancy.

TAFENOQUINE, a synthetic analog of primaquine, is currently being tested. It is highly effective against both liver and blood stages of malaria. Because of its long half-life (14 days versus 6 hours for primaquine), tafenoquine may prove to be a valuable chemoprophylactic drug (Lell et al., 2000). As with primaquine, tafenoquine can produce acute hemolytic anemia in patients with G6PD deficiency.

MEFLOQUINE is a quinoline-methanol derivative of quinine that can be used for treatment or prevention in most areas with multidrug resistant malaria. Resistance to mefloquine occurs frequently in parts of Southeast Asia, however, and sporadic resistance has been reported in areas of Africa and South America. Mefloquine causes a relatively high incidence of neuropsychiatric side effects when used at treatment doses and to a lesser degree when used for prophylaxis. In one large study in Asia, mefloquine was associated with stillbirth when given in pregnancy (Nosten et al., 1999).

HALOFANTRINE is a phenanthrene-methanol compound with activity against the bloodborne stages of the malaria parasite. It is especially useful in areas where multidrug-resistant falciparum malaria is present. Cardiac conduction abnormalities (specifically, prolongation of the PR and QT intervals on a standard electrocardiogram) are halofantrine's major drawback (Nosten et al., 1993). Taking halofantrine immediately following mefloquine or quinine therapy also increases the risk of cardiac complications. Halofantrine and mefloquine may exhibit clinical cross-resistance (Wongsrichanalai et al., 1992; ter Kuile et al., 1993).

CLINDAMYCIN is an antibiotic with weak antimalarial activity. It should only be used in combination with a fast-acting schizonticide, such as quinine, especially when treating patients with little or no immunity to malaria (Pukrittayakamee et al., 2000b; Parola et al., 2001). Clindamycin is considered safe for use in pregnant women and very young children (Pukrittayakamee et al., 2000a).

ARTEMISININ COMPOUNDS include the compounds artesunate, artemether, arteether, and dihydroartemisinin derived from the sesquiterpene lactone principle (artemisinin) of the plant *Artemisia annua*. In severe malaria, artemisinin compounds produce faster parasite clearance and resolution of fever than quinine. Artemisinins also reverse coma more quickly than quinine (Taylor et al., 1993; Salako et al., 1994). However, used alone for periods under 5 to 7 days, recrudescence rates are high. For nonsevere malaria, artemisinins are most successful when used in combination with a second drug (Nosten et al., 1994). The best documented combination is mefloquine plus 3 days of artesunate.

The safety of artemisinins in early pregnancy is of particular concern since the drugs have produced fetal resorption in experimental animals. Despite reassuring clinical data on over 600 carefully followed pregnancies treated with artemisinins in the second and third trimesters of pregnancy, there are unresolved concerns about their effects in early human gestation.

A fixed-dose preparation of lumefantrine and artemether is commercially sold under the trade name of Coartem or Riamet. Lumefantrine (previously known as benflumetol) is an aryl-amino alcohol antimalarial compound. Although chemically related, lumefantrine does not appear to have the same cardiac effects as halofantrine (van Vugt et al., 1999).

Coartem is marketed in two packages: a six-dose (24-tablet) package intended for nonimmune patients and a four-dose (16-tablet) package for use by semi-immune patients. Until studies show conclusive efficacy of the four-dose regimen in semi-immune populations, all patients should receive the six-dose regimen (van Vugt et al., 2000). Until further safety data become available, lumefantrine is not recommended for treatment of pregnant women.

ATOVAQUONE PLUS PROGUANIL (MALARONE) is a fixed-dose combination containing 250 mg of atovaquone (a hydroxynaphthoquinone) and 100 mg of proguanil in a single adult-sized pill taken daily for prophylaxis. An adult treatment course of Malarone is 1,000 mg of atovaquone and 400 mg of proguanil daily for 3 days. Malarone has also been combined with artesunate for treatment of uncomplicated multidrug-resistant falciparum malaria (van Vugt et al., 2002). Malarone is also thought to be effective against bloodborne forms of *P. vivax* (Looareesuwan et al., 1996a).

PYRONARIDINE has been used in China for over 20 years. While it was reportedly 100 percent effective in a single trial in Cameroon, the drug was only 63 to 88 percent effective in Thailand (Ringwald et al., 1996; Looareesuwan et al., 1996b). Further testing is required before pyronaridine can be recommended for widespread use.

PIPERAQUINE is an orally active bisquinoline discovered in the early 1960s and developed for clinical use in China in 1973. In vitro testing in several laboratories has shown that piperaquine approximates chloroquine's effects against sensitive parasites and is significantly more effective than chloroquine in treating resistant *P. falciparum*. In China, Vietnam and Cambodia, piperaquine is now available as a fixed combination with dihydroartemisinin (it has also been combined with trimethoprim and primaquine). Prospective clinical trial data are pending.

Appendix 9-A References

Baird JK, Fryauff DJ, Basri H, Bangs MJ, Subianto B, Wiady I, Purnomo, Leksana B, Masbar S, Richie TL, Jones TR, Tjitra E, Wignall FS, Hoffman SL. 1995. Primaquine for prophylaxis against malaria among nonimmune transmigrants in Irian Jaya, Indonesia. *American Journal of Tropical Medicine and Hygiene* 52(6):479-484.

Bloland PB, Williams H. 2002. *Malaria Control During Mass Population Movements and Disasters*. Committee on Population. National Research Council of the National Academies, Roundtable on the Demography of Forced Migration. Washington, DC: The National Academies Press.

Bloland PB, Ettling M, Meek S. 2000. Combination therapy for malaria in Africa: Hype or hope? *Bulletin of the World Health Organization* 78:1378-1388.

Doherty JF, Sadiq AD, Bayo L, Alloueche A, Olliaro P, Milligan P, von Seidlin L, Pinder M. 1999. A randomized safety and efficacy trial of artesunate plus sulfadoxine-pyrimethamine vs. sulfadoxine-pyrimethamine alone for the treatment of uncomplicated malaria in Gambian children. *Transactions of the Royal Society of Tropical Medicine and Hygiene* 93(5):543-546.

Greenberg AE, Ntumbanzondo M, Ntula N, Mawa L, Howell J, Davachi F. 1989. Hospital-based surveillance of malaria-related paediatric morbidity and mortality in Kinshasa, Zaire. *Bulletin of the World Health Organization* 67:189-196.

Greenwood BM. 1987. Asymptomatic malaria infections. Do they matter? *Parasitology Today* 3:206-214.

Kachur SP, Abdulla S, Barnes K, Mshinda H, Durrheim D, Kitua A, Bloland P. 2001. Letter to the editors. *Tropical Medicine and International Health* 6:324-325.

Kazadi WM, Vong S, Makina BN, Mantshumba JC, Kabuya W, Kebela BI, Ngimbi NP. 2003. Assessing the Efficacy of chloroquine and sulfadoxine-pyrimethamine for treatment of uncomplicated *Plasmodium falciparum* malaria in the Democratic Republic of Congo. *Tropical Medicine and International Health* 8(10):868-75.

Lell G, Faucher J-F, Missinou MN, Bormann S, Dangelmaier O, Horton J, Kremsner PG. 2000. Malaria chemoprophylaxis with tafenoquine: A randomized study. *Lancet* 255:2041-2045.

Looareesuwan S, Viravan C, Webster HK, Kyle DE, Hutchinson DB, Canfield CJ. 1996a. Clinical studies of atovaquone, alone or in combination with other antimalarial drugs for the treatment of acute uncomplicated malaria in Thailand. *American Journal of Tropical Medicine and Hygiene* 54(1):62-66.

Looareesuwan S, Olliaro P, Kyle D, Werndorfer W. 1996b. Pyronaridine. *Lancet* 347:1189-1190.

Miller KD, Lobl HO, Satrial RF, Kuritsky JN, Stern R, Campbell CC. 1986. Severe cutaneous reactions among American travelers using pyrimethamine-sulfadoxine (fansidar) for malaria prophylaxis. *American Journal of Tropical Medicine and Hygiene* 35:451-458.

Molyneux ME, Taylor TE, Wirima JJ, Borgstein J. 1989. Clinical features and prognostic indicators in paediatric cerebral malaria: A study of 131 comatose Malawian children. *Quarterly Journal of Medicine* 71:441-459.

Mutabingwa T, Nzila A, Mberu E, Nduati E, Winstanley P, Hills E, Watkins W. 2001. Chlorproguanil-dapsone for treatment of drug-resistant malaria in Tanzania. *Lancet* 358:1218-1223.

Nosten F, ter Kuile FO, Luxemburger D, Woodrow C, Kyle DE, Chongsuphajaisiddhi T, White NJ. 1993. Cardiac effects of antimalarial treatment with haolfantrine. *Lancet* 341 (8852):1054-1056.

Nosten F, Luxemburger C, ter Kuile FO, Woodrow C, Eh JP, White NJ. 1994. Treatment of multidrug-resistant *Plasmodium falciparum* malaria with 3-day artesunate-mefloquine combination. *Journal of Infectious Diseases* 170:971-977.

Nosten F, Vincenti M, Simpson J, Yei P, Kyaw Lay Thwai, De Vries A, Chongsuphajaisiddhi T, White NJ. 1999. The effects of mefloquine treatment in pregnancy. *Clinical Infectious Diseases* 28(4):808-815.

Nosten F, van Vugt M, Price R, Luxemburger C, Thway KI, Brockman A, McGready R, ter Kuile F, Loosareesuwan S, White NJ. 2000. Effects of artesunate-mefloquine combination on incidence of *Plasmodium falciparum* malaria in western Thailand: A prospective study. *Lancet* 356(9226):297-302.

Parola P, Ranque S, Badiaga S, Niang M, Blin O, Charbit JJ, Delmont J, Brousqui P. 2001. Controlled trial of 3-day quinine-clindamycin treatment versus 7-day quinine treatment for adult travelers with uncomplicated falciparum malaria imported from the tropics. *Antimicrobial Agents and Chemotherapy* 45:932-935.

Price RN, Nosten F, Luxemburger C, van Vugt M, Phaipun I, Chongasuphajaisiddi T, White NJ. 1997. Artesunate/mefloquine treatment of multi-drug resistant falciparum malaria. *Transactions of the Royal Society of Tropical Medicine and Hygiene* 91:574-577.

Pukrittyakamee S, Chantra A, Simpson JA, Vanijanonta S, Clemens R, Loosareesuwan S, White NJ. 2000a. Therapeutic responses to different antimalarial drugs in vivax malaria. *Antimicrobial Agents and Chemotherapy* 44:1680-1685.

Pukrittayakamee S, Chantra A, Vanijanonta S, Clemens R, Loosareesuwan S, White NJ. 2000b. Therapeutic responses to quinine and clindamycin in multidrug-resistant falciparum malaria. *Antimicrobial Agents and Chemotherapy* 44:2395-2398.

Radloff PD, Phillipps J, Nkeyi M, Hutchinson D, Kremsner PG. 1996. Atovaquone and proguanil for *Plasmodium falciparum* malaria. *Lancet* 347:1511-1513.

Ringwald P, Bickii J, Basco L. 1996. Randomised trial of pyronaridine versus chloroquine for acute uncomplicated falciparum malaria in Africa. *Lancet* 347:24-27.

Salako LA, Walker O, Sowunmi A, Omokhodion SJ, Adio R, Oduola AM. 1994. Artemether in moderately severe and cerebral malaria in Nigerian children. *Transactions of the Royal Society of Tropical Medicine and Hygiene* 88(Suppl 1):S13-S15.

Steffen R, Fuchs E, Schildknecht J, Naef U, Funk M, Schlagenhauf P, Phillips-Howard P, Nevill C, Stürchler D. 1993. Mefloquine compared with other malaria chemoprophylactic regimens in tourists visiting East Africa. *Lancet* 341:1299-1303.

Talisuna AO, Bloland P, D'Alessandro U. 2004. History, dynamics, and public health importance of malaria parasite resistance. *Clinical Microbiology Reviews* 17:235-254.

Taylor TE, Wills BA, Kazembe P, Chisale M, Wirima JJ, Ratsma EY, Molyneux ME. 1993. Rapid coma resolution with artemether in Malawian children with cerebral malaria. *Lancet* 341(8846):661-662.

Ter Kuile FO, Dolan G, Nosten F, Edstein MD, Luxemburger C, Phaipun L, Chongsuphajaisiddhi T, Webster HK, White NJ. 1993. Halofantrine versus mefloquine in treatment of multidrug-resistant falciparum malaria. *Lancet* 341(8852):1044-1049.

Van Hensbroek MB, Morris-Jones S, Meisner S, Jaffar S, Bayo L, Dackour R, Phillips C, Greenwood BM. 1995. Iron, but not folic acid, combined with effective antimalarial therapy promotes haematological recovery in African children after acute falciparum malaria. *Transactions of the Royal Society of Tropical Medicine and Hygiene* 89(6):672-676.

van Vugt M, Ezzet F, Nosten F, Gathmann I, Wilairatana P, Looareesuwan S, White NJ. 1999. No evidence of cardiotoxicity during antimalarial treatment with artemether-lumefantrine. *American Journal of Tropical Medicine and Hygiene* 61(6):964-967.

van Vugt M, Angus BJ, Price RN, Mann C, Simpson JA, Poletto C, Htoo SE, Looareesuwan S, White NJ, Nosten F. 2000. A case-control auditory evaluation of patients treated with artemisinin derivatives for multidrug-resistant *Plasmodium falciparum* malaria. *American Journal of Tropical Medicine and Hygiene* 62(1):65-69.

van Vugt M, Leonardi E, Phaipun L, Slight T, Thway KL, McGready R, Brockman A, Villegas L, Looareesuwan S, White NJ, Nosten F. 2002. Treatment of uncomplicated multidrug-resistant falciparum malaria with artesunate-atovaquone-proguanil. *Clinical Infectious Diseases* 35:1498-1504.

Von Seidlen L, Milligan P, Pinder M, Bojang K, Anyalebeschi C, Gosling R, Coleman R, Ude JL, Sadiq A, Duraisingh M, Warhurst D, Alloueche A, Targett G, McAdam K, Greenwood B, Walraven G, Olliaro P, Doherty T. 2000. Efficacy of artesunate plus pyrimethamine-sulphadoxine for uncomplicated malaria in Gambian children: A double-blind, randomized controlled trial. *Lancet* 355(9220):352-357.

Watkins WM, Mberu EK, Winstanley PA, Plowe CV. 1997. The efficacy of antifolate antimalarial combinations in Africa: A predictive model based on pharmacodynamic and pharmacokinetic analyses. *Parasitology Today* 13:459-464.

White N. 1999. Antimalarial drug resistance and mortality in falciparum malaria. *Tropical Medicine and International Health* 4:469-470.

WHO. 2003. Assessment and monitoring of antimalarial drug efficacy for the treatment of uncomplicated falciparum malaria Geneva: World Health Organization. WHO/HTM/RBM/2003.50.

Wongsrichanalai C, Webster HK, Wimonwattrawatee T, Sookto P, Chuanak N, Thimasarn K, Wernsdorfer WH. 1992. Emergence of multidrug-resistant *Plasmodium falciparum* in Thailand: In vitro tracking. *American Journal of Tropical Medicine and Hygiene* 47(1):112-116.

PART 3

Advancing Toward
Better Malaria Control

10

Research and Development for New Antimalarial Drugs

INTRODUCTION

As long as malaria persists as a global health problem, new drugs to treat and prevent it will be needed to replace the old ones as they lose effectiveness. Just a few years ago, there were few new drugs in the pipeline and antimalarial resistance was rising. The situation was desperate. It is now healthier than it has been for many decades, with several new combinations and entirely new classes of drug under development. The continued investment in basic science by agencies such as the U.S. National Institutes of Health, the European Commission, and the Wellcome Trust has provided the scientific underpinnings for these developments. But more significantly, genuine progress has resulted from the creation of the Medicines for Malaria Venture (MMV, a public-private partnership devoted to malaria drug development), the continued activities of the Walter Reed Army Institute of Research (WRAIR) in the United States, and the drug development efforts of the World Health Organization (WHO) Special Programme on Research and Training for Tropical Diseases (TDR). These organizations and their partners form what is basically a single international network of collaborators in malaria drug development (in contrast to the competitive character of most profit-driven drug development). This is cause for optimism, but current funding is still very modest and inadequate to complete development as products move downstream.

The crisis addressed by the IOM committee in this report relates to the economics of drugs to replace chloroquine as first-line treatment for uncomplicated malaria. However, the broader needs that must be addressed by global R&D also include drugs for patients with severe disease, drugs for children (and others) in coma who are unable to take oral drugs, and safe prophylaxis for pregnant women and possibly infants.

This chapter briefly reviews the history and current landscape of R&D for antimalarial drugs.

ANTIMALARIAL DRUG RESEARCH AND DEVELOPMENT

Between 1975 and 1999, only four of almost 1,400 new drugs developed worldwide were antimalarials, and all were at least in part the products of publicly funded research. The pharmaceutical industry largely disengaged from research and development of new drugs for malaria (and other diseases of the poor) in the 1970s because such drugs offered little potential return on investment (Veeken and Pecoul, 2000). This timing was particularly unfortunate because pharmaceutical science was on the brink of major advances and malaria drug development, in large part, missed out on the application of these advances. On the positive side, a sense of opportunity has been heightened by recent decoding of the *Plasmodium* and *Anopheles* genomes.

Malaria and other "neglected diseases" (including tuberculosis, filariasis, trypanosomiasis, leishmaniasis, dengue, to mention but a few)—unlike AIDS—are rarities in high-income countries. The world's poor cannot providentially benefit from new drugs developed for wealthier markets. In the case of antimalarials, the only real commercial market is travelers (whose needs differ greatly from those living in malaria-endemic areas). That industrialized market totals only US$200-300 million per year, well below the radar screen for industry.

The market for innovative new drugs for neglected diseases is further depressed by poor regulatory infrastructure in many countries, and by competing counterfeit drugs. The net effect is that about 10 percent of global drug R&D resources is directed at diseases accounting for 90 percent of the global disease burden (Global Forum for Health Research, 2002). Malaria is among the most poorly resourced diseases.

The UNICEF/UNDP/World Bank/WHO Special Programme for Training and Research in Tropical Diseases (WHO/TDR)

WHO/TDR's engagement in antimalarial drug development (as well as drugs for other target diseases) began more than 20 years ago. Its funding for malaria drug development historically ranges around US$2-4 million per year. WHO/TDR hosted, matured, and developed an initial portfolio for the Medicines for Malaria Venture (MMV) through 1998-1999 until MMV was established as an independent entity in November 1999.

Early on, WHO/TDR worked with WRAIR and pharmaceutical companies to develop mefloquine and halofantrine. More recently, it has collaborated with pharmaceutical partners to develop injectable artemether and injectable arteether for the treatment of severe malaria. WHO/TDR also sponsored the application for U.S. Food and Drug Administration approval of rectal artesunate in severe malaria (application pending). Other recent accomplishments and ongoing work include:

- Gaining regulatory approval of chlorproguanil-dapsone in collaboration with GlaxoSmithKline (GSK) in 2003
- Developing a fixed-dose combination of chlorproguanil-dapsone plus artesunate with GSK and MMV
- Working with Novartis to extend Coartem use in children down to 5 kg and to develop appropriate, user-friendly, and informative packaging

Public-Private Partnerships and the Medicines for Malaria Venture (MMV)

Public-private partnerships for drug development are relatively new. While they are still few, and not exclusively focused on neglected diseases of poor countries (some have formed around rare, or orphan, diseases), such collaborations are becoming very important, reviving R&D in areas that have lain fallow too long. A number of administrative arrangements are possible, but the key is tapping into a variety of skills and resources from institutions in the public and private sectors, often in a "virtual" organization. One of the most successful public-private partnerships involved in neglected diseases is the Medicines for Malaria Venture (MMV), begun in 1999, and profiled below. A new public-private partnership, the Drugs for Neglected Diseases Initiative (DNDi) has taken on late-stage development of two artemisinin coformulations as pilot projects (although the long-term focus of the DNDi will be on diseases other than malaria, e.g., African sleeping sickness).

MMV is among the first public-private partnership established to tackle a major global disease. The initiative arose from discussions between WHO (primarily through WHO/TDR), a number of other partners, and the International Federation of Pharmaceutical Manufacturers Associations (IFPMA). Early partners in these exploratory discussions were the Global Forum for Health Research, the Rockefeller Foundation, the World Bank, the Swiss Agency for Development and Cooperation, the Association of the British Pharmaceutical Industry, and the Wellcome Trust. The idea was to combine the expertise of the pharmaceutical industry in drug discovery and development, and the public sector, with its depth of expertise in basic biology, clinical medicine, field experience, and above all, its responsibility

TABLE 10-1 Contributions to MMV, 2000-2002 ($US)

Sources	2000	2001	2002
Foundation Capital[3]	1,197,619	2,309,741	——[4]
Bill & Melinda Gates Foundation	5,000,000	5,000,000	5,000,000
Rockefeller Foundation	2,300,000	1,000,000	1,000,000
The Wellcome Trust			518,400
Swiss Government (DEZA/SDC)	612,015		604,230[1]
U.K. Government (DFID)		2,827,850	1,561,700
Dutch Government (NMDC)			——[2]
World Bank via Global Forum	500,000	750,000	500,000
WHO Roll Back Malaria		2,500,000	
Exxon Mobil	100,000	100,000	100,000
Total	9,709,634	14,487,591	9,284,330[2]

[1]A second amount of US$607,700 for 2003 from SDC, received in November 2002, was taken to Deferred Income.

[2]An additional amount of US$954,664 for 2002 from the Netherlands Minister for Development Cooperation was still to be transferred by December 31, 2002, through WHO UNDP/WorldBank/WHO Special Programme for Research and Training in Tropical Diseases (TDR). This explains total Donations Received of US$10,238,994 as taken to income and Expenditure.

[3]The founding capital referenced in the statutes amounted in US$4,000,000 from WHO-Roll Back Malaria, and TDR. The TDR funds represent earmarked funding from the UK Department for International Development, the World Bank, and the Netherlands Minster for Development Cooperation prior to the foundation of MMV.

[4]At December 31, 2001, the amount of US$492,640 was still to be transferred from the World Health Organization. At December 31, 2002, the capital fund showed an outstanding balance of US$53,341.

SOURCE: MMV, 2002.

to the public. MMV was officially launched in November 1999 as a Swiss foundation.

The level of financial contributions to MMV has grown annually, as have expenditures. Donors include the Bill & Melinda Gates Foundation, Rockefeller Foundation, The Wellcome Trust, Swiss Government, U.K. Government, Dutch Government, World Bank via the Global Forum for Health Research, and Exxon Mobil (Table 10-1). As well as direct financial support, contributions in kind have been made by all of the corporate partners in specific projects. Total annual expenditures (not including in-kind support) have been:

- US$3,216,472 in 2000
- US$8,274,147 in 2001
- US$12,575,256 in 2002

The 2002 forecasts for future MMV project needs are US$15 to 18 million in 2003, rising to US$20-25 million in 2004.

THE WALTER REED ARMY INSTITUTE OF RESEARCH

The Military Infectious Disease Research Program[1]

The Walter Reed Army Institute of Research (WRAIR), through the United States Army Medical Research and Materiel Command (USAMRMC), is the leader in the United States for the development of new antimalarial drugs. Drug resistant malaria is considered a major military threat as well as an American public health issue. Military personnel, tourists, consultants, Peace Corps volunteers, and State Department employees traveling to, or residing in, malaria-endemic areas are at risk of illness and death from malaria.

When drug resistant malaria was first encountered by U.S. troops during the Vietnam conflict, the U.S. Army established a malaria research program to develop new prophylactic and therapeutic drugs for military use, coordinated through the Division of Experimental Therapeutics at the Walter Reed Army Institute of Research in Washington, D.C. The program was expected to maintain the expertise and laboratory capability to manage an experimental compound from the chemist's bench, through clinical trials, and on to approval by the Food and Drug Administration. WRAIR's accomplishments are summarized in Table 10-2. Funding for the program reached a peak of more than US$12 million in 1969 (equivalent to about US$70 million in 2003, adjusted for inflation) (Figure 10-1), but dropped off precipitously once the Vietnam conflict ended.

The WRAIR malaria drug development program never closed down completely, but government funding began to increase again only in the early 1990s (from about US$2 million in 1990 to about US$14 million in 2004, in constant 2004 dollars), partly in response to an IOM report on malaria research (IOM, 1991), and other favorable reports. Currently, WRAIR has Department of Defense directives to develop a new malaria prophylactic agent, and an intravenous artesunate formulation for severe and complicated malaria.

Perhaps more importantly, WRAIR has become an integral component of the global malaria drug development network, having established strategic alliances with MMV, and the National Institute of Allergy and Infectious Diseases Challenge Grant Program, as well as the pharmaceutical industry. Through MMV projects, WRAIR is supported by a wide range of

---

[1]Based largely on Milhous and Skillman (2004).

TABLE 10-2 Accomplishments of the WRAIR Malaria Drug
Development Program

Drug	WRAIR Role	Collaborators
Chloroquine-primaquine combination tablets	Clinical trials and FDA approval for prophylaxis	Sterling Winthrop
Sulfadoxine/pyrimethamine (Fansidar)	Clinical trials and FDA approval for prophylaxis	Hoffman-LaRoche
Mefloquine (Lariam)	Invented and developed	WHO Hoffman-LaRoche
Halofantrine (Halfan)	Invented and developed	GlaxoSmithKline
Arteether (Artemotil)	Co-developed, clinical trials (Injectable, limited use because of potential neurotoxicity, discovered by WRAIR scientists in animal models)	WHO, Artecef Approved in the Netherlands only
Doxycycline	Phase II challenge and clinical trials, FDA approval for prophylaxis	Pfizer, FDA
Azithromycin	Efficacy trials for prophylaxis Ongoing research on combinations	NIAID, Pfizer
Atovaquone-proguanil (Malarone)	Dose-ranging studies and efficacy trials	GlaxoSmithKline
Primaquine	Investigation for prophylaxis (intended to lead to application for added FDA-approved indication to label, which now includes only treatment)	Sterling Winthrop Naval Medical Research Institute
Tafenoquine	Discovered and in Phase III for prophylaxis	GlaxoSmithKline NIAID

SOURCE WRAIR.

donors. This has allowed the research to benefit both military (drugs mainly
for nonimmune adults entering malarious areas for short periods or moder-
ate-length stays) and broader global applications that focus on residents of
malaria-endemic countries.

An advantage of the WRAIR program is its in-house capabilities to
take a compound from early discovery through to early clinical testing,
much like a for-profit pharmaceutical company (although on a small scale).

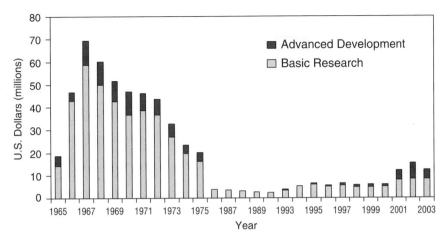

FIGURE 10-1 WRAIR malaria drug program budget from 1965 to 2003 in US$ millions adjusted for inflation.

Final drug development requires teaming with a commercial partner who contributes to financing in the late stages, before or at the time of clinical trials.

Antimalarials in Development[2]

MMV is the main driver of antimalarial drug projects, with many public- and private-sector collaborators. Projects closest to completion are, not surprisingly, several fixed-dose artemisinin combinations. Their likely registration dates, if successful, will be 2006-2007. The large number of fixed-dose combinations in development is currently justified, but as they progress, some may begin to appear more relevant than others. Factors that will influence this are: efficacy, safety, cost, stability, speed of development, and availability. Combinations in development include:

- Chlorproguanil-dapsone-artesunate (Lapdap-artesunate) by GSK with WHO/TDR, and MMV. Phase 2 studies initiated.
- Pyronaridine-artesunate by Shin Poong, Korea, in collaboration with WHO/TDR and MMV (MMV funded). Phase 1 planned for early 2004.
- Piperaquine-dihydroartemisinin (Artekin II) by Holleykin, China. Already marketed in Asia, but not registered in Europe or Africa. Following

---

[2]Based largely on Ridley (2003).

assistance from WHO/TDR, and WHO-RBM an agreement has now been established between Hollekin and MMV for development to international standards. Clinical studies in progress, but further GLP preclinical work still required.

- Mefloquine-artesunate, a proven combination as a non-fixed treatment regimen, is being developed as a fixed-dose combination. A consortium involving the Drugs for Neglected Diseases Initiative (DNDi), TROPIVAL (Bordeaux), and Far Manginhos of Brazil are involved with EU funding, and some WHO/TDR technical support. Phase 1 clinical studies in progress.
- Amodiaquine-artesunate, another proven combination as a non-fixed treatment regimen, is in development by the same consortium as above. A commercial partner is being sought for manufacture and production. Phase 1 clinical studies in progress.

In addition to the combinations cited above, there are several new single agent drugs in development that also may ultimately be used in combination. Some of these agents may be dropped as studies progress and problems appear. Projects include:

- Artemisone, a new artemisinin derivative being developed by Bayer with MMV support. Its *potential* advantage over existing artemisinins is lower neurotoxicity, and enhanced efficacy. This compound may be registered by 2007.
- A new quinoline antimalarial, similar to amodiaquine, being developed by GSK, and the University of Liverpool with support from MMV, and some technical assistance from WHO/TDR. This compound resembles amodiaquine but potentially has an improved safety profile, and is highly active against chloroquine-resistant strains. This compound may be registered by 2008.
- Fosmidomycin, a new class of antimalarial, is under development by Jomaa Pharmaceuticals in Germany. This also may be used in combination with other agents. The major issue is whether it can be given as a 3-day regimen.
- A new class of synthetic endoperoxide, invented at the University of Nebraska, and initially supported by WHO/TDR, is now being developed by a consortium funded and managed by MMV and is licensed to Ranbaxy of India. A compound entered into full preclinical development late in 2003. The advantage of these compounds is that they have longer half-lives than the artemisinins, and so could serve as better partners than artemisinins for longer half-life drugs. A compound in this category could be registered by 2008.

Several earlier phase drug discovery activities funded by MMV also are under way. Thus, entirely new classes of antimalarials may start to come on to the market soon after 2010.

Several enhanced formulations of existing drugs also are under development.

- Paediatric Coartem formulation by Novartis in collaboration with MMV, and TDR (MMV funded).
- Rectal artesunate, developed by WHO/TDR, for use as a single administration for malaria patients unable to take antimalarial medication by mouth, before they are referred for hospital treatment.
- Artesunate i.v. formulation for severe malaria; a collaboration between WRAIR, and MMV.

WRAIR has its own suite of new antimalarial drugs. Several families of compounds have progressed into preclinical development, including:

- Pyrroloquinazolines: new analogs that show none of the toxicity common to the parent drug, and yet retain oral potency against highly resistant malaria in animal studies. Should enter clinical studies in 2005.
- Third generation anti-folates: these show no cross-resistance in studies against multidrug resistant *P. falciparum*. They are under development in collaboration with Jacobus Pharmaceuticals.
- Imidazolinedione derivatives: these compounds are unique in that they specifically kill liver stages of malaria but have no activity against blood stages. Because they are not in the 8-aminoquinolone drug class, they are not expected to create hemolysis in G6PD-deficient people. May enter clinical studies in 2005.
- Tryptanthrins: a well-known, extremely potent class of chemicals with *in vitro* activity against trypanosomiasis as well as malaria. Difficulties with oral bioavailability have historically impaired progress with this drug class.
- New macrolides: azithromycin nearly meets criteria as an effective malaria prophylactic drug. Many analogs have been identified with superior in vitro potency against multidrug-resistant malaria. PLIVA Pharmaceuticals is collaborating with WRAIR to develop these new analogs.
- Chalcones: WRAIR is just beginning assessments of this drug class in collaboration with LICA Pharmaceuticals.
- Methylene blue: this compound very rapidly kills malaria in animal studies, and appears to be nontoxic at effective doses. It may be a good partner for a combination antimalarial regimen. Its potential utility in malaria prophylaxis still being explored.

- Mefloquine analogs: an in vitro assay to predict neurotoxicity has been established, in order to identify several potent mefloquine analogs which do not have in vitro neurotoxic effects.
- Tafenoquine: Phase 2 studies have been completed in partnership with GlaxoSmithKline Pharmaceuticals. This product has a very long half-life, and may be effective for prophylaxis when taken monthly.
- Azithromycin/chloroquine and azithromycin/quinine: these combinations are known to be safe and effective in children and in pregnant women. Pfizer Pharmaceuticals is collaborating with WRAIR in clinical trials in Thailand and Kenya.

CONCLUSIONS

Given the remarkably limited resources, the progress in antimalarial drug development over the past 5 years or so has been impressive. Direct expenditures total less than US$50 million in 2004, even including a large proportion of in-kind expenditures. For most of the products in development, however, the costliest phases—clinical trials—are yet to come. The global community must plan to increase funding resources for the core groups, MMV and WRAIR (mainly the responsibility of the U.S. government). As more projects mature beyond early development, the pharmaceutical industry also will need to step up in-kind contributions in the developmental areas it does best.

It is not a useful exercise to compare expenditures on antimalarial R&D to commercial drug development (which totals some hundreds of millions of dollars per successful product), but something of the scale should be kept in mind when global investments in antimalarials are considered. During the course of this study, the committee did not independently calculate an "appropriate" amount of investment in antimalarial R&D, but has concluded that current levels are less than optimal, and that increased funds will definitely be required merely to maintain the momentum of existing development activities. MMV, which manages about half the antimalarial R&D worldwide, has estimated its needs at US$30 million per year for development and early clinical studies (Personal communication, R. Ridley, WHO, March 2004). As compounds progress through to advanced clinical and field trials, at least an additional US$10 million per year will be needed (this also assumes continuing contributions in kind from industrial partners not included in these figures). The recently established European and Developing Countries Clinical Trials Partnership (whose funding goal over the next five years is 600 million Euros, including 200 million from the founding European Commission (European Union, 2004) could play a key role in this phase. Equal amounts totaling US$30 million per year plus extra funding for clinical trials and industry investments will be needed for the WRAIR program to remain productive.

REFERENCES

European Union. 2004. *EDCTP at a Glance*. [Online]. Available: http://europa.eu.int/comm/research/info/conferences/edctp/pdf/edctp-at-a-glance_en.pdf [accessed April 12, 2004].

Global Forum for Health Research. 2002. The 10/90 report of research 2001-2002. Geneva: Global Forum for Health Research.

IOM. 1991. *Malaria: Obstacles and Opportunities*. Oakes SC, Mitchell VS, Pearson GW, Carpenter CCJ, eds. Washington, DC: National Academy Press.

Medicines for Malaria Venture. 2002. *Annual Report, 2002*. Geneva: MMV.

Milhous W, Skillman DR. 2004. (unpublished manuscript). The military infectious disease research program: Strategic plan for antimalarial prophylaxis. Washington, DC: Walter Reed Army Institute of Medical Research.

Ridley RG. 2003. Overview of malaria drug development. Background paper prepared for World Bank/IOM expert consultation on the procurement and financing of antimalarial drugs, September 15-16, 2003, Washington, DC.

Veeken H, Pecoul B. 2000. Drugs for 'neglected diseases': A bitter pill. *Tropical Medicine and International Health* 5(5):309-311.

11

Maximizing the Effective Use of Antimalarial Drugs

INTRODUCTION

The success or failure of any public health program is largely determined by the public's effective use of the services offered. This principle is especially relevant in treating malaria because prompt use of efficacious drugs greatly reduces the incidence of severe and complicated disease (Salako et al., 2001). Merely making an efficacious treatment available is not enough to reduce malaria mortality, however—the treatment also must be used optimally. Even the most highly efficacious treatment, if not used correctly, can fail to cure the illness, and may facilitate the development of drug resistance.

In real life, many human factors thwart access and use of curative medications in resource-poor settings, including traditional beliefs, illiteracy, mistrust and fatalistic attitudes. In the case of malaria, economic barriers to the purchase of drugs; complex treatment and dosing regimens; limited understanding of how or why to adhere to recommended regimens; and adverse side effects compound the problem (Fungladda et al., 1998; Bloland et al., 2000; Yepez et al., 2000). A false sense of security also affects choice and use of antimalarial treatments, particularly in sub-Saharan Africa. Most residents in malaria-endemic areas of Africa do not appreciate the rising toll of chloroquine-resistant *P. falciparum* because, for many years, chloroquine worked so well. In some cases, chloroquine's loss of activity is also obscured by its partial antipyretic effects, which suggest to some patients that the drug is curing them as opposed to merely relieving symptoms.

> There's a tremendous confidence in the public in the old drug [chloroquine], even though the old drug is failing. That's part of the problem.
>
> Don DeSavigny, Tanzania Essential Health Interventions Project

Another major problem is the inadequacy of public health infrastructure to serve basic health care needs in Africa and other resource-poor settings (Kager, 2002; Moerman et al., 2003). This inadequacy is reflected in a lack of electricity, clean water, or reliable medicines in many public health facilities (Gilson et al., 1994; Israr et al., 2000) as well as poorly trained and poorly motivated staff, leakage of drugs for private resale, unauthorized patient charges, mismanagement of patient user fees, distance to facilities, lack of drugs and other desired services, and lengthy waiting times (Bloland et al., 2003). As a result, private-sector sources—ranging from licensed pharmacies to informal drug kiosks and itinerant drug sellers—have assumed an increasingly important role. In some studies, as many as 60 percent or more of patients seeking help for febrile illness received their medicines from the private sector (McCombie, 1996; WHO/UNICEF, 2003).

This chapter reviews specific barriers to access and use of antimalarial drugs in falciparum-endemic areas, as well as promising strategies to enhance appropriate drug use in the future. When negative and positive factors are added together, the net approximates the ultimate goal of "programmatic effectiveness" (Box 11-1).

OVERCOMING ECONOMIC BARRIERS

The high cost of treatment—real or perceived—is a major barrier to accessing malaria drugs and treatment (Ndyomugyenyi et al., 1998). In addition to direct drug costs, indirect costs such as transportation and time affect utilization. When chloroquine was still effective, many mothers in Ghana who believed in its efficacy failed to use it simply because they lacked access to health services, pharmacies, or urban markets where they could buy the product (Glik et al., 1989). Similarly, in Papua New Guinea, patients' willingness to seek malaria care at primary health facilities was strongly influenced by the distance they had to travel to reach those facilities (Muller et al., 1998).

In another study from Ghana, the cost of treatment influenced where

BOX 11-1
What Is Programmatic Effectiveness?

Development of rational malaria treatment policies in endemic countries relies on consideration of a variety of data, including economic, behavioral, biomedical, and political (Bloland and Ettling, 1999). Among the relevant biomedical data, evidence from carefully conducted in vivo assessments of malaria therapy efficacy using established methodologies are critical for guiding appropriate drug choice, and for timing policy change (WHO, 2003).

Ultimately, however, the central purpose of formulating rational malaria treatment policies is to reduce malaria mortality. Making an appropriate drug available is merely the first step. The optimal use of that drug involves many additional steps. The patient (or their parent) must also:

- recognize the need for treatment with Western medicine;
- believe that the recommended treatment is useful, choose to use it, and know where to get it;
- perceive that treatment is safe, of reasonable quality, available, and affordable;
- at the time of dispensing, receive an appropriate amount of medicine from the provider—whether public sector- or private sector-based—along with adequate information on how to take the treatment correctly; and
- actually take the medicine completely and correctly.

This more holistic view of malaria therapy, i.e., one that takes into account all of the factors that determine treatment success in practice, underlies the concept of "programmatic effectiveness." Programmatic effectiveness recognizes that even the most highly efficacious treatment, if not used correctly, can fail to cure the illness, and possibly contribute to the development of resistance.

In one of the few studies that have tried to measure programmatic effectiveness of malaria therapy, the authors identified a series of 7 critical factors leading to successful treatment (Krause and Sauerborn, 2000). They then measured the frequency with which each factor was satisfied in an actual health setting in Burkina Faso and found that the overall programmatic effectiveness of malaria treatment was only about 3% (i.e., only 3% of patients were successfully treated, according to their definitions). More important, increasing the efficacy of the malaria treatment from 85% to 100% increased overall programmatic effectiveness by less than 1%.

This example illustrates that optimizing a single factor while ignoring other factors may yield minimal improvements overall. In the case of malaria, simply optimizing drug efficacy by providing ACTs without attempting to optimize the environment in which treatment occurs may result in far less influence on overall morbidity and mortality rates than expected. Infusing ACTs in the same environment in which chloroquine, sulfadoxine/pyrimethamine, and other drugs have failed could even be counterproductive. An unprecedented investment in highly efficacious ACTs must be accompanied by investments aimed at improving the environment in which they will be used in order to maximize their benefits minimize the potential for harm resulting from misuse.

Peter Bloland, U.S. Centers for Disease Control and Prevention

malaria care was sought. Interestingly, individuals with higher incomes were more likely to purchase drugs privately and self-medicate for malaria; users acknowledged that the convenience of local purchase and the option of taking a partial course of medication affected their decision to self-treat. This study also found that patients were more likely to visit private or mission facilities (where overall quality was perceived to be higher) when user fees rose at local government clinics (Asenso-Okyere et al., 1997).

Other studies have shown that it is not necessarily the *price* paid for treatment that is most important but *how* it is paid. In Tanzania, for example, many subjects who reported they could not afford Western medicines (including antimalarials) still bought relatively costly traditional medicines. The inconsistency was partly explained by healers' willingness to accept credit or payment in kind as opposed to requiring cash for their products and services. While some public and mission hospitals also extend credit, they do so less frequently than traditional healers (Muela et al., 2000).

Price is an important factor in choosing both a treatment and a treater, but it interacts with a host of other variables. Even when drugs are free through public-sector sources, they are not necessarily accessible. Patients and their families may seek malaria treatment outside the public sector because private outlets are easier to reach, and their products are perceived to be of higher quality. Consumers also may obtain drugs from private facilities for the simple reason that antimalarial drugs are frequently out of stock at public clinics. A global subsidy to flood the public *and* private marketplace with highly effective artemisinin combination therapies (ACTs) in even the most peripheral areas where drug resistant *P. falciparum* is being transmitted would circumvent these economic barriers, as discussed in detail in Chapter 3.

MAKING ANTIMALARIALS SAFER AND MORE USER-FRIENDLY

Packaging That Promotes Appropriate Use

In many parts of the world, especially sub-Saharan Africa, antimalarial pills are still dispensed in unmarked paper envelopes, and syrups constitute the major form of treatment for children under five. Prepackaged tablets are one means by which to ensure proper dosing and adherence to a full course of antimalarial treatment. The Special Programme for Research and Training in Tropical Diseases (TDR) advocates a simple, dose-wise packaging of antimalarials to help patients take the correct drug dosage at the correct time (TDR/RBM, 2002). Well designed drug packages increase adult compliance, on average, 20 percent (Yeboah-Antwi et al., 2001), and the effect in children (Pagnoni et al., 1997) may be even greater. In Ghana, a 91 percent adherence rate was found in children aged 0-5 years who were given prepacked tablets compared with a 42 percent adherence rate in users of antimalarial syrup. The tablets, in contrast to the syrup, did not require measuring, and the daily dose was clearly indicated. Most important, the cost of treating children with tablets was roughly 25 percent that of treating them with syrup (Ansah et al., 2001). Prepackaged tablets also have been associated with reduced drug wastage at health facilities and reduced patient waiting times at dispensaries (Yeboah-Antwi et al., 2001).

> The adherence is actually better to tablets in children. With syrups the mothers get confused. To a mother . . . a spoon is a spoon is a spoon. So you get anything from a one ml spoon to nine ml spoon being used to administer the drug. But if you package it . . . people value it.
>
>   Irene Agyepong, Ghana Health Service

Similar results have been reported elsewhere. In a comparison of blister packaging of antimalarials with other interventions (including public information campaigns and drug quality assessment), blister packaging was most effective at improving adherence (Gomes et al., 1998). Studies in Burma (Shwe et al., 1998) and China (Qingjun et al., 1998) also suggest that blister packs are an effective way to improve adherence to short-course and combination treatments.

A recent qualitative study among urban and rural women in western Uganda found prepacked, unit-dosed malaria treatment for children widely accepted by mothers (Kilian et al., 2003). Ninety-one percent of women said they preferred the prepacked to the conventional type of treatment, and 94 percent were willing to pay between US$0.17 (rural women) and US$0.29 (urban women) more for this treatment. The main reasons for preferring prepacks were safety and cleanliness; ease of application, dosing, and compliance were additional perceived benefits. In Burkina Faso, mothers who received training and packaged drugs recognized and treated malaria promptly and correctly (Sirima et al., 2003).

In sum, evidence that better packaging technology improves adherence is timely and relevant to the introduction of more efficacious antimalarial treatments such as ACTs, particularly in Africa. An emphasis on convenient dosing schedules as well as forms (for example, rectocaps and blister packs) developed in partnership with private industry will be essential to enhanced penetration of new-generation antimalarial drugs.

Poor-Quality and Counterfeit Drugs

The quality of medicines in less developed countries is often poor due to a lack of quality assurance during manufacture, excessive decomposition of active ingredients under hot and humid conditions, and/or counterfeiting. Nonetheless, substandard and expired drugs continue to circulate because of simple economics, lack of adequate drug information, and weak country-level drug regulatory systems. In one study conducted by the Department of Pharmacy of the University of Nairobi, 46 percent of locally manufactured products were substandard when their active ingredient was measured by compendial methods (Kibwage et al., 1992). In another study, almost half of nearly 600 antimalarial, antibacterial, and antituberculosis drugs purchased in Lagos or Abuja, Nigeria did not comply with set pharmacopoeial limits. The sample included chloroquine, sulfadoxine/pyrimethamine (SP), and quinine tablets, and chloroquine and SP syrups, some of which had less than 25 percent active ingredient (Taylor et al., 2001). Failure to dissolve was found in 44 and 13 percent respectively of SP and amodiaquine tablets sold by private wholesale pharmacies in Dar es Salaam, Tanzania (Minzi et al., 2003). These findings validate consumers' concerns about antimalarial drug quality in many malaria-endemic countries.

In contrast to a substandard drug, a counterfeit drug is one that has been incorrectly packaged or constituted in a deliberate attempt to dupe sellers and consumers (Wondemagegnehu, 1995). Among cases in which pharmaceutical preparations contain no active ingredient, a drug other than that stated on the label, or consistently low concentrations of drug, fraud is the most likely cause (Wan Po, 2001). Counterfeit artesunate and mefloquine preparations are widely sold in Cambodia (Rozendaal, 2001). Another recent study from Southeast Asia found that more than a third of tablets labeled "artesunate" purchased from shops in Cambodia, Laos, Burma, Thailand, and Vietnam contained no drug (Newton et al., 2001). Recognizable packaging is one means of increasing the likelihood that drugs are authentic, although it does not eliminate the need to verify quality using, for example, drug testing kits. In Southeast Asia where counterfeit packaging changes frequently, this type of testing must be conducted on a regular basis (Newton et al., 2001).

Labeling and Instructions

Labeling of pharmaceuticals, malaria drugs included, is woefully inadequate in many malaria-endemic settings. When drugs are accompanied by printed information, the information is often written in complicated or technical language, or, in some cases, a language entirely unknown to the

318

SAVING LIVES, BUYING TIME

consumer. And in many cases, the printed information is of no use whatsoever because the consumer is illiterate.

Difficulties reading antimalarial instructions are well documented (Ansah et al., 2001; Okonkwo et al., 2001; TDR/RBM, 2002). In addition, verbal instructions are often inadequate. In Zambia, many children suffering from malaria did not receive the appropriate 3-day course of chloroquine because their caregivers did not receive adequate instruction on how to administer the drug (Baume et al., 2000). In Uganda, only 38 percent of children received chloroquine in compliance with instructions given by health workers or drug shop attendants (Nshakira et al., 2002). Obviously, consumers can only use antimalarials correctly if they receive a full explanation from a health care provider or drug seller, or appropriate written and graphic labeling accompanies the drug.

Good labeling, in fact, is a minor added expense for producers that yields an excellent return on investment. In a three-armed Nigerian study of antimalarial treatment with chloroquine syrup, the addition of a pictorial insert plus good verbal instructions doubled adherence with the correct dosing regimen (Okonkwo et al., 2001). The pictorial insert added only US$0.01 per patient to the base cost of US$.30 for the syrup.

Close-to-Home Treatment

At the Abuja Summit in April 2000, African heads of state agreed that, by 2005, 60 percent of malaria sufferers should have prompt access to affordable, appropriate treatment within 24 hours of the onset of symptoms (WHO, 2000). This recommendation coincided with increasing interest in extending malaria treatment closer to home, or even within the home. Although there is, at present, no single accepted definition of home-based malaria therapy, the general idea is to greatly improve access to efficacious medicines at the most peripheral levels, and to increase community members' knowledge about how to use antimalarial medicines properly (Bloland et al., 2003).

In fact, unsupervised home treatment with antimalarials has been a common practice in certain African countries and settings for many years (Breman and Campbell, 1988; Deming et al., 1989; Ahorlu et al., 1997; Nshakira et al., 2002), especially where local residents are dissatisfied with formal health services. In a recent study in Kenya, home treatment with an antimalarial drug was given to 47 percent of children under 5 years (for 32 percent, this was their only antimalarial treament), 43 percent were taken to a health facility, and 25 percent had no antimalarial treatment (Hamel et al., 2001). In Mali and Nigeria, 76 and 71 percent of mothers, respectively, managed their child's illness at home with antimalarial drugs (Thera et al.,

2000; Fawole and Onadeko, 2001). Urban settings (where population density creates markets responsive to consumer demand) also promote home treatment (Glik et al., 1989; Brinkmann and Brinkmann, 1991; Agyepong and Manderson, 1994). In rural Gambia, in contrast, low rates of home treatment with chloroquine (<10 percent) have been documented in several studies (Menon et al., 1988; von Seidlein et al., 2002; Clarke et al., 2003), possibly due to the restricted availability of antimalarials as well as lower costs for treatment at government health centers. A similar pattern has been reported from Zambia, where private providers also are few, and treatment at government facilities free (Baume et al., 2000).

If the availability of effective antimalarials increased in rural African communities along with stakeholder education, many experts believe that residents could use drugs effectively. One community-based intervention in northern Ethiopia in which mother coordinators provided home treatment reduced under-5 malaria mortality by 40 percent (Kidane and Morrow, 2000). A smaller study in Guinea Bissau found similar treatment outcomes and day 7 chloroquine blood levels in children with symptomatic malaria whose treatment was either supervised in a health center or given at home following adequate caregiver education by health staff (Kofoed et al., 2003). The main disadvantage of self-treatment is the lack of clinical evaluation of patients by trained health professionals, which can result in missed diagnoses and delays in appropriate treatment (Hamel et al., 2001). In addition, presumptive treatment of febrile episodes at home is likely to result in overuse of antimalarial drugs and the attendant risk of escalating drug resistance.

> Malaria is a serious problem. About 95 percent of people in the village get sick with malaria . . . Because health care is very far from the village, most deaths occur at home.
>
> Village official, Mkuranga, Tanzania (2002)

> I think household based treatment is inevitable, it's what people have been doing down the centuries, and they are continuing to do it. And then you have really poor people. They are always doing economic calculations . . . they [calculate] the difference between fish in the soup today or [taking] him to the clinic.
>
> Irene Agyepong, Ghana Health Service (2002)

EDUCATING STAKEHOLDERS

Health Education Messages

Health education messages can provide information and address a variety of misconceptions regarding the use of antimalarials. Common formats include posters, video clips, radio, and other forms of mass media. Other methods include peer education, mothers' clubs, and school-based programs.

In Tanzania, popular misconceptions about SP were undermining adherence to treatment. The Tanzanian health service responded by creating health education messages to counter the belief that SP is ineffective because it lacks chloroquine's immediate antipyretic plus anti-inflammatory effects. Other messages in Tanzania and elsewhere have focused on malaria's symptoms and complications, correct dosing of antimalarial drugs, the use of oral versus injectable antimalarials, and persistent or recurrent symptoms following treatment (Ruebush et al., 1995; Foster, 1995). As with many health education messages (Engleman and Forbes, 1986; Helitzer-Allen et al., 1993; Denis, 1998) however, the Tanzanian malaria campaign was never formally evaluated.

One exception to the dearth of educational evaluations is a study conducted in Cambodia in which posters combined with video clips improved antimalarial adherence rates as much as 20 percent (Denis, 1998). The influence of posters alone was much more modest. Educational benefits were mainly reported among those who visited public and private health practitioners as opposed to consumers who purchased their drugs from vendors. While posters have been used widely in malaria education, this is the only study that has compared their effect on adherence with another form of mass media; namely video.

Training Shopkeepers

Many consumers in Africa, Asia and Latin America seek medical treatment outside the formal heath care sector (Foster, 1995). Although close-to-home treatment is desirable in theory, in practice, private sector vendors are frequently unable to provide appropriate advice, complete doses, or even the correct category of drug for a specific complaint (Bloland et al., 2003). One way of improving quality of private-sector treatment is to train drug sellers and shopkeepers. In western Nigeria, primary health care training of patent medicine vendors improved knowledge about malaria as well as other infectious disorders and malnutrition (Oshiname and Brieger, 1992). In Kenya, 500 private drug sellers were enrolled in a 2-4 day training workshop mounted by the Ministry of Health in conjunction with a public information campaign. The effort resulted in a short-term increase in the appropriate use of over-the-counter chloroquine of 62 percent (Marsh et al., 1999). One year later, however, there was a 20 percent turnover in outlets and/or trained staff (Marsh et al., 2004).

A promising new trend for improving the quality of private-sector malaria prescribing is networks of licensed or franchised drug shops that can dispense quality treatment advice and medications with a high degree of oversight (for examples, see http://msh.org/features/gates/kenya-release.html or http://www.cfwshops.org/about.html).

Educating Health Professionals

It should not be assumed that community-based health care providers—in particular midwives, traditional birth attendants, and health workers—are well informed about malaria. However, with regular training and updates, they can serve as potent advocates for proper case management and adherence to treatment guidelines (Ndyomugyenyi et al., 1998). Medical assistants working in health posts are another target group for ongoing education and auditing. In Ghana, one study found a surprising discrepancy among clinic providers between knowledge and practice of malaria treatment (evidenced by over- and under-dosing of chloroquine) as well as a tendency to yield to patient demands for injections and polypharmacy (Ofori-Adjei and Arhinful, 1996). In-service training did not alter these poor prescribing practices over the long term despite medical assistants' knowledge of correct treatment paradigms. The authors argue for an increased awareness of the sociocultural context of antimalarial drug use when designing educational programs for health providers and patients.

Targeting Family Decision Makers and Traditional Healers

Understanding local knowledge, perceptions, and practices of malaria management has become an increasing focus of research during the last decade. In a recent study based on semi-structured interviews with community members in Mbarara, Uganda, causes of malaria—in addition to "fever due to mosquitoes"—were reported to be drinking of dirty or unboiled water, breathing bad air, staying near somebody with malaria, witchcraft, avenging spirits, and eating fresh maize or sweet fruit such as mangoes, pineapples, and passion fruit. Even those who said that mosquitoes cause or transmit malaria had erroneous ideas about the route of transmission. Most believed that malaria was acquired by drinking mosquito eggs or larvae in dirty water as opposed to a mosquito bite (Nuwaha, 2002).

Despite misconceptions about its cause, many people know malaria's common clinical features. Kenyan and Ghanaian mothers had sufficiently good knowledge to recognize mild to moderate malaria (Ruebush et al., 1995; Ahorlu et al., 1997). In Uganda, not only were convulsions, anemia, and splenomegaly linked to malaria, interviewees also discussed complications of malaria in pregnancy, in particular abortions (Nuwaha, 2002). However, many caregivers in Africa still blame convulsions—a prominent finding in severe malaria—on supernatural causes (Mwenesi et al., 1995; Ahorlu et al., 1997; Nuwaha, 2002). When spiritual causes are invoked, traditional healers, as opposed to medical professionals, are frequently consulted. Educating traditional healers about febrile convulsions and severe malaria is a particularly important means of rerouting children with seizures and impaired consciousness to effective antimalarials.

Another ethnographic study conducted in Tanzania found parents and traditional healers unanimous in their belief that febrile seizures require traditional treatments, at least initially, and that these treatments are effective (Makemba et al., 1996). While traditional healers did refer some patients who were not improving to the District Hospital, the referral typically came late in the course of illness. In Uganda, traditional medicine also was endorsed for treatment of convulsions and splenomegaly (Nuwaha, 2002). Squeezing juice from herbs into the nose and mouth was a common way of treating a convulsing or unconscious child, while splenomegaly was often treated with therapeutic marks and herbs squeezed into cuts overlying the splenic area.

> Let's imagine that we are in a remote area in Africa and a mother has a sick child, and this child has severe malaria, convulsions, etc. that really scares the person. Very often, she doesn't decide immediately or alone [if she will take the child for treatment]. She will either consult the mother-in-law, the neighbor, or the father.
>
> The other important element that comes into the decision is whether or not she is financially able to pay for the transport. So there are several steps in the decision-making process that require a back and forth for the woman and the child that delay the treatment.
>
> Magda Robalo, WHO AFRO (2002)

In focus group discussions, health workers and mothers in Tanzania were clear about the signs and symptoms of *homa ya malaria*, a Swahili term consistent with mild malaria. However mothers also believed that cerebral malaria was a childhood convulsive disorder called *degedege* caused by evil spirits. According to discussants from urban, suburban, and rural settings, effective treatments for *degedege* included urinating on affected children, or fuming them with elephant dung. Injections, on the other hand, were thought to have the power to kill some *degedege* sufferers. The role of grandmothers and mothers-in-law as key decision makers regarding cases of *degedege* was an important finding of the study, suggesting that these individuals be specifically targeted with information and teaching regarding severe malaria (Comoro et al., 2003).

School-Based Education

The education sector already knows the importance of health to schoolchildren as evidenced by the child-friendly schools of UNICEF (United Nations Children's Fund), the health promoting schools of the World Health Organization (WHO), and the International School Health Initiative of the World Bank. Malaria is a disease particularly well suited to public health partnerships with teachers, principals, and designers of school curricula. Although malaria in areas of stable transmission is most common and severe in children who are not yet attending school, it still remains an important cause of mortality (10-20 percent of all cases) and morbidity in schoolchildren (Bundy et al., 2000). In addition, malaria can significantly influence educational outcomes, accounting for roughly three to eight percent of all reasons for absenteeism (Colbourne, 1955; Trape et al., 1987, 1993), 13 to 50 percent of school days missed per year due to preventable medical causes (Bundy et al., 2000), as well as residual neurologic sequelae impairing cognitive and developmental potential in one to five percent of children infected early in life (Snow et al., 1999).

Children in rural African households assume significant responsibility at a young age—for example, looking after siblings, fetching water or firewood, and cooking (van der Geest and Geissler, 2003). They also participate in the collection and preparation of herbal medicines and are sent to buy pharmaceuticals (Sternberg et al., 2000; Prince and Geissler, 2001; Prince et al., 2001). Primary schoolchildren's knowledge of medicines and self-treatment were investigated between 1996 and 1998 among the Luo of western Kenya and the Iteso of eastern Uganda. These studies showed that children of primary school age possess knowledge of both herbal remedies and "hospital" medicines and that they use medicines to treat themselves as well as their younger siblings. However, few children questioned knew the correct dosage of chloroquine for the treatment of malaria or the difference between antimalarials, antipyretics, and analgesics (Geissler et al., 2001).

Children can be important agents for change for themselves and their families. Similarly, school health education can have a significant yield in terms of community-wide understanding of malaria control and treatment. It has been suggested that school-based teaching of medicine could start from standard four (age 10 to 12), focusing on treatments for simple malaria, cough and cold, diarrhea, eye disorders, and pain (van der Geest and Geissler, 2003). Medicine use should be taught in a participatory manner didactically connected with children's everyday experience—this, in turn, requires modification of educational curricula and teacher training. Recognition that the educational system could be used to target messages about antimalarials is now receiving broader acceptance (Bloland et al., 2003).

Other Points of Contact

Integrated management of childhood illness (IMCI) is an algorithm that assists health care workers with minimal training and little or no access to diagnostic aids to treat certain childhood illnesses based on clinical signs and symptoms alone (Perkins et al., 1997). Although IMCI protocols may result in considerable misdiagnosis, and unnecessary treatment of malaria, the program offers another point of contact for malaria education for patients, families, and providers. Intermittent preventive treatment (IPT) (reviewed in Chapter 8) is a WHO-endorsed strategy that aims to provide full treatment doses of antimalarial drugs to pregnant women at least once each during the second and third trimesters of pregnancy (WHO, 2002). IPTi is a new program for infants designed to reduce malaria-related morbidity and mortality by the use of periodic antimalarial treatment doses of antimalarial drugs during infancy. If IPT and IPTi become standard in large areas of sub-Saharan Africa, they also will expedite malaria education of stakeholders. Similarly, linking routine childhood immunization to IPTi has the potential to reduce the clinical effect of malaria (Schellenberg et al., 2001) while facilitating the education of stakeholders about malaria control and treatment.

REFERENCES

Agyepong IA, Manderson L. 1994. The diagnosis and management of fever at household level in the greater Accra region, Ghana. *Acta Tropica* 58(3-4):317-330.

Ahorlu CK, Dunyo SK, Afari EA, Koram KA, Nkrumah FK. 1997. Malaria-related beliefs and behaviour in southern Ghana: Implications for treatment, prevention and control. *Tropical Medicine and International Health* 2(5):488-499.

Ansah EK, Gyapong JO, Agyepong IA, Evans DB. 2001. Improving adherence to malaria treatment for children: The use of pre-packed chloroquine tablets vs. chloroquine syrup. *Tropical Medicine and International Health* 6(7):496-504.

Asenso-Okyere WK, Osei-Akoto I, Anum A, Appiah EN. 1997. Willingness to pay for health insurance in a developing economy. A pilot study of the informal sector of Ghana using contingent valuation. *Health Policy* 42(3):223-237.

Baume C, Helitzer D, Kachur SP. 2000. Patterns of care for childhood malaria in Zambia. *Social Science and Medicine* 51(10):1491-1503.

Bloland PB, Ettling M. 1999. Making malaria-treatment policy in the face of drug resistance. *Ann Trop Med Parasitol* 93(1):5-23.

Bloland PB, Ettling M, Meek S. 2000. Combination therapy for malaria in Africa: Hype or hope? *Bulletin of the World Health Organization* 78(12):1378-1388.

Bloland PB, Kachur SP, Williams HA. 2003. Trends in antimalarial drug deployment in Sub-Saharan Africa. *Journal of Experimental Biology* 206(Pt 21):3761-3769.

Breman JG, Campbell CC. 1988. Combating severe malaria in African children. *Bulletin of the World Health Organization* 66(5):611-620.

Brinkmann U, Brinkmann A. 1991. Malaria and health in Africa: The present situation and epidemiological trends. *Tropical Medicine and Parasitology* 42(3):204-213.

Bundy DA, Lwin S, Osika JS, McLaughlin J, Pannenborg CO. 2000. What should schools do about malaria? *Parasitology Today* 16(5):181-182.

Clarke SE, Rowley J, Bogh C, Walraven GE, Lindsay SW. 2003. Home treatment of 'malaria' in children in rural Gambia is uncommon. *Tropical Medicine and International Health* 8(10):884-894.

Colbourne MJ. 1955. The effect of malaria suppression in a group of Accra school children. *Transactions of the Royal Society of Tropical Medicine and Hygiene* 49(4):556-569.

Comoro C, Nsimba SE, Warsame M, Tomson G. 2003. Local understanding, perceptions and reported practices of mothers/guardians and health workers on childhood malaria in a Tanzanian district—Implications for malaria control. *Acta Tropica* 87(3):305-313.

Deming MS, Gayibor A, Murphy K, Jones TS, Karsa T. 1989. Home treatment of febrile children with antimalarial drugs in Togo. *Bulletin of the World Health Organization* 67(6):695-700.

Denis MB. 1998. Improving compliance with quinine + tetracycline for treatment of malaria: Evaluation of health education interventions in Cambodian villages. *Bulletin of the World Health Organization* 76(Suppl 1):43-49.

Engleman SR, Forbes JF. 1986. Economic aspects of health education. *Social Science and Medicine* 22(4):443-458.

Fawole OI, Onadeko MO. 2001. Knowledge and home management of malaria fever by mothers and care givers of under five children. *West African Journal of Medicine* 20(2):152-157.

Foster S. 1995. Treatment of malaria outside the formal health services. *American Journal of Tropical Medicine and Hygiene* 98(1):29-34.

Fungladda W, Honrado ER, Thimasarn K, Kitayaporn D, Karbwang J, Kamolratanakul P, Masngammueng R. 1998. Compliance with artesunate and quinine + tetracycline treatment of uncomplicated falciparum malaria in Thailand. *Bulletin of the World Health Organization* 76(Suppl 1):59-66.

Geissler PW, Meinert L, Prince R, Nokes C, Aagaard-Hansen J, Jitta J, Ouma JH. 2001. Self-treatment by Kenyan and Ugandan schoolchildren and the need for school-based education. *Health Policy and Planning* 16(4):362-371.

Gilson L, Alilio M, Heggenhougen K. 1994. Community satisfaction with primary health care services: An evaluation undertaken in the Morogoro region of Tanzania. *Social Science and Medicine* 39(6):767-780.

Glik DC, Ward WB, Gordon A, Haba F. 1989. Malaria treatment practices among mothers in Guinea. *Journal of Health and Social Behavior* 30(4):421-435.

Gomes M, Wayling S, Pang L. 1998. Interventions to improve the use of antimalarials in South-east Asia: an overview. *Bulletin of the World Health Organization* 76(Suppl 1):9-19.

Hamel MJ, Odhacha A, Roberts JM, Deming MS. 2001. Malaria control in Bungoma district, Kenya: A survey of home treatment of children with fever, bednet use and attendance at antenatal clinics. *Bulletin of the World Health Organization* 79(11):1014-1023.

Helitzer-Allen DL, McFarland DA, Wirima JJ, Macheso AP. 1993. Malaria chemoprophylaxis compliance in pregnant women: A cost-effectiveness analysis of alternative interventions. *Social Science and Medicine* 36(4):403-407.

Israr SM, Razum O, Ndiforchu V, Martiny P. 2000. Coping strategies of health personnel
during economic crisis: A case study from Cameroon. *Tropical Medicine and International Health* 5(4):288-292.

Kager PA. 2002. Malaria control: Constraints and opportunities. *Tropical Medicine and
International Health* 7(12):1042-1046.

Kibwage IO, Ogeto JO, Maitai CK, Rutere G, Thuranira J, Ochieng A. 1992. Drug quality
control work in Daru: Observations during 1983-1986. *East African Medical Journal*
69(10):577-580.

Kidane G, Morrow RH. 2000. Teaching mothers to provide home treatment of malaria in
Tigray, Ethiopia: A randomised trial. *Lancet* 356(9229):550-555.

Kilian AH, Tindyebwa D, Gulck T, Byamukama W, Rubaale T, Kabagambe G, Korte R.
2003. Attitude of women in western Uganda towards pre-packed, unit-dosed malaria
treatment for children. *Tropical Medicine and International Health* 8(5):431-438.

Kofoed PE, Lopez F, Aaby P, Hedegaard K, Rombo L. 2003. Can mothers be trusted to give
malaria treatment to their children at home? *Acta Tropica* 86(1):67-70.

Krause G, Sauerborn R. 2000. Comprehensive community effectiveness of health care. A
study of malaria treatment in children and adults in rural Burkina Faso. *Annals of
Tropical Paediatrics* 20(4):273-282.

Makemba AM, Winch PJ, Makame VM, Mehl GL, Premji Z, Minjas JN, Shiff CJ. 1996.
Treatment practices for degedege, a locally recognized febrile illness, and implications
for strategies to decrease mortality from severe malaria in Bagamoyo District, Tanzania.
Tropical Medicine and International Health 1(3):305-313.

Marsh VM, Mutemi WM, Muturi J, Haaland A, Watkins WM, Otieno G, Marsh K. 1999.
Changing home treatment of childhood fevers by training shop keepers in rural Kenya.
Tropical Medicine and International Health 4(5):383-389.

Marsh VM, Mutemi WM, Willetts A, Bayah K, Were S, Ross A, Marsh K. 2004. Improving
malaria home treatment by training drug retailers in rural Kenya. *Tropical Medicine and
International Health* 9(4):451-460.

McCombie SC. 1996. Treatment seeking for malaria: A review of recent research. *Social
Science and Medicine* 43(6):933-945.

Menon A, Joof D, Rowan KM, Greenwood BM. 1988. Maternal administration of chloroquine: An unexplored aspect of malaria control. *Journal of Tropical Medicine and Hygiene* 91(2):49-54.

Minzi OM, Moshi MJ, Hipolite D, Massele AY, Tomson G, Ericsson O, Gustafsson LL.
2003. Evaluation of the quality of amodiaquine and sulphadoxine/pyrimethamine tablets sold by private wholesale pharmacies in Dar Es Salaam Tanzania. *Journal of Clinical
Pharmacy and Therapeutics* 28(2):117-122.

Moerman F, Lengeler C, Chimumbwa J, Talisuna A, Erhart A, Coosemans M, D'Alessandro
U. 2003. The contribution of health-care services to a sound and sustainable malaria-
control policy. *The Lancet Infectious Diseases* 3(2):99-102.

Muela SH, Mushi AK, Ribera JM. 2000. The paradox of the cost and affordability of traditional and government health services in Tanzania. *Health Policy and Planning*
15(3):296-302.

Muller I, Smith T, Mellor S, Rare L, Genton B. 1998. The effect of distance from home on
attendance at a small rural health centre in Papua New Guinea. *International Journal of
Epidemiology* 27(5):878-884.

Mwenesi H, Harpham T, Snow RW. 1995. Child malaria treatment practices among mothers
in Kenya. *Social Science and Medicine* 40(9):1271-1277.

Ndyomugyenyi R, Neema S, Magnussen P. 1998. The use of formal and informal services for antenatal care and malaria treatment in rural Uganda. *Health Policy and Planning* 13(1):94-102.

Newton P, Proux S, Green M, Smithuis F, Rozendaal J, Prakongpan S, Chotivanich K, Mayxay M, Looareesuwan S, Farrar J, Nosten F, White NJ. 2001. Fake artesunate in Southeast Asia. *Lancet* 357(9272):1948-1950.

Nshakira N, Kristensen M, Ssali F, Whyte SR. 2002. Appropriate treatment of malaria? Use of antimalarial drugs for children's fevers in district medical units, drug shops and homes in eastern Uganda. *Tropical Medicine and International Health* 7(4):309-316.

Nuwaha F. 2002. People's perception of malaria in Mbarara, Uganda. *Tropical Medicine and International Health* 7(5):462-470.

Ofori-Adjei D, Arhinful DK. 1996. Effect of training on the clinical management of malaria by medical assistants in Ghana. *Social Science and Medicine* 42(8):1169-1176.

Okonkwo PO, Akpala CO, Okafor HU, Mbah AU, Nwaiwu O. 2001. Compliance to correct dose of chloroquine in uncomplicated malaria correlates with improvement in the condition of rural Nigerian children. *Transactions of the Royal Society of Tropical Medicine and Hygiene* 95(3):320-324.

Oshiname FO, Brieger WR. 1992. Primary care training for patent medicine vendors in rural Nigeria. *Social Science and Medicine* 35(12):1477-1484.

Pagnoni F, Convelbo N, Tiendrebeogo J, Cousens S, Esposito F. 1997. A community-based programme to provide prompt and adequate treatment of presumptive malaria in children. *Transactions of the Royal Society of Tropical Medicine and Hygiene* 91(5):512-517.

Perkins BA, Zucker JR, Otieno J, Jafari HS, Paxton L, Redd SC, Nahlen BL, Schwartz B, Oloo AJ, Olango C, Gove S, Campbell CC. 1997. Evaluation of an algorithm for integrated management of childhood illness in an area of Kenya with high malaria transmission. *Bulletin of the World Health Organization* 75(Suppl 1):33-42.

Prince R, Geissler PW. 2001. Becoming "one who treats": A case study of a Luo healer and her grandson in western Kenya. *Anthropology and Education Quarterly* 32(4):447-471.

Prince RJ, Geissler PW, Nokes K, Maende JO, Okatcha F, Gringorenko E, Sternberg R. 2001. Knowledge of herbal and pharmaceutical medicines among Luo children in Western Kenya. *Anthropology and Medicine* 8:211-235.

Qingjun L, Jihui D, Laiyi T, Xiangjun Z, Jun L, Hay A, Shires S, Navaratnam V. 1998. The effect of drug packaging on patients' compliance with treatment for *Plasmodium vivax* malaria in China. *Bulletin of the World Health Organization* 76(Suppl 1):21-27.

Rozendaal J. 2001. Fake antimalaria drugs in Cambodia. *Lancet* 357(9259):890.

Ruebush TK, Kern MK, Campbell CC, Oloo AJ. 1995. Self-treatment of malaria in a rural area of Western Kenya. *Bulletin of the World Health Organization* 73(2):229-236.

Salako LA, Brieger WR, Afolabi BM, Umeh RE, Agomo PU, Asa S, Adeneye AK, Nwankwo BO, Akinlade CO. 2001. Treatment of childhood fevers and other illnesses in three rural Nigerian communities. *Journal of Tropical Pediatrics* 47(4):230-238.

Schellenberg D, Menendez C, Kahigwa E, Aponte J, Vidal J, Tanner M, Mshinda H, Alonso P. 2001. Intermittent treatment for malaria and anaemia control at time of routine vaccinations in Tanzanian infants: A randomised, placebo-controlled trial. *Lancet* 357 (9267):1471-1477.

Shwe T, Lwin M, Aung S. 1998. Influence of blister packaging on the efficacy of artesunate + mefloquine over artesunate alone in community-based treatment of non-severe falciparum malaria in Myanmar. *Bulletin of the World Health Organization* 76(Suppl 1):35-41.

Sirima SB, Konate A, Tiono AB, Convelbo N, Cousens S, Pagnoni F. 2003. Early treatment of childhood fevers with pre-packaged antimalarial drugs in the home reduces severe malaria morbidity in Burkina Faso. *Tropical Medicine and International Health* 8(2):133-139.

Snow RW, Craig M, Deichmann U, Marsh K. 1999. Estimating mortality, morbidity and disability due to malaria among Africa's non-pregnant population. *Bulletin of the World Health Organization* 77(8):624-640.

Sternberg RJ, Nokes K, Geissler PW. 2000. The relationship between academic and practical intelligence: A case study in Kenya. *Intelligence* 29:401-418.

Taylor RB, Shakoor O, Behrens RH, Everard M, Low AS, Wangboonskul J, Reid RG, Kolawole JA. 2001. Pharmacopoeial quality of drugs supplied by Nigerian pharmacies. *Lancet* 357(9272):1933-1936.

TDR/RBM. 2002. Scaling up home management of malaria. *TDR News* 67.

Thera MA, D'Alessandro U, Thiero M, Ouedraogo A, Packou J, Souleymane OA, Fane M, Ade G, Alvez F, Doumbo O. 2000. Child malaria treatment practices among mothers in the district of Yanfolila, Sikasso region, Mali. *Tropical Medicine and International Health* 5(12):876-881.

Trape JF, Zoulani A, Quinet MC. 1987. Assessment of the incidence and prevalence of clinical malaria in semi-immune children exposed to intense and perennial transmission. *American Journal of Epidemiology* 126(2):193-201.

Trape JF, Lefebvre-Zante E, Legros F, Druilhe P, Rogier C, Bouganali H, Salem G. 1993. Malaria morbidity among children exposed to low seasonal transmission in Dakar, Senegal and its implications for malaria control in tropical Africa. *American Journal of Tropical Medicine and Hygiene* 48(6):748-756.

van der Geest S, Geissler PW. 2003. Editorial: Should medicines be kept away from children? African considerations. *Tropical Medicine and International Health* 8(2):97-99.

von Seidlein L, Clarke S, Alexander N, Manneh F, Doherty T, Pinder M, Walraven G, Greenwood B. 2002. Treatment uptake by individuals infected with *Plasmodium falciparum* in rural Gambia, West Africa. *Bulletin of the World Health Organization* 80(10):790-796.

Wan Po AL. 2001. Too much, too little, or none at all: Dealing with substandard and fake drugs. *Lancet* 357(9272):1904.

WHO. 2000. Severe falciparum malaria. *Transactions of the Royal Society of Tropical Medicine and Hygiene* 94(Suppl 1):S1-S90.

WHO. 2002. *Strategic Framework for Malaria Control During Pregnancy in the WHO Africa Region.* Geneva: World Health Organization.

WHO. 2003. *Assessment and Monitoring of Antimalarial Drug Efficacy for the Treatment of Uncomplicated Falciparum Malaria.* Geneva: World Health Organization. WHO/HTM/RBM/2003.50.

WHO/UNICEF. 2003. *The Africa Malaria Report 2003.* Geneva: World Health Organization.

Wondemagegnehu E. 1995. *Counterfeit and Substandard Drugs in Myanmar and Viet Nam.* Geneva: World Health Organization.

Yeboah-Antwi K, Gyapong JO, Asare IK, Barnish G, Evans DB, Adjei S. 2001. Impact of prepackaging antimalarial drugs on cost to patients and compliance with treatment. *Bulletin of the World Health Organization* 79(5):394-399.

Yepez MC, Zambrano D, Carrasco F, Yepez RF. 2000. [The factors associated with noncompliance with antimalarial treatment in Ecuadorian patients]. [Spanish]. *Revista Cubana de Medicina Tropical* 52(2):81-89.

Acronyms and Abbreviations

ACAME	an association of francophone West African countries' central medical stores
ACSI-CCCD	Africa Child Survival Initiative—Combating Childhood Communicable Diseases Project
ACT	artemisinin combination therapy
ACTMalaria	Asian Collaborative Training Network for Malaria
AL	artemether-lumefantrine
A+M	artesunate plus mefloquine
AMI	Amazon Malaria Initiative
APLs	adaptable program loans
AQ	amodiaquine
AS	artesunate
ATM	artemether
ATS	artemisinin
AUC	area under the curve
BOMA	Burden of Malaria in Africa
Bsph	*Bacillus sphaericus*
Bti	*Bacillus thuringiensis subsp. israelensis*
CHAZ	Churches Health Association of Zambia
CIF	cost, insurance, freight
CMH	Commission on Macroeconomics and Health
CMS	Central Medical Stores (Cambodia)

CNM	National Malaria Center (Cambodia)
CNS	central nervous system
COMESA	Common Market for Eastern & Southern Africa
CQ	chloroquine
CRHCS	East and Southern Africa Commonwealth Regional Health Community Secretariat
CRPF	chloroquine-resistant *Plasmodium falciparum*
CRPV	chloroquine-resistant *Plasmodium vivax*
CSA	chondroitin sulphate A
DALY	disability-adjusted life-year
DDT	dichloro-diphenyl-trichloroethane
DDU	duty delivery unpaid
DEET	N,N-diethyl-m toluamide (an insect repellant)
DFWP	duty-free wholesaler price
DHA	dihydroartemisinin
DHFR	dihydrofolate reductase-thymidilate synthase
DHPS	dihydropteroate synthase
DNA	deoxyribonucleic acid
DNDi	Drugs for Neglected Diseases Initiative
DOTS	directly-observed therapy, short course (refers to treatment for tuberculosis)
DSS	Demographic Surveillance Site (or System)
EANMAT	East African Network for Monitoring Antimalarial Treatments
ECG	electrocardiogram
EDB	Essential Drugs Bureau (Cambodia)
EIR	entomologic inoculation rate
EMVI	European Malaria Vaccine Initiative
EPI	Expanded Programme on Immunization
G6PD	glucose-6-phosphate dehydrogenase
G8	Group of Eight [leading industrialized countries]
GAVI	Global Alliance for Vaccines and Immunization
GDF	TB Global Drug Facility
GDP	gross domestic product
GFATM	Global Fund to Fight AIDS, Tuberculosis, and Malaria
GMR	a private South African company that manages medical stores
GNI	gross national income
GSK	GlaxoSmithKline

HIPC	highly indebted poor countries
HIV	human immunodeficiency virus
HMS	hyperreactive malarial splenomegaly
HRP-2	histidine-rich protein 2
IDA	International Development Association
IFPMA	International Federation of Pharmaceutical Manufacturers Association
IMCI	Integrated Management of Childhood Illness
INN	International Nonproprietary Name
IOM	Institute of Medicine (of The National Academies)
IPT	intermittent preventive treatment
IPTc	intermittent preventive treatment in children
IPTi	intermittent preventive treatment in infants
IPTp	intermittent preventive treatment in pregnant women
IRS	indoor residual spraying
ITC	insecticide-treated curtain
ITN	insecticide-treated (bed) net
kdr	knock down resistance
LICUS	low income countries under stress
MARA	Mapping Malaria Risk in Africa
MDA	mass drug administration
MDGs	Millennium Development Goals
MDR	multidrug resistance
MEWS	malaria early warning system
MIC	minimum inhibitory concentration
MIM	Multilateral Initiative on Malaria
MMSS	Malaria Medicines and Supplies Service
MMV	Medicines for Malaria Venture
MoH	Ministry of Health
MPC	minimum parasiticidal concentration
MQ	mefloquine
MSH	Management Sciences for Health
MSL	Medical Stores Ltd.
MSP-1	merozoite surface protein-1
MTCT	maternal to child transmission
MVI	Malaria Vaccine Initiative
NGO	nongovernmental organization
NIH	National Institutes of Health (U.S.)

OTC	over-the-counter
PAHO	Pan American Health Organization
PATH	Program for Appropriate Technology in Health
PCR	polymerase chain reaction
PF	parasitologic failure
Pfcrt	*Plasmodium falciparum* chloroquine resistance transporter gene
Pfdhfr	dihydrofolate reductase gene
Pfdhps	dihydropteroate synthase gene
PfEMP-1	*P. falciparum* erythrocyte membrane protein-1
Pfmdr	*Plasmodium falciparum* multidrug resistance gene
Pgh1	P-glycoprotein homologue
pLDH	parasite enzyme lactate dehydrogenase
PNA	Pharmacie Nationale d'Approvisionnement
PQ	piperaquine
PRA	Pharmacie Regionale d'Approvisionnement
PRSCs	poverty reduction support credits
PRSP	poverty reduction strategy paper
QBC	quantitative buffy coat test
R&D	research and development
RACTAP	Réseau d'Afrique Centrale des Thérapeutiques Antipaludiques (Central African network)
RBC	red blood cell
RBM	Roll Back Malaria
RDT	rapid diagnostic test
RNA	ribonucleic acid
RTS,S	a recombinant protein vaccine which pairs hepatitis B surface antigen with DNA encoding a large portion of *P. falciparum* circumsporozoite protein
SACs	structural adjustment credits
SADCC	Southern African Development Coordination Conference
SALs	structural adjusted loans
SEACAT	South East African Combination Antimalarial Therapy [Evaluation]
SIT	sterile insect technology
SP	sulfadoxine/pyrimethamine
SWAp	sector-wide approach

T 1/2	half-life
TB	tuberculosis
TDR	the UNDP/World Bank/WHO Special Programme for Research and Training in Tropical Diseases
TEHIP	Tanzania Essential Health Interventions Project
TNF-alpha	tumor necrosis factor alpha
TTF	therapeutic treatment failure
UNICEF	United Nations Children's Fund
UNDP	United Nations Development Programme
USAID	U. S. Agency for International Development
USAMRMC	United States Army Medical Research and Materiel Command
VA	verbal autopsy
VAT	value added tax
VLSS	Vietnam Living Standards Surveys
WANMAT	West African Networks for Monitoring Antimalarial Treatments
WHO	World Health Organization
WHOPES	WHO Pesticide Evaluation Scheme
WRAIR	Walter Reed Army Institute of Research
ZK	Zambia Kwacha (currency)

Glossary

acidosis. a disturbance of the body acid-base balance in which there is excessive acidity of the blood. **metabolic acidosis** results from excess acid due to abnormal metabolism (as in severe malaria), excessive acid intake, renal retention, or excessive loss of bicarbonate (as in severe diarrhea); **respiratory acidosis** results from inadequate elimination of carbon dioxide.

agranulocytosis. a condition marked by a sharp drop in circulating white blood cells, often drug- or radiation-induced.

anaphylaxis. an unusual or exaggerated allergic reaction, sometimes leading to shock and death, triggered by a foreign protein or other substance.

anemia. decrease in number of red blood cells and/or quantity of hemoglobin. Malaria causes anemia through rupture of red blood cells during merozoite release as well as other mechanisms, e.g., suppressing red cell production by bone marrow.

anopheline. referring to *Anopheles* mosquitoes.

antenatal care. concerned with the care and treatment of a pregnant woman and her unborn child.

anthropophilic. attracted to humans, especially as a source of food (e.g., malaria-carrying mosquitoes).

antibody. a protein produced by the immune system in response to the introduction of a substance (an antigen) recognized as foreign. The chief purpose of an antibody is to interact with other components of the immune system and render the antigen harmless.

antigen. a molecule capable of eliciting an immune response.

antigenic diversity. the ability of an organism to vary its antigenic features.

antigenic variation. same as **antigenic diversity.**

antipyretic. an agent that reduces fever.

arthralgia. pain in one or more joints.

aspartate aminotransferase. an enzyme produced by the liver. When present in abnormally high levels in the blood, it may indicate inflammation or disease of the liver or another organ.

ataxia. a staggering gait or other inability to coordinate voluntary muscular movements. This finding is symptomatic of certain nervous disorders especially involving the cerebellum.

attenuate (as in vaccine). to reduce the virulence of a pathogenic agent.

auditory evoked potential. electrical brain wave activity measured in response to acoustic stimulation (as sound). Evoked potentials are used as diagnostic tools to investigate potential damage to the central nervous system caused, for example, by a disease like multiple sclerosis or by a drug.

brain stem. the part of the brain composed of the midbrain, pons, and medulla oblongata connecting the spinal cord with the forebrain and cerebrum.

bioassay. a method of determining the relative strength of a substance (as a drug) by comparing its effect on a test organism with that of a standard preparation.

blister pack. a form of medication packaging in which individual doses of one or more types of pill are encased in separate airtight plastic pockets, often accompanied by dosing instructions. Blister packs typically contain all of the doses needed for a single course of treatment.

cardiotoxic. having a toxic effect on the heart.

cell-mediated immunity. an immune process in which subpopulations of effector T cells defend against viruses and intracellular protozoal infections, such as malaria.

centrifuge. a machine that uses centrifugal force to separate substances of different densities, remove moisture, or simulate gravitational effects.

chemoprophylaxis. the use of drugs to prevent infection or progression of infection to illness.

chromosome. any of the usually linear intracellular bodies that contain the genes or hereditary factors of eukaryotic organisms, bacteria, or certain DNA viruses (e.g., bacteriophages).

cinchonism. side effects from quinine or quinidine, reversible with lower dosages or termination of the drugs. Effects include ringing in the ears, headache, nausea, diarrhea, altered auditory acuity, and blurred vision. The term derives from cinchona bark, the natural source of quinine.

clinical cure. elimination of malaria symptoms, sometimes without eliminating all parasites.

coformulation. a fixed-dose combination of two or more drugs, i.e., two (or more) drugs in one pill. This is distinguished from combinations of drugs in separate pills, either blister-packed together or from separate containers.

coma. decreased state of consciousness from which a person cannot be aroused.

cost effective. economical, based on the tangible benefits produced by the money spent.

cost effectiveness. a measure of the value received (effectiveness) for the resources expended (cost). Usually considered as a ratio, the cost effectiveness of a drug or procedure, for example, relates the cost of that drug or procedure to the health benefits resulting from it. In health terms, it is often expressed as the cost per year of life saved or as the cost per quality-adjusted life-year saved.

culicine. referring to mosquitoes of the genus *Culex*.

cytoadherent [parasites]. red blood cells containing mature malaria schizonts that attach to endothelial cells lining small blood vessels.

cytokine. a regulatory protein released by cells of the immune system that acts as an intercellular mediator in the generation of an immune response. Examples of cytokine classes include interleukins and lymphokines.

cytotoxic. toxic to cells.

DDT. 1,1,1-trichloro-2,2-bis(p-chlorophenyl) ethane, or chlorophenothane, a pesticide.

degedege. Swahili term for a febrile illness with convulsions (often cerebral malaria) sometimes perceived as a nonmalarial condition with supernatural causes.

dipstick [test]. shorthand term for rapid diagnostic test (RDT), usually performed by immersing a commercially prepared strip into a body fluid.

DNA. deoxyribonucleic acid, a carrier of genetic information (i.e., hereditary characteristics) found chiefly in the nucleus of cells.

drug pressure. intense exposure of a population to a given drug, usually an antimicrobial agent.

dysdiadochokinesis. the inability to halt one motor action and substitute its opposite action, usually the result of a neurologic disease.

electrocardiogram (ECG). a graphic tracing of the electrical current produced during the contraction of heart muscle.

electrocardiograph. an instrument for recording the changes of electrical activity occurring during heart contraction, often used to diagnose abnormalities of cardiac conduction.

Emax. maximum effect exerted by a drug. In the case of antimalarial drugs, it usually represents the log decrease in total plasmodial burden following exposure to a given agent.

endemic. describing the presence of a disease in a community.

   holoendemic. affecting essentially all the inhabitants of an area.

   hyperendemic. causing a high but steady rate of infection over time.

   hypoendemic. causing a low but steady rate of infection over time.

endothelial cells. cells that line the cavities of the heart, blood and lymph vessels.

entomological inoculation rate (EIR). the measurement of frequency with which a human is bitten by an infectious mosquito; or the average number of infective bites a resident of a malarious area receives over a year or other time period.

enzyme. any of numerous complex proteins that are produced by living cells and catalyze specific biochemical reactions.

eosinophilia. abnormal increase in the number of eosinophils (a type of white blood cell) in the blood, characteristic of allergic states and various parasitic infections.

epidemic. rapid and/or widespread outbreak of a disease through a community in which the disease is normally absent or present at a low level.

epidemiology. study of the distribution and determinants of a disease in populations.

erythrocyte. a red blood cell.

erythrocytic. relating to red blood cells.

erythrocytic stage. stage of the malaria parasite's life cycle infecting and developing within red blood cells.

exoerythrocytic stage. stage of the malaria parasite's life cycle infecting, developing, or remaining latent in liver cells (hepatocytes).

essential drug (or medicine). one of a group of drugs which together comprise safe, effective treatment for the majority of communicable and non-communicable diseases currently affecting the world's population. The 12th Model List of Essential Drugs, prepared by a WHO expert committee in 2002, contains 325 individual drugs.

externality. an economic side-effect: externalities are costs ("negative externalities") or benefits ("positive externalities") arising from an economic activity that affect somebody other than the people engaged in the economic activity and are not reflected fully in prices. Relating to malaria, when a large proportion of people in a community purchase and use insecticide-treated nets (ITNs), even those who do not purchase them gain some protection, a positive externality.

falciparum malaria. malaria caused by the species *Plasmodium falciparum*
febrile. describing an elevated body temperature.
first-line treatment. initial treatment for a specific disease or condition.

gamete. a mature male or female germ cell usually possessing a single set of chromosomes and capable of initiating formation of a new diploid individual by fusion with a gamete of the opposite sex.
gametocytocidal. capable of killing gametocytes.
gametocyte. sexual stage of malaria parasite that forms in red blood cells. Macrogametocytes (female) and microgametocytes (male) form in individual erythrocytes, are ingested by female mosquitoes, and unite in the mosquito's stomach.
gene amplification. a process in response to certain cell development signals or environmental stresses that leads to an increased number of gene copies. In humans, this process is seen most often in malignant cells.
genetically modified mosquito. a mosquito with added or altered genes that either destroy developing malaria parasites or render the mosquito an inhospitable or refractory host for malaria.
genotype. the genetic makeup, as distinguished from the physical appearance, of an organism or a group of organisms; the combination of alleles located on homologous chromosomes that determines a specific characteristic or trait.
glucose-6-phosphate dehydrogenase (G6PD) deficiency. a common enzyme deficiency within the human red cell, affecting an estimated 400 million people worldwide. The deficiency confers some resistance to malaria, but also can lead to hemolytic anemia of varying severiy, especially following exposure to certain drugs including the antimalarial drug primaquine.

half-life. the time required for half of the amount of a substance (as a drug or radioactive tracer) in a physiologic or ecologic system to be eliminated or disintegrated by natural processes.
hematocrit. the ratio of the volume of packed red blood cells to the volume of whole blood as determined by a centrifugation instrument: a measure of possible anemia.
heme dimerization. the stage in the biochemical breakdown of human hemoglobin within the malaria parasite that yields malaria pigment (hemozoin).
hemoglobin. the protein in red blood cells which carries oxygen.

hemolysis. a condition in which red blood cells prematurely rupture. Examples of hemolytic conditions include sickle cell anemia and malaria.

Hemolytic anemia occurs when the bone marrow is unable to compensate for the premature destruction by increasing production of new red cells.

hemozoin. malaria pigment; an iron-containing breakdown product of hemoglobin which accumulates as cytoplasmic granules in malaria parasites and tissues of infected individuals.

hepatocyte. a liver cell.

hyperparasitemia. parasite count in excess of 250,000 per microliter, or a state in which more than 5% of circulating red blood cells are parasitized. Hyperparasitemic patients have an increased risk of death from microvascular disease as well as metabolic effects from the high parasite load.

hypoglycemia. blood glucose less than the lower value of normal (70-110 mg/dL [3.9-6.1 mmol/L in SI reference units]). Glucose levels of 40 and below constitute severe hypoglycemia, a life-threatening emergency. Hypoglycemia is common in malaria, as malaria parasitized red blood cells utilize glucose 75 times faster than uninfected cells. Treatment with quinine also lowers blood glucose by stimulating insulin secretion.

hyponatremia. serum sodium less than the normal lower limit, which is 135-147 mEq/L (135-147 mmol/L in SI reference units). Serum sodium levels approaching 120 and below constitute severe hyponatremia, a medical emergency. Hyponatremia can be seen in malaria, and is indicative of complicated malaria.

hypnozoite. a stage of malaria parasites found in liver cells. After sporozoites invade liver cells, some develop into latent forms called hypnozoites. They become active months or years later, producing a recurrent malaria attack. Only *P. vivax* and *P. ovale* produce hypnozoites in humans.

immune system. a natural defense mechanism of the body, in which specialized cells and proteins in the blood and other body elements interact to eliminate or neutralize infectious microorganisms and other foreign substances.

immunity. the body's ability to control or lessen a malaria attack with antibodies and other protective reactions developed in response to previous malaria attacks. Semi-immune individuals live in malaria endemic areas and are repeatedly infected. Immunity minimizes their symptoms and decreases parasitemia.

immunochromatography. an antibody-based process that uses capillary flow through an absorbent membrane to separate components; used in research and as a basis for diagnostic tests.

incidence. as used in epidemiology, the number of new cases of a disease occurring within a specified period. An incidence *rate* is a measure of the frequency with which new cases occur in a population over a period of time. The denominator is the population at risk and the numerator is the number of new cases occurring during a given time period.

indoor residual spraying (IRS). spraying long-lasting insecticide on indoor walls or rafters in order to kill resting insects, specifically female malaria vectors that rest indoors following blood meals.

integrated control. disease control that involves more than one type of intervention. For malaria, this could involve the combination of drug treatment for symptomatic cases, prevention through ITNs, and environmental measures to reduce mosquito breeding.

insecticide-treated bednet (ITN). a fine meshed net that has either been treated with a long-lasting insecticide or manufactured with insecticide directly incorporated into its fibers, hung over a bed to protect sleepers from insect bites. **Insecticide-treated curtains (ITC)** are hung in windows and doorways.

intermittent preventive treatment (IPT). antimalarial drug treatment during pregnancy to prevent clinical disease. This approach is now being extended to infants and may also be incorporated into childhood immunization schedules in malaria-endemic regions.

intraerythrocytic. situated within red blood cells.

intramuscular. situated within or administered into a muscle.

intrauterine growth restriction (IUGR). failure of appropriate fetal growth, usually defined as a baby weighing below the 10th percentile of expected weight for gestational age. Malaria during pregnancy can cause IUGR.

intravascular. situated within a blood vessel.

intravenous. administered into a vein, as in intravenous fluids for treatment of dehydration.

in vitro. biological processes that occur in isolation from the whole organism, such as in a test tube or in cell culture.

in vivo. biological processes that occur within the body of a living organism.

jaundice. yellowish discoloration of the whites of the eyes, skin, and mucous membranes caused by deposition of bile salts in these tissues. It may be seen in various liver diseases, such as hepatitis, that affect the processing of bile as well as hemolysis (excessive destruction of red blood cells). Also called icterus.

knock down resistance (kdr). a form of resistance to pyrethroid insecticides caused by a genetic point mutation. kdr is found in anopheline malaria vectors as well as other mosquitoes and some other insects.

larvicide. an agent for killing insect larvae (in the case of malaria, mosquito larvae).

ligand. an attachment site or a molecule that binds to a complementary site on another molecule.

light microscope. a conventional laboratory microscope that uses ordinary light (as opposed to parallel beams of electrons, for example, in an electron microscope) to illuminate an object.

lysis. a process of disintegration or dissolution (as of cells).

meningitis. inflammation of the meninges of the brain and the spinal cord, most often caused by a bacterial or viral infection and characterized by fever, vomiting, intense headache, and stiff neck.

merozoite. the stage of the malaria parasite, in the human host, that infects red blood cells.

metabolic acidosis. resulting from excess acid due to abnormal metabolism (as in severe malaria), excessive acid intake, or renal retention or from excessive loss of bicarbonate (as in severe diarrhea).

microhematocrit (tube). a procedure for determining the ratio of the volume of packed red blood cells to the volume of whole blood by centrifuging a minute quantity of blood in a capillary tube coated with heparin.

monotherapy. use of a single drug to treat a disease.

molecular markers. genetic markers, usually proteins or DNA sequences, detected by biochemical methods.

multigravidae. women who have had several previous pregnancies.

mutagenicity. the capacity to induce mutations in DNA.

myalgia. muscle pain.

neutropenia. a decrease in white blood cells chiefly affecting neutrophils.

oocyst. cyst located in the outer stomach wall of a female anopheline mosquito where sporozoite development takes place. When mature, the oocysts rupture and release sporozoites. Sporozoites subsequently migrate to salivary glands to be injected into the host when mosquitoes feed.

ookinete. the fertilized form of the malaria parasite in the mosquito's body.

outbreeding. increasing in numbers faster than a competing population.

parasitemia. condition in which parasites are present in the blood with or without clinical symptoms.

paroxysm. a sudden attack or increase in intensity of a symptom, usually occurring in intervals. Malaria is classically described as producing fever paroxysms—sudden severe temperature elevations preceded by chills and followed by profuse sweating.

perennial transmission. year-round (as opposed to seasonal) transmission.

peripartum. occurring before, during or following birth.

pharmacodynamics. a branch of pharmacology dealing with the reactions between drugs and living systems.

pharmacokinetics. the interactions of drugs with people who take them—how the compounds are absorbed, metabolized, distributed and excreted.

phenotype. the visible properties of an organism that are produced by the interaction of the genotype (genetic make-up) and the environment.

Plasmodium. the genus of protozoans that includes all of the malaria parasites affecting humans and other animals; any individual malaria parasite.

point mutation. a gene mutation specifically involving the substitution, addition, or deletion of a single nucleotide base.

polymerase chain reaction (PCR). A method of amplifying low levels of specific DNA sequences, allowing detection of very low levels of antigen in the sample.

polymorphism. the existence of a gene in several allelic forms.

polypharmacy. prescribing of multiple drugs.

premunition. imperfect immunity.

presumptive treatment. administration of anti-malarial drugs in suspected cases before results of laboratory tests are available to confirm diagnosis.

prevalence. the proportion of a population that is affected with a particular disease at a given time.

primigravidae. women who are pregnant for the first time.

prophylaxis. measures designed to prevent disease and preserve health: protective or preventive treatment.

protozoan. a single-celled animal.

public goods. Things that are either consumed by everybody in a society or by nobody at all. They have three characteristics. Public goods are: 1) non-rival—one person consuming them does not stop another person consuming them; 2) nonexcludable—if one person can consume them, it is impossible to stop another person consuming them; and 3) non-rejectable—people cannot choose not to consume them even if they want to. Examples include clean air, a national defense system, and the judiciary.

Global public goods cannot be provided by one country acting alone, but only by the joint efforts of many (strictly, all) countries. The universal use of combination drug treatment (as opposed to monotherapy) for malaria would reduce the likelihood that resistant plasmodia will develop, and would benefit all.

pulmonary edema. abnormal accumulation of fluid in the lungs.

pyrethrin. either of two oily liquid esters—$C_{21}H_{28}O_3$ and $C_{22}H_{28}O_5$—extracted from dried chrysanthemum flowers (the oldest effective insecticide known) that have insecticidal properties and are the active components of pyrethrum.

pyrethroids. any of various synthetic compounds that are related to the pyrethrins and resemble them in insecticidal properties.

quartan malaria. malaria caused by *Plasmodium malariae* and marked by recurrence of bouts of chills and fever at 72-hour intervals.

rapid diagnostic test (RDT). a rapid, convenient and/or inexpensive method of determining whether a patient has a certain disease.

RBC. red blood cell.

reagent. a substance used to detect, measure or synthesize a product because of its chemical or biological activity; a reactor.

recombinant vaccine. a vaccine prepared by recombinant DNA technology in which a host organism (expression vector) is directed to synthesize specific molecules after DNA segments from another organism (such as the malaria parasite) are inserted. In this manner, vaccines that are directed against specific antigens on or within the parasites can be made.

recrudescence. a repeated attack of malaria due to the survival of malaria parasites in red blood cells.

relapse. a repeat attack of malaria specific to *P. vivax* and *P. ovale*, in which the repeat attack represents re-seeding of the bloodstream by latent hypnozoites in the liver.

reticular. of, relating to, or forming a network.

reticulocyte. an immature red blood cell that appears especially during regeneration of lost blood and that has a fine basophilic reticulum formed of the remains of ribosomes. *P. vivax* exclusively parasitizes reticulocytes.

rigor. severe chill, characterized by shaking of the body.

schizont. a multinucleate parasite that represents a mature stage of the asexual malaria parasite.

schizogony. the asexual cycle of sporozoa, particularly the life cycle of the malaria parasite in the red blood cells of man.

sensitivity. the property of a test or case definition defined by the degree to which it correctly identifies those having the disease or condition of interest.

specificity. the property of a test or case definition defined by the degree to which it correctly identifies those *not* having the disease or condition of interest.

splenomegaly. an enlarged spleen. A common finding in malaria patients that can sometimes be detected by physical examination of the abdomen.

sporogony. the portion of the sexual reproduction of the malaria parasite that takes place in the mosquito.

sporozoite. stage of malaria parasites injected into the bloodstream by biting infective mosquitoes. Sporozoites infect liver cells, disappearing from the bloodstream within 30 minutes of entry.

sterile insect technique (SIT). the mass release of sterile male insects to displace the normal male population, thus reducing the number of females who reproduce. Radiation is most often used to sterilize male insects, but genetic techniques have also been developed. SIT has not yet played a role in malaria control, but research is ongoing.

tachycardia. increased heart rate, greater than 100 beats per minute.

tachypnea. increased respiratory rate, greater than 20 breaths per minute.

teratogenic. capable of causing structural abnormalites (i.e., birth defects) during fetal development.

tertian malaria. malaria caused by *Plasmodium vivax* or *Plasmodium ovale*, marked by recurrence of bouts of chills and fever at 48-hour intervals.

thrombocytopenia. low platelet count, defined as less than 150,000 per mL. Low platelet counts can lead to impaired blood clotting, and counts below 50,000 per mL increase the risk of spontaneous bleeding.

tiered pricing. a mechanism for segmenting the global market, used in the case of medicines, so that poor countries pay lower prices than richer ones; also called equitable, or differential, pricing.

trophozoite. the asexual growing stage of the malaria parasite in the human red blood cell, leading to the mature schizont.

vector. an agent that transmits disease from one host to another, e.g., the mosquito that transmits the malaria parasite.

vivax malaria. malaria caused by the malaria parasite *Plasmodium vivax*.

wild type [genes]. phenotype, genotype, or gene that predominates in a natural population of organisms or strain of organisms in contrast to that of natural or laboratory mutant forms; also an organism or strain displaying the wild type.

zoophilic/zoophagic. preferring lower animals to humans as a source of food.

zooprophylaxis. the diversion of disease carrying insects from humans to animals.

Index

H

Poverty Reduction Support Loans and
  Credits (PRSCs), 102
R&D, 302–303
Structural Adjustment Loans and
  Structural Adjustment Credits (SALs
  and SACs), 102
World Health Organization (WHO)
  Abuja Conference, 49
  artemisinins, 12, 263
  centralized procurement system, 9, 112–
    113
  control strategies, 199–200, 234
  endorsement of combination therapy, 5,
    61, 72, 79, 80, 237
  environmental controls, 211
  Global Burden of Disease program, 169
  Global Drug Facility (GDF), 118–119,
    119, 120
  global eradication of chloroquine, 131
  Higher Impact Adjustment Lending, 103
  in vivo antimalarial drug sensitivity
    classification, 277, 277
  IPT recommendations, 218
  ITN approval, 206
  major initiatives, 46, 174
  Medicines for Malaria Venture initiative,
    47
  mefloquine development, 132
  partnership with U.S. Agency for
    International Development, 20
  Pesticide Evaluation Scheme (WHOPES),
    200
  pre-qualification for drug suppliers, 40
  quality assurance strength, 116
  school-based education, 323
  severe malaria, defined, 150
  Special Programme on Research and
    Training in Tropical Diseases (TDR),
    10, 46–49, 48, 203, 301, 302–303,
    304, 306, 307–309, 315
  support for Cambodian Pharmaceutical
    Enterprise, 38
  treatment benchmarks, 66

World Health Report, 67
World Trade Organisation, 99
World War I, 131
World War II, 127, 130, 132, 198, 200,
  206
WRAIR. See Walter Reed Army Institute of
  Research
Wright's stain, 220

Y

Ya chud, 31
Yorktown, Virginia, 126

Z

Zaire, 205, 232
Zambia
  ACT as first-line therapy, 236
  availability of antimalarials, 42
  Central Board of Health, 36
  chloroquine-resistant *P. falciparum*, 132
  control methods, 229
  drug financing, 44–45
  drug pricing, 43, 44
  economic and health indicators, 35
  health care expenditures, 98
  home treatment, 319
  illegal drug flows, 42
  Kafue, 44
  Lusaka, 40, 41, 44
  malaria in, 34
  Medical Stores Ltd., 36
  private sector drug flows, 40–41
  public sector drug flows, 36, 38
Zambian National Formulary, 41
Zanzibar, 235, 236
Zhou En Lai, 133
Zimbabwe, 24, 36, 98, 222
Zoophagic, 141
Zoophilic, 141
Zooprophylaxis, 210